OXFORD ASSESS AND PROGRESS

Series Editors

Kathy Boursicot

Reader in Medical Education and Deputy Head of the Centre for
Medical and Healthcare Education,
St George's, University of London

David Sales

Consultant in Medical Assessment

OXFORD ASSESS AND PROGRESS

CLINICAL
MEDICINE

Alex Liakos

Martin Hill

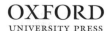

OXFORD
UNIVERSITY PRESS

OXFORD
UNIVERSITY PRESS

Great Clarendon Street, Oxford OX2 6DP

Oxford University Press is a department of the University of Oxford.
It furthers the University's objective of excellence in research,
scholarship, and education by publishing worldwide in

Oxford New York

Auckland Cape Town Dar es Salaam Hong Kong Karachi
Kuala Lumpur Madrid Melbourne Mexico City Nairobi
New Delhi Shanghai Taipei Toronto

With offices in

Argentina Austria Brazil Chile Czech Republic France Greece
Guatemala Hungary Italy Japan Poland Portugal Singapore
South Korea Switzerland Thailand Turkey Ukraine Vietnam

Oxford is a registered trade mark of Oxford University Press
in the UK and in certain other countries

Published in the United States
by Oxford University Press Inc., New York

© Oxford University Press 2010

British Library Cataloguing in Publication Data

Data available

Library of Congress Cataloging in Publication Data

Data available

Typeset by Macmillan Publishing Solutions
Printed in China
on acid-free paper
through Asia Pacific Offset

ISBN 978–0–19–956212–1

5 7 9 10 8 6

Oxford University Press makes no representation, express or implied,
that the drug dosages in this book are correct. Readers must therefore
always check the product information and clinical procedures with the
most up-to-date published product information and data sheets provided
by the manufacturers and the most recent codes of conduct and safety
regulations. The authors and the publishers do not accept responsibility
or legal liability for any errors in the text or for the misuse or
misapplication of material in this work. Except where otherwise stated,
drug dosages and recommendations are for the non-pregnant adult who
is not breast-feeding.

SERIES EDITOR PREFACE

The Oxford Assess & Progress Series is a groundbreaking development in the extensive area of self assessment texts available for medical students. The questions were specifically commissioned for the series, written by practising clinicians, extensively peer reviewed by students and their teachers, and quality assured to ensure that the material is up to date, accurate, and in line with modern testing formats.

The series has a number of unique features and is designed as much as a formative learning resource as a self assessment one. The questions are constructed to test the same clinical problem solving skills that we use as practising clinicians, rather than just testing theoretical knowledge, namely:

- Gathering and using data required for clinical judgment
- Choosing examination, investigations, and interpretation of the findings
- Applying knowledge
- Demonstrating diagnostic skills
- Ability to evaluate undifferentiated material
- Ability to prioritise
- Making decisions and demonstrating a structured approach to decision making.

Each question is bedded in reality and is typically presented as a clinical scenario, the content of which have been chosen to reflect the common and important conditions that most doctors are likely to encounter both during their training and in exams! The aim of the series is to build the reader's confidence around recognizing important symptoms and signs and suggesting the most appropriate investigations and management, and in so doing aid development of a clear approach to patient management which can be transferred to the wards.

The content of the series has deliberately been pinned to the relevant Oxford Handbook but in addition has been guided by a blueprint which reflects the themes identified in *Tomorrow's Doctors* and *Good Medical Practice* to include novel areas such as history taking, recognition of signs including red flags, and professionalism.

Particular attention has been paid to giving learning points and constructive feedback on each question, using clear fact or evidence based explanations as to why the correct response is right and why the incorrect responses are less appropriate. The question editorials are clearly referenced to the relevant sections of the accompanying Oxford Handbook and/or more widely to medical literature or guidelines. They are designed to guide and motivate the reader, being multi-purpose in nature, covering, for example, exam technique, approaches to difficult subjects, and links between subjects.

Another unique aspect of the Series is the element of competency progression from being a relatively inexperienced student to a more experienced junior doctor. We have suggested the following four degrees of difficulty to reflect the level of training so the reader can monitor their own progress over time, namely:

★	Graduate should know
★ ★	Graduate nice to know
★ ★ ★	Foundation should know
★ ★ ★ ★	Foundation nice to know.

We advise the reader to attempt the questions in blocks as a way of testing knowledge in a clinical context. The Series can be treated as a dress rehearsal for life on the ward by using the material to hone clinical acumen and build confidence by encouraging a clear, consistent, and rational approach, proficiency in recognizing and evaluating symptoms and signs, making a rational differential diagnosis, and suggesting appropriate investigations and management.

Adopting such an approach can aid not only being successful in examinations, which really are designed to confirm learning, but more importantly being a good doctor. In this way we can deliver high quality and safe patient care by recognizing, understanding, and treating common problems, but at the same time remaining alert to the possibility of less likely but potentially catastrophic conditions.

David Sales and Kathy Boursicot,
Series Editors
22 May 2009

A NOTE ON SINGLE BEST ANSWER AND EXTENDED MATCHING QUESTIONS

Single best answer questions are currently the format of choice being widely used by most undergraduate and postgraduate knowledge tests, and hence most of the assessment questions on this book follow this format.

Briefly, the single best answer question presents a problem, usually a clinical scenario, before presenting the question itself and a list of five options. Of these five, there is one correct answer and four incorrect options or 'distractors' from which the reader chooses a response.

Extended matching questions are also known as extended matching items and were introduced as a more reliable way of testing knowledge. They are still currently widely used in many undergraduate and postgraduate knowledge tests, and hence are included in this book.

An extended matching question is organized as one list of possible options followed by a set of items, usually clinical scenarios. The correct response to each item must be chosen from the list of options.

All of the questions in this book, which typically are based on an evaluation of symptoms, signs, or results of investigations either as single entities or in combination, are designed to test *reasoning* skills rather than straightforward recall of facts, and use cognitive processes similar to those used in clinical practice.

The peer-reviewed questions are written and edited in accordance with contemporary best assessment practice and their content has been guided by a blueprint pinned to all areas of *Good Medical Practice*, which ensures comprehensive coverage.

The answers and their rationales are evidence-based and have been reviewed to ensure that they are absolutely correct. Incorrect options are selected as being plausible and indeed may look correct to the less knowledgeable reader. When answering questions, readers may wish to use the 'cover' test in which they read the scenario and the question but cover the options.

K. Boursicot and D. Sales,
Series Editors

PREFACE

As undergraduate finals approach, students drift from the safety of their bible, the *Oxford Handbook of Clinical Medicine* (OHCM), towards a range of disparate self-test resources in a bid to assess their progress. Meanwhile, senior colleagues attempt to reassure, saying, 'Know the OHCM and you'll be fine….' So rich in detail and broad in its range, the challenge of knowing the OHCM is a daunting one. We wrote this book after our own finals to help students meet that challenge.

The vehicles for this are two types of self-assessment question: the single best answer and extended matching question, increasingly the favoured formats in written medical exams. Gone (or going) are the reams of true or false questions that quiz the student on abstract details of clinical specifics. The questions here are all based on clinical scenarios with the student generally required to play the role of the junior doctor.

Each question is accompanied by an explanation behind the answer (Why A?), as well as, crucially, an explanation as to why the answer is none of the other options (Why not B, C, D, or E?). These explanations are linked both to the relevant page in the OHCM and, where appropriate, to illuminating papers or supporting guidelines.

It would be impossible for the questions to cover every topic featured in the OHCM. Whilst some niche topics are addressed, the majority of scenarios are built around either very common clinical areas ('regulars') or situations that could have catastrophic consequences ('unmissables').

Although this book is a self-assessment aid, it is not exam-centric. It acknowledges the fact that the transition from student to junior doctor is a silent one and that preparations for finals must also include practical preparations for working. There is much in these questions that does this. As is the case for a junior doctor, the focus is often not on diagnosis but on ensuring a safe and systematic approach to acute and chronic management, examination findings and techniques, communication, patient safety, ethical dilemmas, and professional practice.

The principle of this book is not simply to reinforce the encyclopaedic knowledge of the OHCM in order to pass exams. It is to hone the student's ability to apply this knowledge confidently in the varying and challenging range of rotations and scenarios that they face post-graduation. In this way, we hope that this book becomes an invaluable reference text and a worthy junior companion to the OHCM.

Alex Liakos and Martin Hill

ACKNOWLEDGEMENTS

We would like to thank the staff of Oxford University Press for their expertise in producing this volume. We are particularly grateful to Caroline Connelly for the trust she placed in us and to Holly Edmundson for her close guidance and attention to detail. We are indebted to the authors of the OHCM for allowing our work to be associated with their seminal book and to use it as a template for our assessment edition. The energy and enthusiasm of our editors David Sales and Kathy Boursicot has been a constant driving force: we are fortunate to have been led by two such authorities in medical assessment. Thanks to the huge number of anonymous reviewers who have questioned and challenged our ideas throughout the writing process, allowing us to improve our original ideas.

Finally but most importantly, all our love and thanks to Hester, Eleni, and Rosa (AL) and Nic and Ethan (MH) who over the last 2 years have given us endless support and patience while repeatedly being told, 'It's almost finished…'

Alex Liakos and Martin Hill

FIGURE ACKNOWLEDGEMENTS

We are grateful to Queen Mary's Hospital, Sidcup, and King's College Hospital, London, for granting us permission to use their images. Many thanks to all those patients who consented to their images being used.

Figure 1.6: reproduced by permission of Steven Fruitsmaak; Figure 3.2: © Dr P. Marazzi/Science Photo Library; Figure 8.2: reproduced with the kind permission of Dr James Holt; Figure 8.6: reproduced with the kind permission of Dr James Holt and the Royal Berkshire Hospital; Figure 10.7: © Dr Abhijit Datir: Figures 12.1 and 12.2: © Resuscitation Council (UK) reproduced with permission. Reproduced with permission from Oxford University Press: Figure 1.5: Myerson *et al.*, *Emergencies in Cardiology*, p336; Figure 1.7: Sundaram *et al.*, *Training in Ophthalmology*, p31, Figure 1.37; Figure 1.11: Myerson *et al.*, *Emergencies in Cardiology*, p145, Figure 2; Figure 1.15: Myerson *et al.*, *Emergencies in Cardiology*, p275; Figure 1.18: Myerson *et al.*, *Emergencies in Cardiology*, p337; Figure 3.3: Sundaram *et al.*, *Training in Ophthalmology*, p157, Figure 4.13; Figure 3.4: Sundaram *et al.*, *Training in Ophthalmology*, p157, Figure 4.15; Figure 8.8: Endacott *et al.*, *Clinical Nursing Skills: Core and Advanced*, p433, Figure 8.6; Figure 12.7: Myerson *et al.*, *Emergencies in Cardiology*, p154.

CONTENTS

NORMAL AND AVERAGE VALUES

	Normal value
Haematology	
White cell count (WCC)	4–11 × 10⁹/L
Haemoglobin (Hb)	M: 13.5–18g/dL F: 11.5–16g/dL
Packed cell volume (PCV)	M: 0.4–0.54L/L F: 0.37–0.47L/L
Mean corpuscular volume (MCV)	76–96fL
Neutrophils	2–7.5 × 10⁹/L
Lymphocytes	1.3–3.5 × 10⁹/L
Eosinophils	0.04–0.44 × 10⁹/L
Basophils	0–0.1 × 10⁹/L
Monocytes	0.2–0.8 × 10⁹/L
Platelets	150–400 × 10⁹/L
Reticulocytes	25–100 × 10⁹/L
Erythrocyte sedimentation rate (ESR)	<20mm/h (but age dependent; see OHCM p356)
Prothrombin time (PT)	10–14s
Activated partial thromboplastin time (aPTT)	35–45s
International normalized ratio (INR)	0.9–1.2
Biochemistry	
Alanine aminotransferase (ALT)	5–35IU/L
Albumin	35–50g/L
Alkaline phosphatase (ALP)	30–150U/L
Amylase	0–180U/dL
Aspartate transaminase (AST)	5–35IU/L
Bilirubin	3–17µmol/L

Calcium (total)	2.12–2.65mmol/L
Chloride	95–105mmol/L
Cortisol	450–750nmol/L (am) 80–280nmol/L (midnight)
C-reactive protein (CRP)	<10mg/L
Creatine kinase	M: 25–195IU/L F: 25–170IU/L
Creatinine	70–<150µmol/L
Ferritin	12–200µg/L
Folate	2.1µg/L
γ-Glutamyl transpeptidase (GGT)	M: 11–51IU/L F: 7–33IU/L
Lactate dehydrogenase (LDH)	70–250IU/L
Magnesium	0.75–1.05mmol/L
Osmolality	278–305mOsmol/kg
Potassium	3.5–5mmol/L
Protein (total)	60–80g/L
Sodium	135–145mmol/L
Thyroid stimulating hormone (TSH)	0.5–5.7mu/L
Thyroxine (T_4)	70–140nmol/L
Thyroxine (free)	9–22pmol/L
Urate	M: 210–480µmol/L F: 150–39µmol/L
Urea	2.5–6.7mmol/L
Vitamin B_{12}	0.13–0.68mmol/L
Arterial blood gases	
pH	7.35–7.45
PaO_2	>10.6kPa
$PaCO_2$	4.7–6.0kPa
Base excess	±2mmol/L
Urine	
Cortisol (free)	<280nmol/24h
Osmolality	350–1000mOsmol/kg
Potassium	14–120mmol/24h
Protein	<150mg/24h
Sodium	100–250mmol/24h

ABBREVIATIONS

A&E	Accident and Emergency
AAA	abdominal aortic aneurysm
ABC	airway, breathing, circulation
ABCDE	airway, breathing, circulation, disability, exposure
ABG	arterial blood gases
ABPI	ankle brachial pressure index
ACE	angiotensin-converting enzyme
ACTH	adrenocorticotrophic hormone
ADH	antidiuretic hormone
ADHD	attention deficit hyperactivity disorder
AF	atrial fibrillation
AIDS	acquired immunodeficiency syndrome
AIHA	autoimmune haemolytic anaemia
ALP	alkaline phosphatase
aPTT	activated partial thromboplastin time
ARDS	adult respiratory distress syndrome
AST	aspartate aminotransferase
AV	atrioventricular
AV(N)RT	atrioventricular (nodal) re-entrant tachycardia
BASHH	British Association for Sexual Health and HIV
BE	base excess
Bili	bilirubin
BiPAP	bi-level positive airway pressure
BMI	body mass index
BMJ	British Medical Journal
BNF	British National Formulary
BP	blood pressure
bpm	beats per minute
BTS	British Thoracic Society
C	Celsius
Ca^{2+}	calcium
CCB	calcium-channel blocker
CD^{4+}	cluster of differentiation 4
CK	creatine kinase
CKD	chronic kidney disease
CLL	chronic lymphocytic leukaemia
CLO	Campylobacter-like organism
cm	centimetre

CML	chronic myeloid leukaemia
CMV	cytomegalovirus
CN	cranial nerve
CO_2	carbon dioxide
COPD	chronic obstructive pulmonary disease
CPAP	continuous positive airway pressure
CPR	cardiopulmonary resuscitation
Cr	creatinine
CREST	calcinosis, Raynaud's syndrome, esophageal dysmotility, sclerodactyly, telangiectasia
CRP	C-reactive protein
CRT	capillary refill time
CSM	Committee on Safety of Medicines
CT	computed tomography
CTPA	computed tomography pulmonary angiogram
CVP	central venous pressure
DC	direct current
DEXA	dual energy X-ray absorptiometry
DIC	disseminated intravascular coagulation
DKA	diabetic ketoacidosis
dL	decilitre
DNAR	Do Not Attempt Resuscitation
DPG	2,3-diphosphoglycerate
DRE	digital rectal examination
dsDNA	double-stranded deoxyribonucleic acid
DVT	deep vein thrombosis
EC	enteric coated
ECG	electrocardiogram
EEG	electroencephalogram
ERCP	endoscopic retrograde cholangiopancreatography
ESR	erythrocyte sedimentation rate
ESWL	extracorporeal shockwave lithotripsy
FFP	fresh frozen plasma
fL	femtolitre
g	gram
G	gauge
GALS	gait, arms, legs, spine
GCS	Glasgow Coma Scale
(e)GFR	(estimated) glomerular filtration rate
GGT	γ-glutamyl transferase
GMC	General Medical Council
GORD	gastro-oesophageal reflux disease
GP	general practitioner
h	hour

H_2O	water
HAART	highly active antiretroviral treatment
Hb	haemoglobin
HbA1C	glycosylated haemoglobin
hCG	human chorionic gonadotropin
HCO_3^-	bicarbonate
HDU	High-Dependency Unit
HE	hepatic encephalopathy
Hg	mercury
5-HIAA	5-hydroxyindoleacetic acid
HiB	Haemophilus influenzae type B
HIDA	hepatobiliary iminodiacetic acid (scan)
HIT	heparin-induced thrombocytopenia
HIV	human immunodeficiency virus
HIVAN	human immunodeficiency virus-associated nephropathy
HOCM	hypertrophic cardiomyopathy
HONK	hyperosmolar non-ketotic
HR	heart rate
Hz	hertz
Ig	immunoglobulin
IGF-1	insulin-like growth factor 1
IM	intramuscular
INH	inhaler
INR	international normalized ratio
ITP	idiopathic thrombocytopenic purpura
ITU	Intensive Therapy Unit
IV	intravenous
IVU	intravenous urogram
JVP	jugular venous pressure
K^+	potassium
KCl	potassium chloride
kg	kilogram
KUB	kidneys, ureters, and bladder
L	litre
LAD	left anterior descending
LCA	left (main) coronary artery
LCx	left circumflex coronary artery
LDH	lactate dehydrogenase
LMN	lower motor neurone
LMWH	low-molecular-weight heparin
LV	left ventricle
m	metre
MCV	mean corpuscular volume
mg	milligram

PO_4^{3-}	phosphate
PPI	proton pump inhibitor
PR	per rectum
PRN	pro re nata (when required)
PSA	prostate-specific antigen
PT	prothrombin time
PTH	parathyroid hormone
RCA	right coronary artery
RhF	rheumatoid factor
RR	respiratory rate
Rt	right
RUQ	right upper quadrant
RV	right ventricle
s	seconds
SA	sinoatrial
SaO$_2$	arterial oxygen saturation
SC	subcutaneous
SCD	sickle cell disease
SIADH	syndrome of inappropriate antidiuretic hormone secretion
SIRS	systemic inflammatory response syndrome
SPC	Summary of Product Characteristics
SLE	systemic lupus erythematosus
STAT	immediately
T	temperature
T$_3$	triiodothyronine
(f)T$_4$	(free) thyroxine
T-score	T-score (from T statistic) of bone mineral density measurement
TDD	total daily dose
TIA	transient ischaemic attack
TIBC	total iron-binding capacity
TSH	thyroid-stimulating hormone
U	unit
U&E	urea and electrolytes
UK	United Kingdom
Ur	urea
USS	ultrasound scan
V/Q scan	ventilation /perfusion scan
VF	ventricular fibrillation
VT	ventricular tachycardia
VTE	venous thromboembolic disease
WCC	white cell count
WHO	World Health Organization

HOW TO USE THIS BOOK

Oxford Assess and Progress, Clinical Medicine has been carefully designed to ensure you get the most out of your revision and are prepared for your exams. Here is a brief guide to some of the features and learning tools.

Organization of content

Chapter editorials will help you unpick tricky subjects, and when it's late at night and you need something to remind you why you're doing this, you'll find words of encouragement!

Single Best Answer (SBA) questions are indicated with this symbol ⚡ and Extended Matching Questions (EMQs) questions with this ⚡. Answers can be found at the end of each chapter. First the SBA answers ⚡, and then the EMQ answers ⚡.

How to read an answer

Unlike other revision guides on the market, this one is crammed full of feedback, so you should understand exactly why each answer is correct, and gain an insight into the common pitfalls.

With every answer there is an explanation of why that particular choice is the most appropriate. For some questions there is additional explanation of why the distracters are less suitable. Where relevant you will also be directed to sources of further information, such as the *Oxford Handbook of Clinical Medicine*, websites and journal articles.

→ http://www.nice.org.uk/nicemedia/pdf/word/CG43NICEGuideline.doc

Progression points

The questions in every chapter are ordered by level of difficulty and competence, indicated by the following symbols:

★   *Graduate 'should know'*—you should be aiming to get most of these correct.

★ ★   *Graduate 'nice to know'*—these are a bit tougher but not above your capabilities.

★ ★ ★   *Foundation Doctor 'should know'*—these will
      really test your understanding.

★ ★ ★ ★ *Foundation Doctor 'nice to know'*—give these a go
      when you're ready to challenge yourself.

Oxford Handbook of Clinical Medicine

The OHCM page references are given with the answers to some
questions. OHCM 8th edn → p402 Please note that this reference
is the 8th Edition of the OHCM, and that subsequent editions
are unlikely to have the same material in exactly the same place.

The Online Resource Centre

Bonus questions will be released monthly in the run up to final
medical examinations. Visit the website to sign up for alerts as
new questions are added.

 www.oxfordtextbooks.co.uk/orc/liakos_hill/

CHAPTER 1

CARDIOVASCULAR MEDICINE

The stethoscope is the symbol of graduation from the classroom to the ward. For many medical students, the act that christens this new tool happens under the gaze of a consultant cardiologist:

'Can you hear that? A clear ejection systolic murmur, heard loudest over the aortic area, with radiation to the carotids, grade 3/6.'

At this stage, even being told that there is a murmur does not guarantee that we will be able to hear it. The great news from clinical practice is that it is very rarely incumbent on a junior doctor to diagnose a *new* heart murmur (except, of course, in the setting of a pyrexia of unknown origin, in which case we need to entertain the possibility of a new murmur and take serial blood cultures with an endocarditis in mind). Most 'cardiac' patients come armed with reams of correspondence from eminent cardiologists describing their defect in the minutest detail – and if even they've missed it, there's always the echocardiogram report.

However, it is of course desirable to be able to detect these murmurs and always good practice to train our ear by listening to them, but even more important to understand their implications and suggest appropriate treatments.

Cardiology for the junior doctor is a lot more than the difference between an Austin Flint and a Graham Steell murmur. It should provide the foundation for almost all clinical assessments during which the following details will need to be gathered:

History

- Chest pain or shortness of breath
- Palpitations or collapse

- Exercise tolerance
- Orthopnoea or paroxysmal nocturnal dyspnoea
- Raised cholesterol level
- Diabetes
- Hypertension
- Ischaemic heart disease
- Smoking
- Family history

Examination
- General appearance
- Observations
- Peripheral perfusion
- Radial pulse
- Jugular venous pressure
- Eyes
- Praecordium
- Lungs
- Liver
- Legs

Investigations
- Full blood count
- Urea and electrolytes
- Blood sugar
- Cardiac enzymes
- Serial ECGs
- Chest X-rays
- Echocardiograms
- ECG exercise tests
- 24h tapes
- Angiography

The aim of this chapter is to build confidence in applying this approach to the most common clinical scenarios that junior doctors can expect to meet. The stress is not necessarily on diagnosis, but on developing clinical prowess and the ability to recognize the signs of cardiac impairment, and suggesting the most appropriate investigations and treatments to stabilize the patient.

Initially and most importantly, this means confronting pulmonary oedema, arrhythmias and acute coronary syndromes, and latterly more idiosyncratic situations such as malignant hypertension and heart muscle disease. As is the theme for the rest of this book, the aim is to develop a consistent approach that allows a clear way of thinking. In this way, we can make our patients safe by understanding and treating common and important problems, as well as staying one step ahead by thinking outside of the box and being open to more exotic possibilities. ∎

CARDIOVASCULAR MEDICINE
SINGLE BEST ANSWERS

1. A 53-year-old man is suffering from increasingly frequent bouts of chest pain. The pain has been provoked by exercise for the past 18 months. It is associated with shortness of breath and sweating, but passes as soon as he takes a moment to rest. He has stopped smoking and is currently taking aspirin 75mg PO once daily and atenolol 50mg PO once daily. Which is the *single* most appropriate management? ★

A Amlodipine

B Bendroflumethiazide

C Losartan

D Ramipril

E Simvastatin

2. An 84-year-old man has central chest pain that has gradually worsened over the last month. He finds it is made worse on exertion – especially climbing the stairs to his flat. He has type 2 diabetes and a hiatus hernia.

```
T 37.1°C, HR 95bpm, BP 165/95mmHg.
```

An ECG and a chest X-ray are both reported as 'normal'. Which is the *single* most likely diagnosis? ★

A Angina

B Gastro-oesophageal reflux disease

C Heart failure

D Myocardial infarction

E Oesophageal spasm

3. A 30-year-old man is woken from sleep by central chest pain and breathlessness. The pain radiates through to his back making him sit up in bed. He is otherwise fit and well, aside from having had a sore throat 2 weeks previously.

```
T 37.8°C, HR 110bpm, BP 125/90mmHg.
```

His chest X-ray is reported as 'normal' and an ECG is performed (Figure 1.1). Which is the *single* most likely diagnosis? ★

A Acute pericarditis

B Hypertrophic obstructive cardiomyopathy (HOCM)

C Infective endocarditis

D Myocardial infarction (MI)

E Pulmonary embolus (PE)

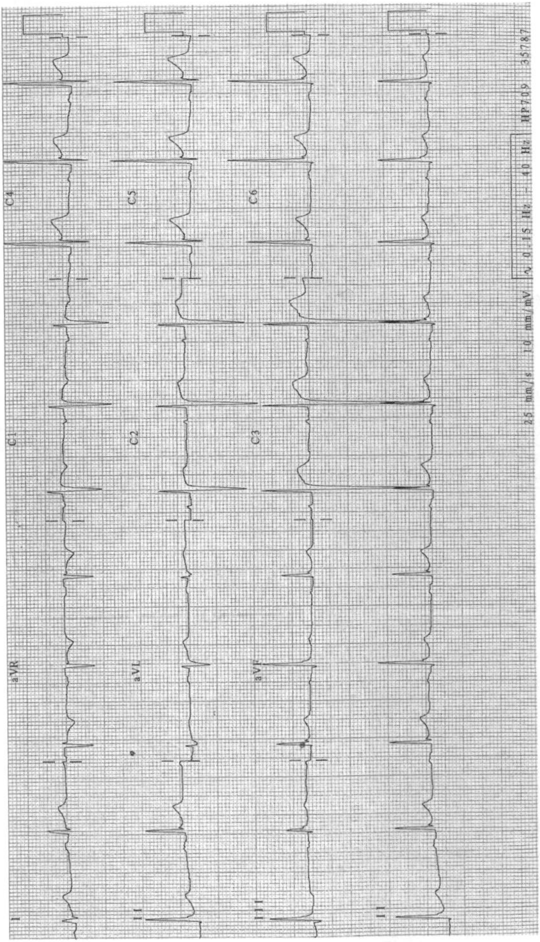

Figure 1.1

6

4. A 68-year-old woman has had palpitations and felt short of breath for the last few months. She has rheumatoid arthritis and takes methotrexate. The doctor examining her detects an ejection systolic murmur. This is difficult to hear so he asks her to carry out a manoeuvre to make it clearer. Which is the *single* most appropriate instruction to give to accentuate the murmur? ★

A Lean backwards on the couch

B Lean to your left side

C Squat down

D Take a deep breath in

E Try to breath out as if you were straining

5. A 20-year-old woman has had palpitations for 6h. She has had similar episodes before but they have never lasted this long. An ECG shows a regular rhythm of 160bpm with inverted P waves in leads II, III, and aVF, and narrow QRS complexes. Although vagal manoeuvres do not work, after adenosine 6mg IV, normal sinus rhythm at 90bpm is restored. Which is the *single* most likely origin of her tachycardia? ★

A Atrium

B Atrioventricular (AV) node

C Bundle of His

D Sinoatrial (SA) node

E Ventricle

6. A 71-year-old man has had a central chest pain radiating to his left arm for 1h. While an ECG is being recorded, some observations are carried out.

```
T 37.1°C, HR 44bpm, BP 110/65mmHg,
RR 22/min.
```

Which is the *single* most likely occluded coronary artery? ★

A Left anterior descending artery (LAD)

B Left circumflex coronary artery (LCx)

C Left main coronary artery (LCA)

D Posterior descending artery (PDA)

E Right coronary artery (RCA)

7. A 65-year-old man has had a central chest pain radiating to his left arm for 2h. He has had increasingly regular chest pain over the last 2 weeks. He has type 2 diabetes and takes metformin. An ECG is performed (Figure 1.2). Which is the *single* most likely occluded coronary artery? ★

A Left anterior descending artery (LAD)

B Left circumflex coronary artery (LCx)

C Left main coronary artery (LCA)

D Posterior descending artery (PDA)

E Right coronary artery (RCA)

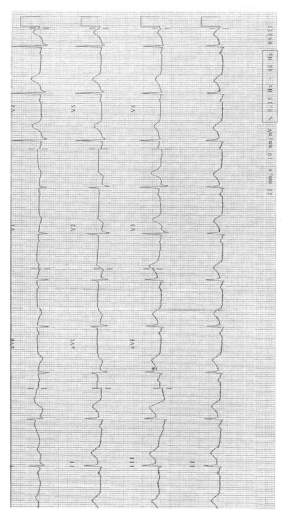

Figure 1.2

8. A 78-year-old man is recovering after an ST elevation myocardial infarction (STEMI). In the past hour, his pulse rate has increased from 100 to 130bpm and his respiratory rate from 20 to 30/min. The junior doctor is called. The patient has a productive cough and is sitting forward with his hands on his knees. Which *single* treatment is most likely to reverse this man's deterioration? ★

A Bendroflumethiazide 2.5mg PO

B Bumetanide 1mg PO

C Furosemide 80mg IV

D Heparin 5000U IV

E Metoprolol 50mg IV

9. A 72-year-old man has felt dizzy and short of breath for the past couple of hours. He is very conscious of his heart beating and is extremely anxious. He has hypertension and was discharged from hospital 3 months previously after a non-ST-elevation myocardial infarction (NSTEMI).

```
T 36.6°C, HR 140bpm, BP 115/80mmHg.
Chest: clear.
```

An ECG is performed (Figure 1.3). Which would be the *single* most appropriate immediate management? ★

A Adenosine

B Amiodarone

C Digoxin

D Lidocaine

E Synchronized cardioversion

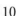

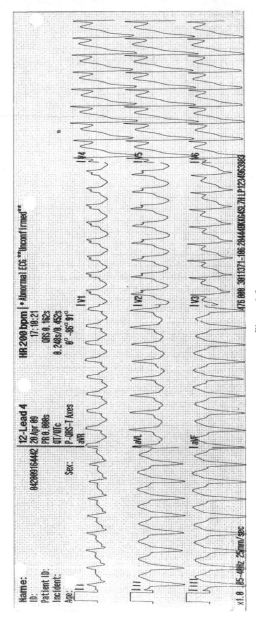

Figure 1.3

?

11

10. A 72-year-old woman feels her heart beating fast. She becomes anxious and increasingly uncomfortable and wants to see a doctor. She has a chest infection for which she is receiving co-amoxiclav 1.2g IV three times daily. The nursing staff contact the junior doctor and discuss the patient over the telephone. Which single question would be most useful in the immediate assessment of this patient? ★

A Is the heart beat regular or irregular?

B Is she confused?

C Is she short of breath?

D What is her blood pressure?

E What is her temperature?

11. A 74-year-old man has felt progressively short of breath over the last year. He has had recurrent attacks of bronchitis over 6 months and friends have said his voice sounds increasingly hoarse, despite being a lifelong non-smoker. The doctor examining him detects a mid-diastolic murmur that is difficult to hear, but she asks him to carry out a manoeuvre to make it clearer. Which is the *single* most appropriate instruction to give to accentuate the murmur? ★

A Lean backwards on the couch

B Lean to your left side

C Sit up and lean forwards

D Take a deep breath in

E Try to breathe out as if you were straining

12. A 52-year-old man has had pain in his upper chest for the last 1h. It came on after he had climbed the stairs to his office and since then, he has found his breathing constricted and has felt hot and uncomfortable. He recalls a similar episode a month ago after running for a bus. He is a non-smoker and takes no regular prescription medications.

```
12h troponin I <0.05µg/L.
```

An ECG is performed (Figure 1.4). Which is the *single* most appropriate initial investigation of this man's symptoms? ★

A Coronary angiogram

B Dobutamine stress test

C Echocardiogram

D Exercise ECG

E 24h ECG monitoring

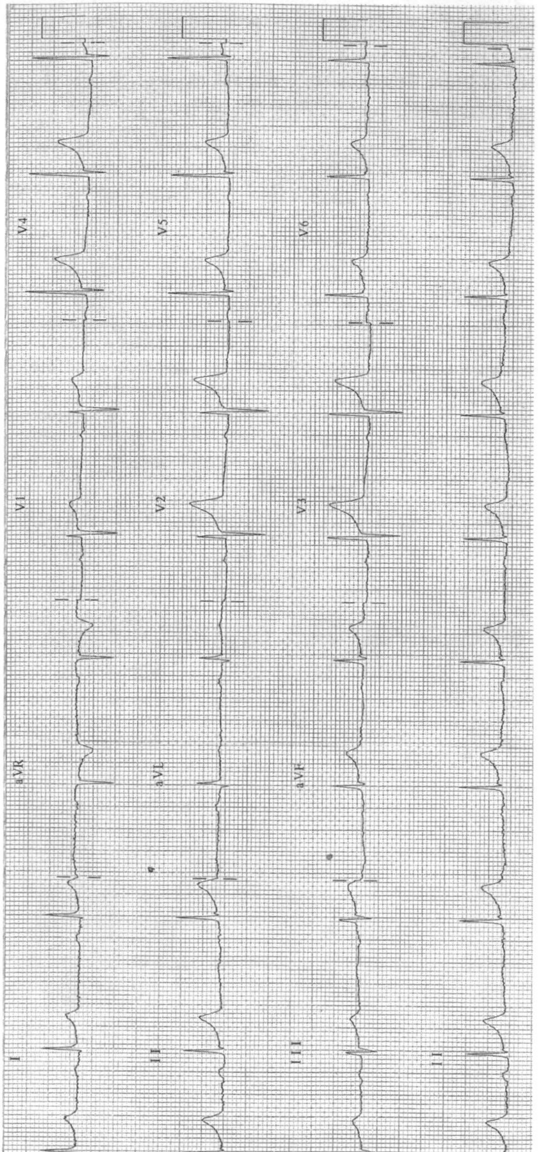

Figure 1.4

14

13. A 44-year-old man has had a sudden-onset chest pain radiating to his jaw, plus sweating and nausea. An ECG is performed and shows ST elevation in the V1–V6, I, and aVL leads. Which is the *single* most likely occluded coronary artery? ★

A Left anterior descending artery (LAD)

B Left circumflex coronary artery (LCx)

C Left main coronary artery (LCA)

D Posterior descending artery (PDA)

E Right coronary artery (RCA)

14. A 66-year-old woman has been feverish for the past 2 weeks, particularly at night. She has been brought into the Emergency Department by her husband who woke to find her shivering. She has type 2 diabetes and had a prosthetic mitral valve fitted 9 months previously.

```
T 38.4°C, HR 110bpm, BP 95/50mmHg.
Urine dipstick: blood 2+.
```

Which *single* additional fact from the woman's recent history would most support the likely diagnosis? ★

A She did a 10km charity run

B She has had the 'flu vaccine

C She recently started taking insulin

D She spent 2 weeks in southern Europe

E She underwent dental surgery

15. A 32-year-old man has felt generally unwell for the last month or so. He has had sweats at night and has lost 3kg. He is otherwise fit and well but does confess to injecting illicit drugs.

```
T 38.1°C, HR 100bpm, BP 105/80mmHg.
```

There is a pansystolic murmur loudest at the left sternal edge. Which *single* investigation is most likely to support the diagnosis? ★

A Arterial blood gas

B Creatine kinase

C Sputum sample

D Urea and electrolytes

E Urinalysis

16. A 24-year-old man has felt increasingly short of breath over 3 months. He has no family history of cardiac disease. He has a harsh ejection systolic murmur and a double apex beat. Which is the *single* most likely description of his pulse characteristic? ★

A Anacrotic

B Bisferiens

C Bounding

D Collapsing

E Jerky

17.

A 26-year-old woman has a routine medical prior to travelling abroad for voluntary medical service.

```
T 36.6°C, HR 90bpm, BP 115/80mmHg.
```

Her heart sounds are normal with no murmurs. An ECG is performed (Figure 1.5). Which is the *single* most likely diagnosis? ★

A First-degree heart block

B Left bundle branch block

C Normal

D Sinus arrhythmia

E Wolff–Parkinson–White syndrome

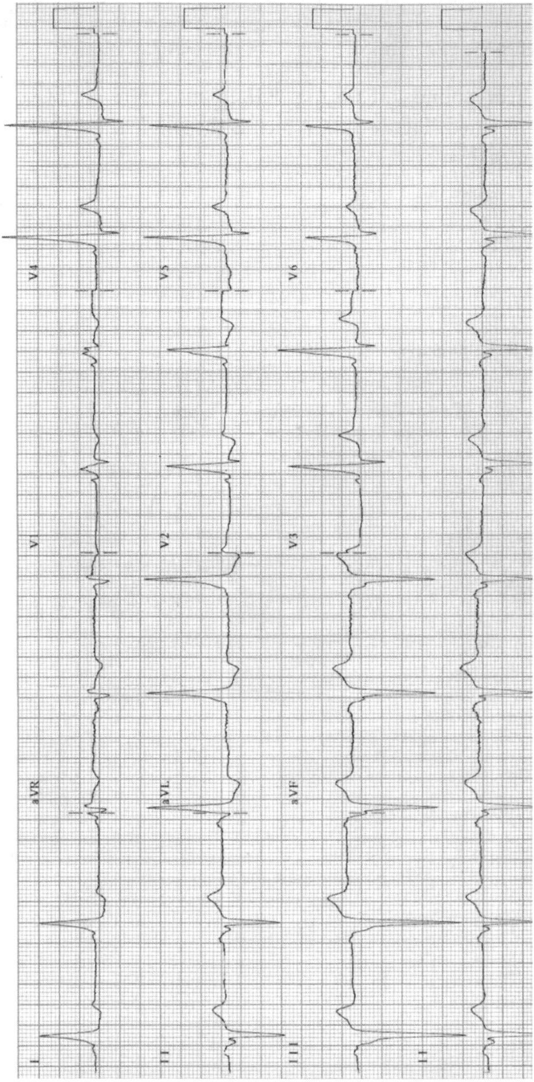

Figure 1.5

18. A 77-year-old woman has felt intermittently dizzy for the last 6 months. She has not fallen but has felt as if she might faint, especially when exerting herself. Which *single* description of her pulse is most likely to support the diagnosis? ★

A Collapsing

B Irregularly irregular

C Jerky

D Slow-rising

E Thready

19. A 73-year-old man has had a cough and been short of breath for 3 months. He has been sleeping in a chair and now finds it difficult to leave the house at all. He has pitting oedema up to the mid-thigh and his JVP is evident just below the angle of the jaw. An echocardiogram shows that his left ventricular ejection fraction is 15%. Which is the *single* most likely description of his pulse characteristic? ★

A Anacrotic

B Bisferiens

C Collapsing

D Jerky

E Pulsus alternans

$20.$ A 45-year-old man suffers sudden central chest pain while at rest. It spreads across his chest and up to his neck. After 20min, the pain has not eased and he is increasingly sweaty and short of breath. This is the third such episode in the last 3 months.

```
12h troponin I <0.05µg/L.
```

Which would be the *single* most accurate classification of this event? ★

A Acute coronary syndrome

B Non-ST elevation myocardial infarction

C ST elevation myocardial infarction

D Stable angina

E Unstable angina

$21.$ The on-call junior doctor receives a call from a nurse about a 55-year-old man who is experiencing palpitations on one of the medical wards. These started 5min ago and the nurse has taken an ECG and asked for the patient to be reviewed. His heart rate is 140bpm. It is a busy night shift and there are five patients waiting to be seen in A&E. Which *single* additional detail from the nurse should prompt an immediate review of the patient (i.e. within the next 5min)? ★

A He is currently being loaded with digoxin

B SaO_2 98% on 10L O_2

C Systolic BP 90mmHg

D Temperature 38.1°C

E The patient is extremely anxious

22. A 45-year-old man has had back pain for the last 3 weeks and visits his GP. He is a non-smoker with no family history of heart disease. His BMI is 25kg/m²

```
BP 115/75mmHg.
```

Whilst examining him, the doctor notices his eyes (Figure 1.6). Which is the *single* most appropriate initial management? ★

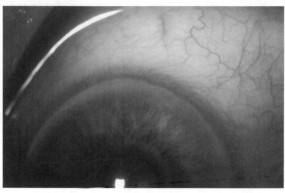

Figure 1.6

A Advise him to lose weight

B Check renal, liver, and thyroid function

C Start bezafibrate 200mg PO twice daily

D Start a low-fat diet

E Start simvastatin 40mg PO once daily

23. The junior doctor on-call receives a bleep from a nurse during a busy night shift. A 53-year-old man with type 1 diabetes has had central chest pain over the last 10min. He has been admitted electively under the general surgeons for a laparoscopic inguinal hernia repair. The nurse has already performed an ECG. Which *single* additional detail from the nurse should prompt an immediate review of the patient (i.e. within the next 5min)? ★

A Blood glucose 15.2mmol/L

B He has vomited twice since the pain has started

C His operation is tomorrow morning

D HR 98bpm

E SaO$_2$ 96% on air

24. A 73-year-old woman has been short of breath for the past 3 weeks. She now needs to sleep with four pillows rather than two and has swollen ankles by the end of the day. She uses a regular steroid inhaler for asthma but has never been in hospital for any reason. Which is the *single* most likely diagnosis? ★

A Acute exacerbation of asthma

B Angina

C Cardiac failure

D Pneumonia

E Pulmonary embolus

25. A 44-year-old man has a spell of central chest pain that lasts 20min. He describes it as 'aching' and spreading up to his neck. He has type 2 diabetes and hypertension.

T 36.4°C, HR 90bpm, BP 140/80mmHg, SaO$_2$ 99% on 15L O$_2$.

An ECG is performed (Figure 1.7). Which is the *single* most likely diagnosis? ★

A Acute myocarditis

B Acute pericarditis

C Lateral ischaemia

D Myocardial infarction

E Unstable angina

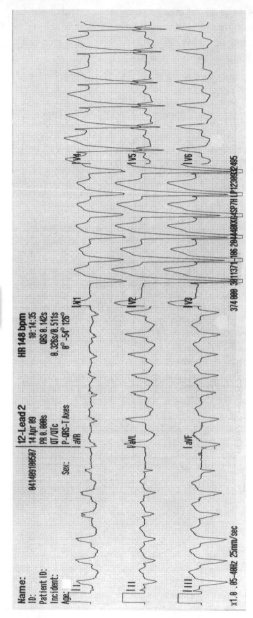

Figure 1.7

24

26. A 72-year-old woman has noticed that her abdomen has swollen over the past 6 months. It has become uncomfortable and she has felt increasingly short of breath. She has been on home nebulizers for chronic obstructive pulmonary disease (COPD) for many years.

T 37.2°C, HR 90bpm, BP 135/90mmHg, RR 20/min.

Bilateral ankle oedema pitting to the knee.

JVP: visible 5cm above the sternal angle.

Abdomen: distended but non-tender with no organomegaly.

Shifting dullness is demonstrated.

Which is the *single* most likely cause of this woman's abdominal distension? ★

A Budd–Chiari syndrome

B Chronic persistent hepatitis

C Constrictive pericarditis

D Cor pulmonale

E Portal hypertension

$27.$ A 62-year-old man is dizzy and complains of palpitations. He has become drowsy and is making little sense to the nursing staff who bleep the on-call doctor. He is being treated for a urinary tract infection with co-amoxiclav 1.2g IV three times daily.

```
T 38.1°C, HR 150bpm, BP 110/70mmHg, SaO₂ 97%
on air.
```

An ECG is performed (Figure 1.8). Which is the *single* most appropriate management? ★

A Amiodarone 400mg IV STAT

B Digoxin 500mcg IV STAT

C Direct current (DC) cardioversion

D Metoprolol 50mg IV STAT

E Temporary cardiac pacing

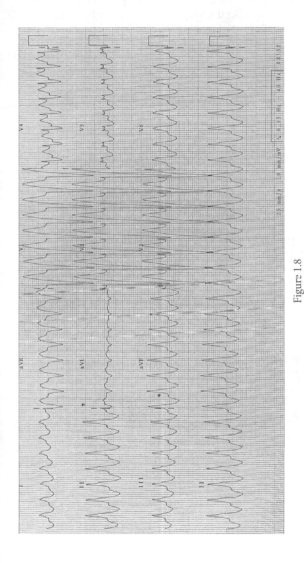

Figure 1.8

28. A 36-year-old woman has been lethargic and felt increasingly dizzy over the last 2 months. She is usually well but does report long and very heavy periods, especially in the last 6 months.

```
T 36.6°C, HR 110bpm, BP 95/65mmHg.

Bilateral ankle oedema pitting to
the mid-calf.

JVP: visible 5cm above the sternal angle.

Chest: fine end-inspiratory crepitations at
both bases.
```

Which is the *single* most appropriate next step? ★ ★

A Furosemide 40mg IV

B Human albumin solution 20% 200mL IV

C Iron sucrose 200mg IV

D Packed red cells 2U IV

E Vitamin K 10mg IV

29. A 52-year-old man suffers sudden central chest pain while watching television. He describes it as a 'suffocating' sensation that rose up to his neck and made it difficult to breathe. He arrives at the Emergency Department at 22.00 within 2h of the onset of the pain. An ECG is performed (Figure 1.9).

```
Troponin I <0.05µg/L.
```

The following morning he looks pale, clammy and anxious. Which is the *single* most appropriate course of action? ★ ★

A Angiogram

B Creatine kinase level

C Echocardiogram

D Exercise tolerance test

E Repeat troponin level

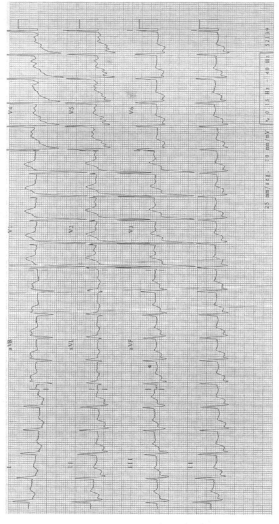

Figure 1.9

30. A 70-year-old man has had palpitations and been short of breath for the last 24h. He has hypertension and was recently discharged from hospital after a myocardial infarction. An ECG is performed (Figure 1.10). The on-call registrar suggests giving the man adenosine 6mg IV. Which *single* description most accurately explains why it works? ★ ★

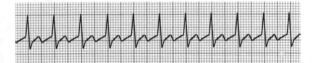

Figure 1.10

A It blocks the atrioventricular (AV) node, thus unmasking flutter waves

B It increases vagal tone, thus slowing the atrial rate

C It reduces the force of contractions and thus corrects the arrhythmia

D It resets the sinoatrial (SA) node, thus correcting ventricular tachycardia (VT)

E It transiently stops the atria from fibrillating

31. A 30-year-old man has been involved in a road traffic accident. He has sustained injuries to the chest wall and is short of breath. A trauma series of X-rays suggests fluid in the pleura and pericardium. This is confirmed by a transthoracic echocardiogram. The JVP rises with inspiration. Which *single* description most accurately explains the pathological JVP? ★ ★

A Pleural fluid causes pressure to back up onto the right heart

B The right heart cannot increase in size due to restriction

C There must also be a clot in the pulmonary circulation

D There must also be a thrombus in the right subclavian vein

E There must be concurrent valvular damage

32. A 53-year-old man has felt increasingly tired for the last month. He has had mild pain in his abdomen, which he feels is slightly fuller than normal. He says he has 'heart valve problems'. There is a pan-systolic murmur, heard best at the left sternal edge. Which *single* pair of examination findings supports the diagnosis? ★ ★

A Collapsing pulse + nodding head

B Hyperdynamic apex beat + visible carotid pulsation

C Prominent 'a' wave in JVP + widely split S_2

D Prominent 'v' wave in JVP + right ventricular (RV) heave

E Tapping apex beat + malar flush

33. A 55-year-old woman has noticed her heart beating fast. It happens infrequently and is not associated with any other symptoms. She is anxious about the cause of these attacks as she has no other medical problems.

```
HR 80bpm, BP 115/75mmHg.
```

After a normal ECG, a 24h tape is performed (Figure 1.11). Which is the *single* most appropriate treatment? ★ ★ ★

A Amiodarone 100mg PO once daily

B Digoxin 62.5mcg PO once daily

C Flecainide 150mg PO as required

D Metoprolol 25mg PO twice daily

E Sotalol 40mg PO twice daily

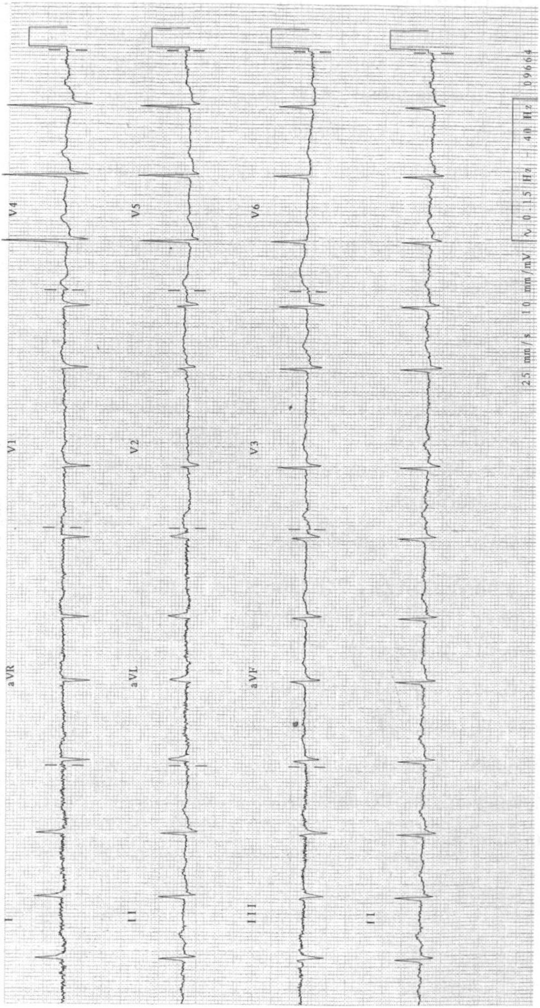

Figure 1.11

34. A 62-year-old woman is recovering on a medical ward after an exacerbation of her asthma. Her regular observations are checked.

```
BP 205/115mmHg.
```

The nursing staff contact the junior doctor and discuss the patient over the telephone. Which *single* question would be most useful in the immediate assessment of this patient? ★ ★ ★

A Are her pupils equal and reactive to light?

B Does she have a headache?

C Has her medication been changed recently?

D Has this happened before?

E What is her heart rate?

35. A 77-year-old man has been increasingly short of breath for the past 6 weeks and over the last few days he has become drowsy and confused. He has chronic atrial fibrillation on warfarin and digoxin but is otherwise well. He was a heavy smoker until 10 years ago and does not drink alcohol.

```
T 37.7°C, HR 140bpm (irreg.), BP 140/90mmHg,
SaO₂ 88% on air.

JVP: visible at the earlobe.

Chest: widespread inspiratory crepitations.

Ankle oedema pitting to the mid-calf.
```

He is given high-flow oxygen and his SaO₂ improve to 97% on 10L. As he is being examined, he becomes tremulous and increasingly agitated. Which is the *single* most likely explanation for the man's agitation? ★ ★ ★

A He has developed a pulmonary embolus

B He has gone into septic shock

C He has gone into ventricular tachycardia (VT)

D He has undiagnosed chronic obstructive pulmonary disease (COPD)

E He is hypoglycaemic

36. A 72-year-old woman has become extremely short of breath over a matter of minutes. She is coughing up frothy sputum and is unable to complete sentences but has no chest pain. She has hypertension and chronic renal impairment that has deteriorated despite recently starting ramipril and losartan. A chest X-ray is performed (Figure 1.12). Which *single* investigation would be most likely to identify the underlying diagnosis? ★ ★ ★

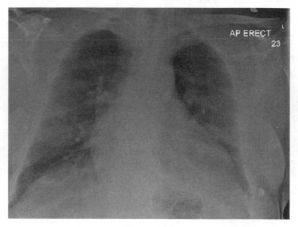

Figure 1.12

A Coronary angiogram

B CT scan of chest

C Doppler ultrasound scan (USS) of renal arteries

D Transthoracic echocardiogram

E USS of kidneys and bladder

37. A CVP line is inserted for fluid resuscitation of a patient with left ventricular failure and acute renal failure. Which *single* X-ray finding is most likely to confirm correct placement of the line? ★ ★ ★

A Both ends of the line can be seen

B The line is lying lateral to the upper thoracic transverse processes

C The line tip is between the first and third sternocostal joints

D The line tip is in the midline above the level of the clavicles

E There is no obvious intra-pleural air

38. A 62-year-old man has collapsed. He had felt fine beforehand apart from a fluttering feeling in his chest. He turned very pale as he fell to the ground, but within seconds his face flushed and full consciousness was regained. This has happened on two previous occasions. An ECG is performed (Figure 1.13). Which is the *single* most appropriate treatment for these episodes? ★ ★ ★

A Amiodarone 200mg PO twice daily

B Flecainide 50mg PO twice daily

C Implantable cardioverter defibrillator

D Permanent pacemaker

E Radiofrequency ablation of aberrant pathway

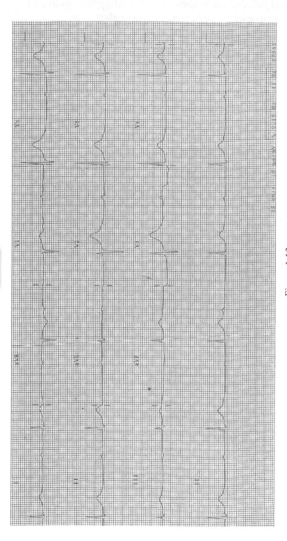

Figure 1.13

39. A 54-year-old woman has collapsed. She cannot remember feeling unwell beforehand and has no residual symptoms afterwards. She has hypertension, type 2 diabetes, depression, and schizophrenia. She takes nifedipine, bendroflumethiazide, metformin, amitriptyline, and olanzapine. Her blood tests are within normal limits. An ECG is performed (Figure 1.14). Which *single* medicine is most likely to have been responsible for her collapse? ★ ★ ★

A Amitriptyline

B Bendroflumethiazide

C Metformin

D Nifedipine

E Olanzapine

Figure 1.14

40. A 32-year-old woman has had worsening central chest pain over the last 7 days. She feels breathless and thinks her ankles are swollen. She is currently taking hydroxychloroquine to control recurrent wrist swelling. A chest X-ray shows an enlarged cardiac silhouette. Which is the *single* most likely description of her pulse characteristic? ★ ★ ★

A Anacrotic

B Bisferiens

C Collapsing

D Pulsus alternans

E Small-volume

41. A 54-year-old man is recovering on a surgical ward after thromboplasty to his right leg. Routine observations are carried out.

```
HR 100bpm, BP 230/135mmHg, SaO₂ 96% on air.
```

Over the next 4h, the man develops central chest pain radiating to his jaw. Serial ECGs show dynamic T-wave changes in the lateral chest leads. His blood pressure remains unchanged. Which is the *single* most appropriate approach to treating the blood pressure? ★ ★ ★

A Do not treat until the patient is pain free

B Intermittent use of a sublingual spray

C Lower with oral therapy over next 24–48h

D Lower urgently with IV therapy

E Use one-off dose of a sublingual tablet

42. A 40-year-old woman has become increasingly short of breath over a 24h period. She also has central chest pain that is made slightly easier if she sits forwards. She has had no previous cardiorespiratory problems but does take prednisolone 20mg PO once daily for a rheumatological condition.

```
T 37.2°C, HR 100bpm, BP 115/75mmHg.
```

She has several mouth ulcers and tender, swollen wrist joints. Which *single* examination finding is most likely to support the diagnosis? ★ ★ ★ ★

A Displaced apex beat

B Flushed cheeks

C Pericardial rub

D Red rash on trunk with clear centres

E Splinter haemorrhages in fingernails

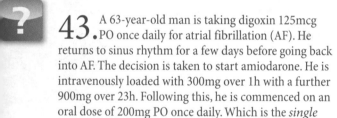

43. A 63-year-old man is taking digoxin 125mcg PO once daily for atrial fibrillation (AF). He returns to sinus rhythm for a few days before going back into AF. The decision is taken to start amiodarone. He is intravenously loaded with 300mg over 1h with a further 900mg over 23h. Following this, he is commenced on an oral dose of 200mg PO once daily. Which is the *single* most appropriate next step in management? ★ ★ ★ ★

A Continue both drugs at their current doses

B Decrease the amiodarone dose to 100mg PO once daily

C Decrease the digoxin dose to 62.5mcg PO once daily

D Increase the amiodarone dose to 400mg PO once daily

E Increase the digoxin dose to 250mcg PO once daily

EXTENDED MATCHING QUESTIONS

Treatment of heart failure

For each patient with heart failure, choose the *single* medication that it would be most appropriate to start from the list of options below. Each option may be used once, more than once, or not at all. ★ ★ ★

A Amiodarone 200mg PO once daily

B Amlodipine 5mg PO once daily

C Aspirin 75mg PO once daily

D Bisoprolol 1.25mg PO once daily

E Clopidogrel 75mg PO once daily

F Digoxin 62.5mcg PO once daily

G Diltiazem 120mg PO once daily

H Furosemide 40mg PO once daily

I Losartan 50mg PO once daily

J Ramipril 2.5mg PO twice daily

K Simvastatin 40mg PO once daily

L Spironolactone 25mg PO once daily

M Verapamil 120mg PO once daily

1. A 77-year-old man attends his quarterly review with his family doctor. He is currently asymptomatic and has not been in hospital for any reason for more than 2 years. He takes a loop diuretic and an angiotensin-converting enzyme (ACE) inhibitor.
HR 75bpm, BP 140/70mmHg.
Echocardiogram: left ventricular ejection fraction 25–30%.

2. A 69-year-old woman has been tired with breathlessness, especially at night, for the past week. This is the third time that such symptoms have required her to be admitted to hospital in the last 9 months. Prior to this, she was started on bumetanide 1mg PO twice daily, ramipril 5mg PO twice daily, bisoprolol 2.5mg PO once daily, and digoxin 125mcg PO once daily.
HR 88bpm, BP 128/75mmHg.

3. A 68-year-old woman feels tired and increasingly short of breath, especially on walking to the local shops. She has recently begun sleeping on multiple pillows at night.
HR 90bpm, BP 175/80mmHg.
Echocardiogram: left ventricular ejection fraction 35%.

4. A 74-year-old man is suffering with a progressive reduction in his exercise tolerance. He can now only manage a few steps before becoming breathless and light-headed. He takes bumetanide 1mg PO twice daily, bisoprolol 5mg PO once daily, and ramipril 10mg PO twice daily.
HR 88bpm (irregular), BP 145/76mmHg.
Echocardiogram: left ventricular ejection fraction 10–15%.

5. A 75-year-old woman has noticed her ankles are swollen at the end of each day. She has also started to get short of breath after walking up several flights of stairs.
HR 78bpm, BP 120/65mmHg.

Treatment of hypertension

For each patient with hypertension, choose the *single* medication that it would be most appropriate to start from the list of options below. Each option may be used once, more than once, or not at all.

A Alfuzosin 5mg PO once daily

B Amlodipine 5mg PO once daily

C Atenolol 25mg PO once daily

D Bendroflumethiazide 2.5mg PO once daily

E Bumetanide 1mg PO once daily

F Diltiazem 60mg PO three times a day

G Furosemide 40mg PO once daily

H Ivabradine 2.5mg PO once daily

I Losartan 25mg PO once daily

J Ramipril 2.5mg PO twice daily

6. A 42-year-old Caucasian man has been asked to return to his family doctor having had elevated blood pressure readings on two previous occasions.
BP 170/100 mmHg.

7. A 66-year-old Caucasian man has his quarterly appointment with his family doctor. He has been taking an angiotensin-converting enzyme (ACE) inhibitor for just over a year and uses allopurinol for gout.
BP 165/95 mmHg.

8. A 38-year-old Afro-Caribbean woman has had repeatedly high blood pressure readings over the last 6 months. She also has type 1 diabetes.
BP 155/95 mmHg.

9. A 32-year-old Caucasian woman sees her family doctor after having a high blood pressure reading at a routine work medical. She is currently trying to get pregnant and is concerned what effect this or any medications could have on the baby.
BP 170/90 mmHg.

10. A 74-year-old woman has had a persistent dry cough for the last 3 months. Prior to this, she was diagnosed with hypertension and started on perindopril 4mg PO once daily.
BP 115/75 mmHg.

Treatment of tachycardia

For each patient with tachycardia below, choose the single most appropriate immediate treatment from the list of options below. Each option may be used once, more than once, or not at all. All the answers are in line with the Resuscitation Council (UK) guidelines 2005 (http://www.resus.org.uk/pages/periarst.pdf). ★ ★ ★

A Adenosine 6mg IV

B Amiodarone 300mg IV

C Asynchronous direct current (DC) cardioversion

D Atenolol 5mg IV

E Carotid sinus massage

F Digoxin 500mcg IV

G Flecainide 50mg PO

H Furosemide 40mg IV

I Magnesium 2g IV

J Sodium chloride 0.9% 1L IV over 4h

K Sotalol 80mg PO

L Synchronized DC cardioversion

M Valsalva manoeuvre

11. A 66-year-old woman with metastatic bowel cancer is undergoing palliative chemotherapy. She had an inferior myocardial infarction 3 years ago but currently has no chest pain. An ECG is performed (Figure 1.15).
HR 160bpm, BP 110/50mmHg, SaO$_2$ 98% on 2L O$_2$.
Chest: good air entry bilaterally.

12. A 48-year-old woman has had palpitations for the last 4h and now feels light-headed. She has no previous cardiac history. She has increased her alcohol consumption over the last few months and was at a party last night but cannot remember how much she drank. An ECG is performed (Figure 1.16).
HR 135bpm, BP 85/65mmHg, SaO$_2$ 96% on 15L O$_2$.

13. A 67-year-old man has felt his heart 'racing' for the last 6h. He suffered from this a few months ago but did not come to hospital. He has no chest pain and otherwise feels well.
HR 180bpm, BP 110/70mmHg, SaO$_2$ 97% on 15L O$_2$.
A rhythm strip shows a regular narrow complex tachycardia. Blowing into the end of a syringe does not affect the rhythm.

14. A 72-year-old man has had palpitations over the last 8h and now has chest pain and feels more short of breath. He has never had any cardiac problems.
HR 180bpm, BP 100/60mmHg, SaO$_2$ 96% on 15L O$_2$.
He has bibasal crepitations and a raised JVP. An ECG is performed (Figure 1.17).

15. A 55-year-old man has had thrombolysis for an inferior myocardial infarction. He is recovering well until he starts to experience palpitations. An ECG is performed (see Figure 1.3, p11).
HR 175bpm, BP 125/70mmHg, SaO$_2$ 98% on air.

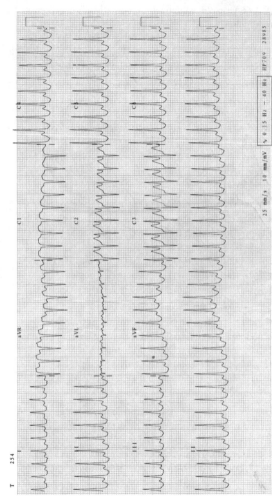

Figure 1.15

48

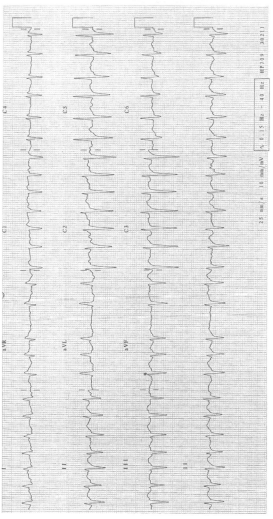

Figure 1.16

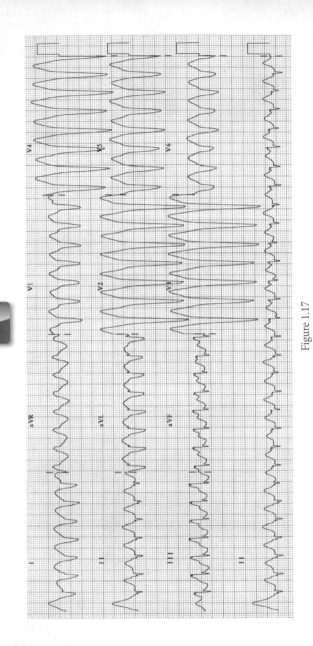

Figure 1.17

Drug side effects

For each scenario, choose the *single* drug from the list of options below most likely to be responsible for the symptoms described. Each option may be used once, more than once, or not at all. ★ ★ ★

A Alfuzosin

B Amlodipine

C Atenolol

D Bendroflumethiazide

E Bumetanide

F Furosemide

G Hydralazine

H Lisinopril

I Losartan

J Methyldopa

K Verapamil

16. An 72-year-old man is given a new antihypertensive medication. Three weeks later, he feels unwell and a blood test shows the following results:
Sodium 139mmol/L, potassium 4.9mmol/L, creatinine 281μmol/L, urea 15.2mmol/L.

17. A 42-year-old woman has type 2 diabetes mellitus and hypertension. She has recently been started on a new antihypertensive medication and has noticed that her blood glucose control is not as good as it was before.

18. A 64-year-old woman has always had cold hands and feet, even in summer. She has recently started an additional antihypertensive medication and has found that her cold peripheries are even worse than usual.

19. A 55-year-old man has noticed that his ankles are more swollen than is usual for him. Two weeks ago, he was started on an antihypertensive medication.

20. An 80-year-old woman has been feeling dizzy and lethargic for the past week. She has recently been started on a second antihypertensive medication, having been on a beta-blocker for many years.
HR 45bpm, BP 75/40mmHg.

Single Best Answers

1. A ★

This man is suffering from stable angina. He is already taking atenolol and should be commenced on the long-acting dihydropyridine, amlodipine.

Beta-blockers, nitrates, and long-acting calcium-channel blocker (CCBs) all prolong the length of exercise available before the onset of angina and ST depression, and decrease the frequency of angina. A number of leading cardiology societies recommend beta-blockers as the first-line therapy in stable angina. However, a large meta-analysis showed no difference in rates of myocardial infarction (MI) or cardiac death between CCBs and beta-blockers. In hypertensive patients, short-acting CCBs (but not the longer-acting dihydropyridines) have showed an increased risk of MI and, at high doses, mortality rate. If patients remain symptomatic current recommendations are to combine the beta-blocker with a nitrate/dihydropyridine CCB or a short-acting CCB and a nitrate.

Ben-Dor I and Battler A (2007) Treatment of stable angina. *Heart* **93**:868–874.

2. A ★

Chest pain that is brought on by exertion is by definition angina. This man has two risk factors for developing the atheromatous vessels that are the main precipitant of angina: hypertension and diabetes.

B AND E   Although he has a hiatus hernia, the fact that his pain is linked to exercise would make it atypical of either reflux disease or spasm.

C The normality of his chest X-ray and the absence of any suggestive symptoms make it improbable that he has heart failure.

D Whilst he may have suffered myocardial damage at some point over the last month, it is unlikely given his normal ECG.

3. A ★

In a young, previously healthy individual who has just had a minor infection, symptoms like this are strongly suggestive of pericardial inflammation. In 9/10 cases, the ECG will be supportive. The pain is eased with simple anti-inflammatory drugs.

B HOCM usually announces itself with a collapse or even sudden death and has a strong family history.

C Endocarditis is unlikely to affect a previously healthy individual without risk factors (e.g. IV drug use, replacement valves); those who present with it are usually rather unwell with a new heart murmur but a normal ECG.

D MI in a young man is unlikely.

E The sudden nature and distribution of the pain make a PE possible, but the surrounding story is not supportive.

4. C ★   OHCM 8th edn → p44

This is aortic stenosis, with squatting increasing venous return and accentuating the murmur, although admittedly this might be difficult in a woman of this age with RA.

A This would have no effect.

B This would be used to detect mitral stenosis.

D This reduces the blood flow to the left side of the heart, softening murmurs on this side of the circulation.

E This is known as the Valsalva manoeuvre and decreases venous return and accentuates mitral valve prolapse and hypertrophic obstructive cardiomyopathy.

5. B ★

The clues here are in the ECG and the fact that the tachycardia resolves with adenosine. Inverted P waves in the inferior leads are suggestive of retrograde atrial conduction. This phenomenon is common to junctional tachycardias, which would also fit with the patient – the fact that she has had them before – and the fact that it resolves once the AV node is blocked by adenosine.

Junctional tachycardias originate from the region of the AV node. They are either atrioventricular re-entry tachycardias (AVRTs) or atrioventricular nodal re-entry tachycardias (AVNRTs). AVNRTs are the most common, usually affecting young, healthy individuals with no organic heart disease. They are caused by having two distinct pathways in the region of the AV node – a fast and a slow one.

In AVRT, there is an accessory pathway that actually bypasses the AV node and activates the ventricles prematurely. The most common type is Wolff–Parkinson–White syndrome.

6. E ★

This man has had a myocardial infarction (MI) and is bradycardic. The most likely cause of bradycardia is an inferior MI as, in 60% of cases, the RCA supplies the sinoatrial (SA) node (the LCA supplying the other 40%).

→ http://en.ecgpedia.org/wiki/Myocardial_Infarction#The_location_of_the_infarct

7. E ★

This is an inferior myocardial infarction caused by an occlusion in the RCA.

In the LCA, the left main stem divides into the left anterior descending and left circumflex arteries. The LAD supplies two-thirds of the interventricular septum, the anterior portion of the left ventricle (LV) and the apex of the heart. The LCA can branch again into the left marginal artery supplying the left atrium, the obtuse margin of the heart, and the posterior LV wall.

The RCA supplies blood to the right ventricle and 25–35% of the blood to the LV. In 90% of people, it supplies the atrioventricular (AV) node, in 60% the sinoatrial (SA) node, and in 85% of people it gives off the PDA, which supplies the inferior wall, ventricular septum, and posteromedial papillary muscle.

→ http://en.ecgpedia.org/wiki/Myocardial_Infarction#The_location_of_the_infarct

8. C ★

This man is displaying the signs of severe acute heart failure, common after an MI, and requires intravenous diuresis. Sudden changes in physiology after a cardiac event should raise the suspicion of failure and can be confirmed by eliciting the signs of fluid overload (jugular venous pressure, gallop rhythm, fine lung crackles).

9. B ★

The ECG shows ventricular tachycardia (VT). Guidelines state that if the patient is not cardiovascularly compromised – as in this case where he is maintaining a good blood pressure – the first-line treatment is amiodarone followed by lidocaine (although care should be exercised in using lidocaine in those with impaired left ventricular function). In those that are compromised (chest pain, signs of heart failure, systolic BP<90mmHg, reduced level of consciousness), the first-line treatment is with synchronized cardioversion.

→ http://www.resus.org.uk/pages/tachalgo.pdf

10. D ★

When the doctor receives the phone call from the ward about this patient, it is vital that he establishes immediately whether the palpitations are causing her haemodynamic compromise. He can do this by checking for the presence of any of the following four factors:

1) Systolic BP <90mmHg

2) Chest pain

3) Heart failure

4) HR >150bpm

If any are present, then he should be heading to the ward immediately with a view to discussing sedation and direct current (DC) cardioversion with his senior, obviously having seen the patient himself first.

A This may separate an atrial fibrillation (AF) (irregular) from a ventricular tachycardia (VT)/supra-ventricular tachycardia (regular).

B AND E   These are unlikely to add much in a known case of chest infection.

C This does not discriminate between anxiety and worrying cardiovascular compromise.

11. B ★   OHCM 8th edn → p44

This man has an enlarged left atrium due to mitral stenosis, which is causing difficulty clearing bronchial secretions, and a hoarse voice due to its effects on the recurrent laryngeal nerve.

A The would have no effect.

C This is for aortic regurgitation.

D This accentuates right-sided murmurs.

E This is the Valsalva manoeuvre, which increases intrathoracic pressure, decreases venous return, and hence reduces blood flow through the heart.

12. D ★

The history is suggestive of angina, which can often have a normal ECG. The next stage is to stress the myocardium and see how it responds. If it responds to stress negatively (i.e. causes ischaemic changes on the ECG), angiography may be required to assess the degree and site of coronary artery damage. It is important to remember that in the setting of unstable angina (i.e. pain while at rest), stress testing is contraindicated.

13.A ★

This is an anterior myocardial infarction caused by an occlusion in the LAD.

In the LCA, the left main stem divides into the left anterior descending and left circumflex arteries. The LAD supplies two-thirds of the interventricular septum, the anterior portion of the left ventricle (LV), and the apex of the heart. The LCA can branch again into the left marginal artery supplying the left atrium, the obtuse margin of the heart, and the posterior LV wall.

The RCA supplies blood to the right ventricle and 25–35% of the blood to the LV. In 90% of people, it supplies the atrioventricular (AV) node, in 60% the sinoatrial (SA) node, and in 85% of people it gives off the PDA, which supplies the inferior wall, ventricular septum, and posteromedial papillary muscle.

14.E ★

Signs of sepsis plus heart valve replacement raise the suspicion of infective endocarditis. Recent evidence suggests that there is no clear association between interventional procedures and infective endocarditis, and therefore antibiotic prophylaxis is no longer recommended in these patients. However, with this history together with the presentation, this is the most likely source of bacteraemia.

→ http://www.nice.org.uk/Guidance/CG64#documents

15.E ★

The scenario is suggestive of subacute infective endocarditis. Although the history is non-specific, IV drug use along with systemic inflammatory response syndrome (SIRS) and tricuspid regurgitation prompt urgent referral to a cardiologist for an ECHO. Whilst vasculitis may not be evident in the form of physical findings, it may be revealed by microscopic haematuria.

16.E ★   OHCM 8th edn → pp40, 146

This man has hypertrophic cardiomyopathy (HOCM), the leading cause of sudden death in young adults. Half of cases have no family history and are usually sporadic mutations of the gene producing the β-myosin heavy chain.

A An anacrotic or 'slow-rising' pulse occurs in aortic stenosis.

B This occurs in mixed aortic stenosis and regurgitation.

C This is caused by CO_2 narcosis, sepsis, and liver failure.

D This is caused by aortic regurgitation.

In Wolff–Parkinson–White syndrome, an accessory pathway –
the bundle of Kent – is situated between the atria and the
ventricles. In comparison with the atrioventricular (AV) node,
this pathway is able to conduct electrical impulses rapidly,
leading to extremely fast rates and a risk of sudden death.
The rapid conduction between the atria and ventricles
causes a slurred upstroke (delta wave) and a short
PR interval.

There are many causes of faints in the older population,
but in the search for a diagnosis, a feel of the radial pulse
may give an early clue. If it rises slowly ('anacrotic') and is
associated with a narrow pulse pressure and an ejection systolic
murmur, then it may be a stenosed aortic valve that is the cause of
the exertional dizziness. Cases like this should serve as a reminder
that there is more to be learnt from the radial pulse than just the
heart rate.

A A collapsing or 'waterhammer' pulse is found in aortic
incompetence and is more likely to present with breathlessness or
heart failure.

B This describes atrial fibrillation or a regular output
punctuated by multiple ectopics: an ECG would help to
differentiate the two. This is the best differential diagnosis
as it can present with faintness, but would be more likely also
to cause palpitations.

C This is found in hypertrophic cardiomyopathy (HOCM), which
would be very unlikely in this age group.

E This indicates a barely palpable pulse as may be found
in shock.

This man has severe congestive heart failure and his pulse has
alternating weak and strong beats.

A An anacrotic or 'slow-rising' pulse occurs in aortic stenosis.

B This occurs in mixed aortic stenosis and regurgitation.

C This is caused by aortic regurgitation.

D This occurs in hypertrophic cardiomyopathy (HOCM).

Cardiovascular medicine

The term acute coronary syndrome encompasses the cardiac events on the spectrum from unstable angina (in which pain occurs at rest without causing myocardial damage) via non-ST elevation myocardial infarction (NSTEMI) to ST-elevation myocardial infarction (STEMI). It does not include stable angina, which develops during exertion but settles with rest. Purely on the basis of a cardiac sounding history and a convincing examination, scenarios can be labelled as acute coronary syndrome while ECGs and cardiac markers are awaited. These can then be used to classify the event more specifically. In this man's case, there was cardiac-sounding pain at rest with no ST elevation on the ECG and negative cardiac markers (Figure 1.18).

Alpert JS, Thygesen K, Antman E, and Bassand JP (2000). Myocardial infarction redefined – a consensus document of The Joint European Society of Cardiology/American College of Cardiology Committee for the redefinition of myocardial infarction. *J Am Coll Cardiol* **36**:959–969.

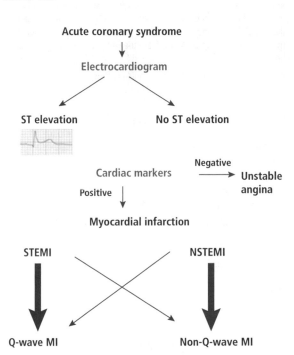

Acute coronary syndrome

↓

Electrocardiogram

ST elevation   **No ST elevation**

Cardiac markers   Negative → **Unstable angina**

Positive ↓

Myocardial infarction

STEMI   **NSTEMI**

Q-wave MI   **Non-Q-wave MI**

Figure 1.18

21. C ★

In the context of a tachyarrhythmia, his blood pressure is unstable (systolic BP <90mmHg = 'haemodynamically unstable') and this should prompt an immediate review of the patient. Concurrent fever would obviously need investigation and treatment soon in the course of the night shift. The need for high-flow oxygen would also need to be reviewed soon, whilst the patient's anxiety could be monitored for a while prior to a review.

22. B ★

The image shows corneal arcus, a sign – especially in those under 60 – of hyperlipidaemia (in those over 60 it can be a normal finding). The key is finding the cause of the high lipid levels. If they are primary, then they will need treatment – initially with lifestyle measures and then with medications. However, it is important to first rule out secondary causes of hyperlipidaemia, i.e. liver, kidney, and thyroid disease.

23. B ★

The blood glucose is high but the raised heart rate could be due to anxiety and in isolation would not prompt an urgent review. The oxygen saturation is satisfactory, although in a patient with chest pain supplementary oxygen should be given. The fact that he has vomited might point towards this pain being cardiac rather than another aetiology.

24. C ★

This woman has the classic symptoms of heart failure: breathlessness, orthopnoea, reduced exercise tolerance, and peripheral oedema.

The gradual decline means that this cannot be something as acute as a pulmonary embolus or an exacerbation of asthma. This woman may well be wheezing, however, as not only does she have asthma but her heart failure will give her an element of cardiac asthma on examination. There is no suggestion that this is an infective process and no mention of exertion-related pain to support angina.

25. D ★

The story is consistent with acute myocardial damage and is confirmed by the ECG, which shows ST elevation in the inferior leads. Upsloping ST segments would be more indicative of a pericarditis, as would the background of an upper respiratory tract infection.

Lateral ischaemia would be represented by T-wave inversion in chest leads V3–V6, whilst unstable angina may have a normal ECG but describes cardiac chest pain that occurs at rest.

26.D ★

This lady has cor pulmonale or right ventricular failure due to chronic hypoxic pulmonary vasoconstriction. Right ventricular hypertrophy, raised right atrial pressures (raised JVP), and raised systemic venous pressure can cause ascites and peripheral oedema. Peripheral oedema in someone with COPD should always prompt assessment of right heart function.

A This can present with ascites and abdominal pain but symptoms and signs of liver failure including hepatomegaly would be expected.

B There is no mention of jaundice.

C This is a good differential for someone with features of right heart failure, but in someone with COPD, it is less likely to be the cause than cor pulmonale.

E This can present with ascites but usually presents with organomegaly on a background of liver cirrhosis most likely due to chronic alcohol use.

27.C ★

Guidelines state that in cases of haemodynamic compromise, ventricular tachycardia (VT) (as depicted on the ECG) should be cardioverted. Compromise is usually indicated by either hypotension (systolic BP<90mmHg), tachycardia (HR>150bpm), heart failure, or chest pain. However, it is also strongly indicated by a disturbance of consciousness as in this case and so requires immediate cardioversion.

A This is for stable VT (as well as refractory ventricular fibrillation (VF) and certain types of atrial fibrillation (AF)).

B AND D These are for acute AF.

E This is for symptomatic bradycardias and suppression of drug-resistant tachyarrhythmias.

→ http://emedicine.medscape.com/article/159075-treatment

28.D ★ ★

This is symptomatic anaemia (Hb usually <5g/dL) causing heart failure. In treating the low Hb, it is important to transfuse slowly in conjunction with a diuretic, e.g. furosemide 10–40mg IV with alternate units.

A This woman is in a severe relative hypovolaemic state and does not need diuresis (although, as stated above, furosemide does have a *supportive* role in transfusion).

B This might transiently improve the situation but has no oxygen-carrying capacity so blood is preferred.

C Oral iron replacement would be useful if the symptoms were mild, but if she was unable to tolerate this and symptoms persisted, the IV route would be useful.

E This might help if a clotting disorder was found to be the cause of the menorrhagia but would not improve her symptoms of heart failure.

29. E ★★   OHCM 8th edn → p113

A, C, and D may all be indicated at some stage, but the key to deciding which management path to take rests on whether the myocardium has sustained any damage. This man has suffered chest pain at rest and has ECG changes, but to direct treatment appropriately, another troponin reading is needed (to decide whether this event is unstable angina or a non-ST-elevation myocardial infarction). The initial troponin was taken only 2h after the onset of pain, when it is unlikely to have risen even in the presence of infarction; therefore, before any management decisions can be made, it needs to be repeated from 12h after the onset of pain (as it reaches a peak 12–24h after myocardial infarction).

Creatine kinase (B) does rise in myocardial infarction but also in other situations (post-trauma, myocarditis, pericarditis, normal in Afro-Caribbeans). It can be supportive of the diagnosis but does not guide treatment.

Ferguson J, Beckett GJ, Stoddart M, Walker SW, and Fox KAA (2002) Myocardial infarction redefined: the new ACC/ESC definition, based on cardiac troponin, increases the apparent incidence of infarction. *Heart* **88**:343–347.

→ http://ukpmc.ac.uk/articlerender.cgi?artid=987995

30. A ★★   OHCM 8th edn → p818

Adenosine is used in atrial flutter (depicted here with 2:1 block) as it causes a transient heart block at the AV node, slows the ventricles, and reveals the underlying atrial rhythm.

31. B ★★   OHCM 8th edn → p40

This paradoxical rise is Kussmaul's sign. Anything – any sort of fluid or an abnormal pericardium (in this case, a pericardial effusion) –

that stops the heart from expanding during inspiration also stops the jugular venous pulse from falling as it should.

32. D ★ ★

This is tricuspid regurgitation causing tender hepatomegaly.
A pansystolic murmur is found with mitral and tricuspid regurgitation and ventricular septal defects. The 'v' wave occurs towards the end of the pulse and represents atrial filling against a closed tricuspid valve. RV heave is usually caused by RV hypertrophy and causes the examining hand to be forced off the chest wall during systole.

A This indicates aortic regurgitation, the so-called 'waterhammer' pulse and de Musset's sign.

B This indicates volume overload causing ventricular dilatation and Corrigan's sign.

C The 'a' wave represents atrial systole and occurs just before the carotid pulsation. Prominence is seen in pulmonary hypertension/stenosis. A widely split S2 is seen when A2 occurs early or P2 is delayed, as in this case where the most likely cause is pulmonary stenosis.

E A palpable first heart sound and facies are typical of mitral stenosis.

33. C ★ ★ ★

In patients who have paroxysmal atrial fibrillation (AF), guidance is that a 'pill in pocket' strategy (i.e. a medicine to be taken as required) should be considered if the following criteria are met:

• There is no history of left ventricular dysfunction, or valvular or ischaemic heart disease.

• There are infrequent symptomatic episodes of paroxysmal AF.

• Systolic BP >100mmHg and resting HR >70bpm.

• Patients can understand how and when to take the medication.

Flecainide is a class Ic anti-arrhythmic agent and can be used in this way due to its rapidity of action. Studies have shown that it is effective in 80% of arrhythmic episodes in those with paroxysmal AF and so reduces the need for hospitalization.

A Amiodarone can be used if beta-blockers have been unable to suppress paroxysms in those with poor left ventricular function.

B Digoxin is not used in paroxysmal AF but as a rate control in permanent AF for 'sedentary' patients.

D Metoprolol (or another 'standard' β-blocker) would be the first choice in paroxysmal AF where a pill-in-the-pocket strategy is not thought appropriate.

E Sotalol would be the next choice after a standard β-blocker if
suppression of symptoms has not been achieved.

→ http://www.nice.org.uk/nicemedia/pdf/word/
CG036niceguidelineword.doc

(NICE Clinical Guideline 36 (2006). *Atrial Fibrillation: The
Management of Atrial Fibrillation.*)

Alboni P, Botto GL, Baldi N, *et al.* (2004). Outpatient treatment of
recent onset atrial fibrillation with the 'pill-in-the-pocket' approach.
N Engl J Med **351**: 2384–2391.

→ https://content.nejm.org/cgi/reprint/351/23/2384.pdf?ck=nck

34.B ★ ★ ★

In severe hypertension, it is vital to establish whether the raised
blood pressure is causing end-organ dysfunction, as, if it is, it will
need emergency treatment. This is obvious in cases of myocardial
infarction, pulmonary oedema, and aortic dissection, but can be
present in rather more covert ways. One of these is hypertensive
encephalopathy, which classically presents with a headache, change
in consciousness, and some minor neurological dysfunction. In this
case, therefore, the junior doctor should establish over the phone
whether the patient has a headache: if she does, then he should
head directly to the ward to perform an urgent assessment of her
Glasgow Coma Scale (GCS) score, neurology, and fundi.

A This is a reasonable examination to perform but is not as crucial
as fundoscopy as it will not help to assess end-organ damage.

C This is useful in finding the cause of the problem, but should take
a back seat while the problem is being dealt with.

D This would provide valuable information and help stratify the risk
of this being an emergency, but is not a rate-limiting step.

E This should clearly be asked, but is not the key to the case.

Varon J & Marik P (2000). The diagnosis and management of
hypertensive crises, *Chest* **118**:214–227.

→ http://www.chestjournal.org/content/118/1/214.long

35.D ★ ★ ★

The drowsiness and confusion that preceded his admission to
hospital coupled with his agitation after high-flow oxygen therapy
suggest that this man has acute on chronic hypercapnoea. Although
no formal diagnosis is reported, he does have a significant smoking
history and is likely to have COPD. The difficulty for the junior doctor
in this situation is dealing with the obvious presentation – heart
failure – but being sensitive to what is developing in front of him

and responding appropriately, in this case using controlled oxygen therapy and monitoring the pH and pCO_2.

36. C ★ ★ ★

This woman has gone into flash pulmonary oedema due to renal artery stenosis. The main clue is the worsening renal function after treatment with an angiotensin-converting enzyme (ACE) inhibitor and an angiotensin II receptor antagonist. Whilst a Doppler USS is not the gold standard diagnostic tool (renal angiography would be), it is certainly the first-line choice if renal artery stenosis is suspected. Although a plain USS may show a smaller kidney on the affected side, the Doppler studies are needed to show disturbance in blood flow.

37. C ★ ★ ★   OHCM 8th edn → p788

This is a common task for the on call junior doctor. A post-insertion X-ray should always be requested to check for two main things: (i) that there are no complications from the procedure and (ii) that the line is lying in the correct place for use. The most common immediate complication that can be screened for on an X-ray is a pneumothorax. If the junior doctor is happy that there are no intrapleural slivers of air and he or she can confirm that the line tip lies between the first and third sternocostal joints – i.e. in the superior vena cava – then he or she can say that there have been no immediate complications from the procedure and that the line is lying in the correct place ready for use.

38. D ★ ★ ★

The history recounts a series of Stokes–Adams attacks. These are transient bradycardias due to lack of conduction through the atrioventricular (AV) node causing decreased cardiac output and loss of consciousness. The ECG shows a lack of correlation between the P waves and the QRS complexes, and a ventricular rate of 25–30/min. Emergency treatment involves continuous cardiac monitoring and transcutaneous pacing with a view to the placement of a definitive transvenous pacemaker, even if the patient is asymptomatic.

A This is the treatment of choice for stable ventricular tachycardia (VT), shock refractory ventricular fibrillation (VF), and various forms of atrial fibrillation (AF), but is contraindicated in AV block.

B This acts on the His–Purkinje system and is therefore used in the treatment of many supra-ventricular tachycardias.

C This is used for ventricular tachyarrhythmias causing syncope.

E This is the definitive treatment for some supraventricular tachyarrhythmias.

→ http://emedicine.medscape.com/article/758454-treatment

39.A ★ ★ ★

The ECG shows a long QT interval (i.e. QT^c >420ms), which has led to the collapse and is most likely to be due to the tricyclic antidepressant amitriptyline.

B Bendroflumethiazide can precipitate electrolyte imbalances. Electrolyte imbalances (hypokalaemia, hypocalcaemia, and hypomagnesaemia) can in turn precipitate prolongation of the QT interval, but in this case, blood tests are normal.

C There are no reports of this in the Summary of Product Characteristics (SPC) for metformin.

D There are no reports of this in the SPC for nifedipine.

E Some antipsychotics are associated with a prolonged QT interval, but from clinical trials, olanzapine is no more likely to cause this than a placebo. A long QT interval is associated with polymorphic ventricular arrhythmias (torsade de pointes) and can cause syncope, seizures, and sudden death.

40.E ★ ★ ★   OHCM 8th edn → pp40, 556

This woman has systemic lupus erythematosus (SLE), which is being treated with hydroxychloroquine, and an associated pericardial effusion, which is causing a cardiac tamponade. This serositis can also cause pleural effusions. The accumulation of fluid in the pericardial space raises intrapericardial pressure, limiting ventricular filling, and leads to a fall in cardiac output and a small-volume pulse.

A An anacrotic or 'slow-rising' pulse occurs in aortic stenosis.

B This occurs in mixed aortic stenosis and regurgitation..

C This is caused by aortic regurgitation.

D This occurs in hypertrophic cardiomyopathy (HOCM).

41.D ★ ★ ★

Treating severe hypertension is a common but difficult clinical problem. The key to management is to appreciate the actual effect that the raised blood pressure is having. If the blood pressure is causing end-organ dysfunction, then it can be said to represent a hypertensive emergency; if it is not, then it is termed a hypertensive urgency. There are certain situations that are indicative of end-organ damage, and therefore, an emergency:

- Acute myocardial infarction/unstable angina
- Acute pulmonary oedema

- Acute renal failure
- Acute aortic dissection
- Hypertensive encephalopathy
- Eclampsia.

The aim in emergencies is to stop ongoing end-organ damage. The most effective way of doing this (without dropping the blood pressure too quickly and adversely affecting cerebral perfusion) is via controlled IV therapy (labetalol is recommended), with the aim of reducing the diastolic blood pressure by 10–15%.

B Sublingual nitrate sprays may be useful for pain relief but will not treat the blood pressure effectively.

C A slower approach can be taken in urgencies with the aim of reducing the blood pressure gradually over a couple of days.

E The use of sublingual therapies such as nifedipine has been condemned due to the seriousness of adverse events reported due to the uncontrolled way in which it drops blood pressure.

Varon J & Marik P (2000). The diagnosis and management of hypertensive crises, *Chest* 118:214–227.

→ http://www.chestjournal.org/content/118/1/214.long

42. C ★ ★ ★ ★ OHCM 8th edn → pp148, 556

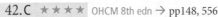

This scenario describes chest pain and breathlessness that has developed against the background of a rheumatological condition. The combination of mouth ulcers and arthritis in a woman of 40 years on maintenance steroids should be suspicious for systemic lupus erythematosus (SLE). One of the other diagnostic criteria for this condition is serositis (i.e. pleuritis or pericarditis). Given this woman's history, that her pain is relieved by sitting forwards, and her low-grade temperature and tachycardia, it is likely that she is suffering from pericarditis or a pericardial effusion, which can be detected clinically by impaired venous return (raised JVP) and a superficial scratching sound on auscultation (pericardial rub).

A This is most commonly a sign of left ventricular hypertrophy.

B This is the malar flush of mitral stenosis and should not be confused with the fixed erythema that occurs over the malar eminences in SLE.

D This is the rash of erythema marginatum that may be found in rheumatic fever.

E This is a vasculitic effect of infective endocarditis.

43. C ★★★★

Digoxin is cleared both renally and metabolically. Chronic cardiac failure and hypothyroidism reduce the efficacy of clearance, leading to elevated levels. Drugs such as amiodarone, verapamil, and quinidine have the same effect and should prompt a reduction in digoxin dose once started to avoid precipitating toxic levels.

Extended Matching Questions

1. D ★★★

After a diuretic and an ACE inhibitor, a beta-blocker should be started, even in asymptomatic left ventricular failure (NICE Guidelines July 2003: 1.2.2.6).

2. L ★★★

If moderately to severely symptomatic despite optimal therapy, spironolactone decreases mortality by 30% (RALES trial) (NICE Guidelines July 2003:1.2.2.9).

3. J ★★★

All patients with heart failure due to left ventricular failure should be started on an angiotensin-converting enzyme (ACE) inhibitor as a first-line therapy (NICE Guidelines July 2003: 1.2.2.2).

4. F ★★★

If left ventricular failure remains severely symptomatic despite optimal treatment, digoxin can improve symptoms – even in those in sinus rhythm (NICE Guidelines July 2003: 1.2.2.11).

5. H ★★★

This is routinely used for the relief of congestive symptoms (NICE Guidelines July 2003: 1.2.2.1).

6. J ★★★

For a hypertensive Caucasian of less than 55 years, the first-line treatment is with an angiotensin-converting enzyme (ACE) inhibitor (NICE guidelines June 2006: 1.4.5).

7. B ★★★

If a patient is on an angiotensin-converting enzyme (ACE) inhibitor but remains hypertensive, add a thiazide or a calcium channel blocker; in this case, a thiazide is contraindicated due to gout (NICE guidelines June 2006: 1.4.6).

8. B ★★★

In any black patient, the first-line treatment is a calcium channel blocker or a thiazide. In this case, she has diabetes; therefore, a calcium channel blocker is advised (NICE guidelines June 2006: 1.4.4).

9. C ★★★

Women with 'child-bearing potential' are advised to begin on a beta-blocker due to the teratogenicity of angiotensin-converting enzyme (ACE) inhibitors (NICE guidelines June 2006: 1.4.11).

10. I ★★★

If an angiotensin-converting enzyme (ACE) inhibitor is not tolerated, try an angiotensin 2 receptor antagonist (NICE guidelines June 2006: 1.4.5).

11. M ★★★

A regular narrow complex tachycardia should initially be treated with a vagal manoeuvre. This increases vagal tone at the atrioventricular (AV) node in order to prevent conduction of impulses from the atria. In order of effectiveness these include the Valsalva manoeuvre, carotid sinus massage, and the 'diving reflex', where the patient's face is submerged in cold water or covered with a towel soaked in cold water.

Skinner D, Swain A, Robertson C, and Peyton JWR (eds) (1997). *Cambridge Textbook of Accident and Emergency Medicine*, p913. Cambridge University Press, UK.

12. L ★★★

Regardless of the cause of the tachyarrhythmia, signs that the patient is unstable include: (i) chest pain; (ii) signs of heart failure; (iii) reduced consciousness level; and (iv) systolic BP <90mmHg. This should prompt urgent electrical cardioversion under sedation or general anaesthetic. The shock delivered is 'synchronized' with the pulse, in contrast to the asynchronous shock used in cardiac arrest when there is no pulse present. 'Stable' atrial fibrillation is treated with either a beta-blocker or digoxin, although if it is less than 48h since the onset, amiodarone can be used.

13. A ★★★

The patient has a supra-ventricular tachycardia but the Valsalva manoeuvre has not terminated the attack. The next step in a stable patient is to try adenosine 6mg IV, followed by up to two doses of 12mg. If this does not terminate the attack, expert help should be sort.

14. L ★★★

Chest pain and signs of heart failure indicate that this patient is unstable. The regular broad complex tachycardia is ventricular tachycardia (VT) and he will require up to three shocks with synchronized DC cardioversion (or adenosine if he has a previously confirmed supra-ventricular tachycardia with right-bundle branch block). If this fails, chemical cardioversion with amiodarone can be tried.

15. B ★★★

This man has a regular broad complex tachycardia (presumed to be ventricular tachycardia) but is haemodynamically stable and therefore chemical cardioversion can be attempted.

16. H ★★★

Renal impairment may occur after starting an angiotensin-converting enzyme (ACE) inhibitor in patients with bilateral renal artery stenosis. These patients rely on angiotensin II to maintain glomerular capillary pressure by vasoconstriction on the efferent more than the afferent arteriole and if this is removed (by ACE inhibition), there is an abrupt fall in glomerular filtration rate.

17. D ★★★

Thiazide diuretics can affect blood glucose control by decreasing both insulin secretion and peripheral insulin sensitivity. They can also lead to electrolyte imbalance, especially hypokalaemia, particularly in patients who have hepatic and renal impairment.

18. C ★★★

Beta-blockers are contraindicated in Raynaud's phenomenon due to peripheral vasoconstriction, which is mediated via peripheral β_2-receptor antagonism.

19. B ★★★

The dihydropyridine calcium channel blockers reduce systemic vascular resistance via peripheral vasodilatation and as a result can cause swollen ankles, headaches and flushing. Verapamil is relatively more selective for the myocardium and has minimal vasodilatatory effects.

20. K ★★★

When co-administered, these drugs, which both have negative inotropic effects on the heart, can lead to a profound bradycardia or even complete depression of ventricular contraction leading to asystole.

CHAPTER 2
CHEST MEDICINE

'Have a listen to the chest and tell me your findings.' Your heart sinks. The post-take ward round is in full swing as this invitation echoes across the bed in your direction. You slowly make your way round to the patient's right-hand side and introduce yourself, stalling for time as you try to think of all the plausible findings from the history that has been presented…

Despite the discomfort that this would cause in all of us, these situations *should* be relatively straightforward. With a thorough history and careful look at the patient from the end of the bed, the diagnosis can be clinched long before we even start listening to the chest: unilateral expansion might suggest a large pneumothorax, stridor and a respiratory rate of 40/min occurs in upper airways obstruction, and a barrel-shaped chest with pursed-lipped breathing are typical features of an exacerbation of chronic obstructive pulmonary disease (COPD). Despite the temptation to rush in with our tubes, there is much information to be gained elsewhere.

This chapter aims to hone our skills in detecting and using this information via the 'regulars' (asthma, COPD) and the 'unmissables' (pulmonary embolism, lung cancer, pneumothorax). Certain situations should sound the alarm for a potential unmissable:

- Painful with a deep breath – pulmonary embolism?
- Suddenly short of breath – a pneumothorax?
- Smoker with a persistent cough – lung cancer?

Add to this the consideration that shortness of breath does not always originate from the respiratory tract and that a respiratory rate may be raised to compensate for a problem elsewhere.

And so, back to the chest. Initially, bronchial breathing, crepitations, variable air entry, and wheeze seem not only difficult to hear but also difficult to differentiate between.

Rest assured, however, that it will soon become possible – simply by practising – to grade the severity of a wheeze, rather than just detect it. Whilst it may seem disheartening to be unable to distinguish coarse and fine crepitations, many of our more senior colleagues disagree on these too. Ultimately, the CT scan has replaced a fair amount of clinical uncertainty over the cause of respiratory disease.

Even in the muddier waters of the occupational, fibrotic, and eponymous respiratory conditions, we have a role to play: although we are unlikely to diagnose a case of Churg–Strauss syndrome or Goodpasture's disease, we can manage the haemoptysis and shortness of breath in the usual way and, by appreciating the nuances of the history and the subtleties of the examination, begin to think beyond the thorax. ■

Chest medicine

SINGLE BEST ANSWERS

1. A 60-year-old man has right-sided chest pain. He is short of breath and is bringing up increasing volumes of foul-smelling rusty sputum. These symptoms have persisted despite having been on intravenous antibiotics for the past 4 days. He says he was given oral tablets the previous week by his doctor but did not complete the course. His observation chart is shown below (Figure 2.1). The medical team are concerned about the man's poor progress and request a chest X-ray. Which *single* X-ray finding would be most supportive of the likely diagnosis? ★

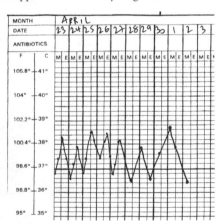

Figure 2.1

A Air within the right pleural space

B Completely obscured right heart border

C Single circular opacity in peripheral right hemithorax

D Tramlines and ring shadows in right hemithorax

E Walled-off cavity in right hemithorax with a fluid level

2. A 30-year-old woman has had an acute severe episode of asthma. This is her first acute episode for over 10 years and she is recovering in hospital. She has a salbutamol 100mcg inhaler that she uses occasionally and a beclometasone 200mcg inhaler that is prescribed for use twice daily. Which *single* measure is most likely to improve this woman's long-term asthma control? ★

A Add montelukast 10mg PO once daily

B Add salmeterol 50mcg INH twice daily

C Ensure up-to-date spirometry and lung function tests

D Organize a review by an asthma specialist in 3 months' time

E Write a plan of how and when to take the inhalers

3. A 52-year-old woman is severely short of breath. She is confused and cannot respond to questions. There is no one accompanying her to shed light on her medical history.

```
T 37.1°C, HR 120bpm, BP 105/65mmHg,
RR 26/min.
```

Her lips appear blue, her neck muscles are being used to assist breathing, and there is a generalized wheeze on her chest. She is put on high-flow oxygen. Which is the *single* most appropriate course of immediate management? ★

A Aminophylline 300mg IV

B Epinephrine (adrenaline) 0.5mg IM

C Hydrocortisone 100mg IV

D Magnesium sulphate 1.2g IV

E Salbutamol 5mg NEB

4. A 28-year-old woman has felt unwell for the last 4 days with coryzal symptoms and worsening breathlessness. She is asthmatic and has used her inhalers without any relief for the last hour. On arrival in the Emergency Department, she is talking in broken sentences and her peak expiratory flow rate (PEFR) is 45% of predicted.

```
HR 115bpm, RR 28/min.
```

She is assessed and given oxygen via a non-rebreather mask while a salbutamol and ipratropium nebulizer is being prepared. An hour after admission, her PEFR is 80% of predicted. Which is the *single* most appropriate management? ★

A Contact the on-call anaesthetist for admission to the High-Dependency Unit

B Discharge home with medication and a follow up in 2 weeks

C Observe in the medical admissions ward for 24h

D Start bi-level positive airway pressure

E Start continuous positive airway pressure

5. A 69-year-old man has had a cough, myalgia, and felt feverish for the last 7 days. He is wheezy and is finding it particularly difficult to breathe. He has asthma and is using his usual inhalers every half an hour but feels that they are not having any effect on his symptoms. Which *single* finding is most consistent with a *severe* attack of asthma? ★

A BP 90/60mmHg

B Inability to complete sentences

C Inaudible air entry bilaterally

D Peak expiratory flow rate (PEFR) <33% of predicted

E SaO$_2$ <75% on air

6. A 36-year-old man with asthma has used a salbutamol 100mcg inhaler once a day for as long as he can remember. However, he is concerned that his symptoms are worsening and that his asthma is not as well controlled as it could be. Which *single* feature from the history would most support the man's concerns? ★

A Chest tightness is brought on by cold weather

B Having to use the salbutamol inhaler every day

C Most breathless early in the morning

D Waking at night with coughing

E Wheezing is brought on by exercise

7. A 30-year-old woman is recovering in hospital after an episode of acute asthma. Overnight, she required hourly salbutamol 5mg nebulizers and after the morning ward round is now receiving them every 2h. She is intermittently using oxygen 3L via a Hudson mask. She has regular admissions to hospital but has a young family and is keen for an early discharge home. Her normal regimen is a salbutamol 100mcg inhaler PRN and beclometasone 200mcg inhaler twice daily. She wants to be discharged by the end of the day. Which is the *single* most appropriate time for this woman to be discharged? ★

A When her nebulizers are stopped

B When she feels ready

C When she has been stable on inhalers for 24h

D When she has been stable on nebulizers for 24h

E When she is no longer requiring oxygen therapy

8. A 32-year-old woman has asthma and is increasingly short of breath in the mornings. She describes her chest feeling tight and says it is hard for her to catch her breath. As a result, she is taking two puffs of her salbutamol 100mcg inhaler at least three times before midday.

```
Peak expiratory flow rate: 310 L/min.
```

Which is the *single* most appropriate next step in her management? ★

A Beclometasone 200mcg INH twice daily

B Prednisolone 40mg PO once daily for 5 days

C Salbutamol 200mcg INH four times daily

D Salmeterol 50mcg INH twice daily

E Seretide® 50/100mcg INH twice daily

9. A 17-year-old woman is leaving home to start further education. She has asthma and uses a salbutamol 100mcg inhaler three or four times a month. She has never had an acute episode before and is worried that she may not be able to recognize one if it were happening, and she asks for guidance as to what to look out for. Which is the *single* most important feature for the doctor to stress? ★

A Dizziness and tingling of peripheries

B Her inhaler does not improve symptoms

C Her inhaler gives her a tremor

D She is breathless after running for a bus

E She is breathless after running up a flight of stairs

10. A 20-year-old man has been diagnosed with asthma and is worried about the prospect of having an 'attack' and its treatment. He is advised firstly to take one puff of his regular inhaler. Which is the *single* most appropriate additional instruction for the man to follow? ★

A Call for the emergency services

B Go into the open air and wait for the attack to pass

C Lie down, loosen clothing, and wait for the attack to pass

D Take one puff every minute and reassess at 5min

E Use the inhaler continuously until symptoms resolve

11. An 18-year-old man has had a cough for the last 6 weeks. It has got worse over the past week such that he is now bringing up large volumes of green- and red-coloured sputum. He has had regular such exacerbations. He uses insulin 12U SC twice daily. Which is the *single* most accurate explanation for his sputum production? ★

A Chronic inflammation of lung parenchyma

B Chronic swelling of airway mucosa

C Permanent dilatation of the bronchioles

D Progressive fibrosis and remodelling of interstitium

E Prolonged bronchial muscle contraction

12. A 41-year-old man has felt unwell for 5 days. He has a cough productive of green sputum with an occasional reddish tinge. He has been feeling hot and cold, particularly at night, and has pain in the right side of his chest. He has smoked ten cigarettes a day for 25 years.

```
T 37.8°C, HR 100bpm, BP 115/80mmHg,
RR 22/min, SaO₂ 93% on air.
```

There are basal crepitations on the right side of the chest. Which is the *single* most likely diagnosis? ★

A Bronchial carcinoma

B Community-acquired pneumonia

C Sarcoidosis

D Tuberculosis

E Wegener's granulomatosis

13. An 83-year-old man is prescribed modified-release morphine tablets twice daily. He is seen in the outpatient lung cancer clinic having run out. A new prescription must be written. Which is the *single* most important detail required on the prescription to satisfy legal requirements? ★

A Date of birth

B Dose in words and figures

C General Medical Council (GMC) number

D Handwritten prescription

E Patient's address

14. A 19-year-old woman has been coughing up copious amounts of sputum over the past week. It has been green with some rusty specks. For the third time this year, she is admitted for a course of IV antibiotics. Which *single* set of examination findings would be most supportive of the likely diagnosis? ★

A Enlarged supraclavicular lymph nodes + focal bronchial breathing

B Finger clubbing + coarse inspiratory crepitations

C Mouth ulcers + unilateral dullness to percussion

D Pitting unilateral calf oedema + pleural rub

E Unilateral ptosis + unilateral reduced air entry

15. A 56-year-old man who has chronic obstructive pulmonary disease (COPD) and uses long-term oxygen therapy at home has not left his house for the last 2 weeks. He has started sleeping for large parts of the day and his wife says that he has also occasionally been confused.

T 36.4C, BP 146/90mmHg, HR 90bpm, SaO_2 89% on 2L O_2.

Arterial blood gases (on 2L O_2): pH 7.1, pCO_2 6.8kPa, pO_2 8.5kPa, base excess 5.5mmol/L, bicarbonate 31mmol/L.

Which is the *single* most appropriate next step? ★

A Increase oxygen to 4L/min

B Nebulized salbutamol 5mg

C Non-rebreather mask at 15L/min

D Trial of non-invasive ventilation (NIV)

E Trial of continuous positive airway pressure (CPAP)

16. A 68-year-old man becomes suddenly short of breath with left-sided chest discomfort. He has chronic obstructive pulmonary disease (COPD) and is on home oxygen, regular nebulizers, and maintenance oral steroids.

T 37.1°C, HR 100bpm, RR 24/min, SaO$_2$ 86% on 2L O$_2$.

A CT pulmonary angiogram rules out a pulmonary embolus. Which *single* examination finding is most likely to support the diagnosis? ★

A Left-sided bronchial breath sounds

B Left-sided hyper-resonant percussion note

C Left-sided hypo-resonant percussion note

D Left-sided increased vocal resonance

E Left-sided stony dull percussion note

17. A 21-year-old woman has had left-sided chest pain for 1 week. It came on gradually, is sharp in nature, and is worse on deep inspiration.

T 36.6°C, HR 85bpm, RR 18/min, SaO$_2$ 99% on air.

The left medial border of the sternum is tender to palpation, but her chest is otherwise clear. Which is the *single* most likely diagnosis? ★

A Acute pericarditis

B Community-acquired pneumonia

C Costochondritis

D Myocardial infarction

E Pulmonary embolus

18. A 70-year-old woman has had griping abdominal pain and constipation for the past month. As well as feeling generally 'achy', she admits to feeling mentally low. She has had a cough for the past 9 months during which time she has lost more than 5kg. She is an ex-smoker. She has been told that there is a 'shadow' on her chest X-ray and that her new symptoms may be related to this. Which is the *single* most likely mechanism that links her new symptoms to the X-ray findings? ★

A A carcinoid tumour is secreting serotonin

B A lung tumour has metastasized to the liver and brain

C A lung tumour is secreting parathyroid hormone

D A urogenital tumour has metastasized to the lung and bone

E An abdominal tumour has metastasized to the lung

19. A 60-year-old man has had a persistent cough for the past year. He has lost 5kg during this time and has had increasing episodes of breathlessness. He has smoked heavily for many years. There are no specific chest signs, but he is cachectic and has a drooping eyelid on the right-hand side. A chest X-ray shows a single nodule in the right apical hemithorax, which it is suggested may be the cause of all of his symptoms. Which is the *single* structure that the nodule is most likely to be compressing? ★

A Accessory nerve

B Cervical sympathetic plexus

C Oculomotor nerve

D Superior vena cava

E Trigeminal nerve (ophthalmic division)

20. A 72-year-old woman is found confused and drowsy in her own home. She has recently been diagnosed with a bronchial carcinoma.

```
Sodium 124mmol/L, potassium 4.4mmol/L,
urinary sodium 35mmol/L.
```

Which is the *single* most likely type of carcinoma? ★

A Adenocarcinoma

B Alveolar cell

C Large cell

D Small cell

E Squamous cell

21. A 66-year-old man has been admitted with an episode of acute confusion. He does not respond as he is having his 4h observations. The attending nurse asks the junior doctor, who is on the ward, for urgent help. As the doctor approaches the man, he can hear gurgling. Which is the *single* most appropriate immediate management? ★

A Ask the nurse to put out a crash call

B Begin chest compressions at 30:2

C Give O_2 15L/min via a non-rebreather mask

D Insert an oropharyngeal airway

E Suction the airway

22. A 70-year-old woman has a swollen left calf. She is admitted to a medical ward. Within 24h of admission, she dies. The junior doctor who attended to her on the ward is subsequently contacted by the hospital's legal department. They are concerned about one of the entries he made in the medical notes.

```
16/6/10 Junior Dr review, Watson #111

Asked to see patient: c/o chest pain

Pain in rt chest for last 2 hours

Came on suddenly - not had this pain before

Worse on inspiration

Rated 7/10, no shortness of breath

No radiation, nothing makes it better

T 36.8°C, HR 110bpm, 110/70mmHg, SaO₂ 95% on
air, RR 24/min

Chest clear, no focal tenderness, HS I+II+0

Plan: ECG, chest X ray, regular paracetamol

Watson #111
```

Which is the *single* reason that is most likely to cause the legal team concern about this entry? ★

A Discussions with seniors either not sought or documented

B Full examination either not performed or documented

C Impression of clinical picture not documented

D No mention made of admitting complaint

E Time of review not documented

23. A 79-year-old woman has become acutely short of breath in hospital. The junior doctor notes that she has had a previous aspiration pneumonia, a pulmonary embolus, and is not for resuscitation. As the junior doctor is examining the woman, her respiratory effort dwindles and then ceases and no pulses are palpable. Which is the *single* most appropriate next step? ★

A Ask a nurse to put out a cardiac arrest call

B Continue to examine for signs of life before confirming death

C Insert a Guedel airway and attempt ventilation

D Insert two large-bore cannulae into the antecubital fossae

E Start cardiac chest compressions immediately

24. The junior doctor on-call receives a bleep from a nurse during a busy night shift. A 63-year-old man has felt increasingly short of breath over the last 10min. He has been admitted with an infective exacerbation of chronic obstructive pulmonary disease (COPD) and has suddenly found it very difficult to breathe. He is on co-amoxiclav 1.2g IV. Which *single* additional detail from the nurse should prompt an immediate review of the patient, i.e. within the next 5min? ★

A He is on non-invasive ventilation (NIV)

B HR 92bpm

C Left-sided chest pain

D SaO_2 92% on 28% O_2

E Temperature 37.9°C

25. A 76-year-old woman has been reported as 'out of breath' for the past 12h. She has been sleepy and very quiet, refusing all meals in her care home. She has chronic obstructive pulmonary disease (COPD) and metastatic breast cancer.

```
T 37.5°C, HR 110bpm, BP 100/70mmHg, SaO₂ 65%
on air, RR 7/min.
```

Which is the *single* most appropriate additional examination or bedside test to aid her treatment? ★

A Abbreviated mental test

B Lower limbs

C Peak flow

D Pupillary

E Respiratory

26. A 72-year-old man has been breathless for 2 days with a cough productive of white sputum. It came on suddenly while he was running for a bus. He now has right-sided chest pain, which is worse on deep breaths in. He has been a smoker for 60 years but is not on any regular medication.

```
T 37.2°C, HR 110bpm, SaO₂ 92% on air.
```

He has a generalized wheeze. Which is the *single* most likely diagnosis? ★

A Acute asthma

B Heart failure

C Infective exacerbation of chronic obstructive pulmonary disease (COPD)

D Myocardial infarction

E Pulmonary embolus

27. A 46-year-old woman has felt breathless for the last 48h and had an episode of haemoptysis this morning. She has recently undergone surgery to remove an ovarian carcinoma.

```
T 37.2°C, BP 110/58mmHg, HR 90bpm, SaO₂ 95%
on 2L O₂.
```

The chest has some dullness to percussion at the right base. Which *single* feature from the history below is consistent with the most likely diagnosis? ★

A 5kg weight loss over the last month

B Breathlessness is maximal on exertion

C Cough productive of green sputum

D Pain worse on taking a deep breath in

E Swinging fevers and sweats, particularly at night

28. A 26-year-old man has a sudden pain over his lower sternum. He feels breathless and nauseous but does not vomit. He has no other medical problems. There is decreased air entry at the right apex. Which is the *single* most likely diagnosis? ★

A Acute pericarditis

B Community-acquired pneumonia

C Costochondritis

D Pneumothorax

E Pulmonary embolus

29. A 19-year-old man becomes suddenly short of breath while playing football. He feels nauseous with left-sided chest discomfort. He smokes ten cigarettes a day and admits to an occasional cough in the morning. He uses bronchodilators for his asthma but has never been admitted to hospital. Which *single* pair of examination findings is most likely to support the diagnosis? ★

A Bronchial breathing + dull to percussion on left

B Decreased expansion + crackles on left

C Decreased expansion + increased vocal resonance on left

D Hyper-resonant to percussion + diminished breath sounds on left

E Stony dull to percussion + decreased vocal resonance on left

30. A 23-year-old woman has suffered an infective exacerbation of her asthma. She has taken a 5-day course of prednisolone 40mg PO once daily and is now ready to be discharged from hospital. This is her first hospital admission because of her asthma since childhood. Her discharge summary and prescription are being prepared. Which is the *single* most appropriate instruction for taking the prednisolone? ★

A Continue the same dose and see her GP in 2 weeks

B No further prednisolone is needed

C Reduce by 5mg every day for the next 8 days

D Reduce by 10mg every day for the next 4 days

E Reduce by 10mg every week for the next month

31. A 66-year-old man is breathless and being treated for an exacerbation of chronic obstructive pulmonary disease (COPD). It has not been possible to obtain a blood gas sample from the radial artery, and repeated attempts have left the patient in a great deal of distress. The registrar has asked the on-call junior doctor to take the blood from the femoral artery. The junior doctor has never performed this skill before.

```
RR 22/min, SaO₂ 96 % on O₂ 5L/min.
```

Which is the *single* most appropriate next step? ★

A Abandon the procedure as the man's oxygen saturation is within acceptable limits

B Analyse a venous sample obtained from the antecubital fossa instead

C Ask another doctor to explain the procedure before trying to take the blood from the femoral artery

D Talk the patient into allowing another attempt at taking the blood from the radial artery

E Tell the registrar that they have no experience of this procedure

32. A 66-year-old man has had abdominal pain with nausea for the past week. He has felt dizzy and fainted on two occasions. He has a chronic cough and was recently diagnosed with a bronchial carcinoma.

```
Lying BP 135/90mmHg, standing BP 90/75mmHg.
```

Which *single* category of complication is most likely to explain this man's new symptoms? ★

A Endocrine

B Local

C Metastasis

D Neurological

E Other

33. A 72-year-old man is said to be in a 'deep sleep' by the nursing staff. He is unrousable and does not even wake when he has his blood sugar checked. He is being treated with IV antibiotics for a lower respiratory tract infection and morphine liquid 5mg PO as required for associated chest pain. He is receiving 30% O_2 10L/min via a Venturi™ mask. The junior doctor who is on the ward is asked to see the man urgently. As the doctor reaches the man's bedside, he hears loud snoring. Which is the *single* most appropriate immediate management? ★

A Head tilt and chin lift manoeuvres

B Insert a nasopharyngeal airway

C Naloxone 500mcg IV STAT

D Reduce the O_2 flow rate

E Urgent cricothyroidotomy

34. A 20-year-old man has suffered his first acute episode of breathlessness. It came on first thing in the morning as he was walking to work. His chest feels tight and he is unable to take long, slow breaths in. He has noticed mild chest tightness in the mornings for the last few weeks. He is otherwise well aside from some well-controlled eczema. There is widespread wheeze on auscultation of his chest. Which is the *single* most appropriate initial investigation to establish the diagnosis? ★

A Arterial blood gas

B Bronchial challenge test

C Chest X-ray

D Skin prick allergy tests

E Spirometry

35. A previously well 22-year-old woman has had difficulty breathing for the past month. She notices it especially in the mornings when she feels pressure on her chest and an inability to take satisfactory deep breaths. After a series of tests, it is suggested to her that she has mild asthma and may need to start using inhalers. She is pregnant and is thus reluctant to take any of the drugs recommended to her. Which *single* non-pharmacological measure is most likely to be of benefit in controlling her symptoms? ★

A Acupuncture

B Air ionizers

C Breathing techniques

D Fish oil supplements

E Immunotherapy

36. A 59-year-old man is brought into the emergency department by ambulance. The crew present their findings:

'This is John, he's 59 with COPD. He's had difficulty breathing especially for the past day or so. On arrival, his sats were 77% on air, pulse 125bpm, BP 110/75mmHg. We gave him a neb, and on 5L of O_2 his sats improved to 97%. He's more comfortable but a bit confused.'

Which is the *single* most appropriate immediate management? ★

A Check his peak flow

B Give him another salbutamol 5mg NEB

C Reduce the O_2 flow rate from 5L to 2L

D Request a chest X-ray

E Start co-amoxiclav 1.2g IV

37. A 31-year-old woman has been increasingly short of breath for the past 3 weeks. She sweats at night, has a non-productive cough, and has lost 5kg.

```
T 37.6°C, HR 95bpm, BP 100/60mmHg, SaO₂ 92%
on air (↓ to 86% on exertion).
```

She is cachectic and has thick white patches on her tongue. Her chest X-ray is shown in Figure 2.2. Which is the *single* most likely diagnosis? ★ ★

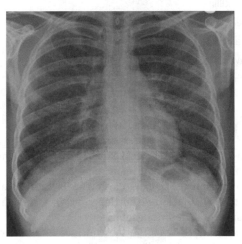

Figure 2.2

A Bronchial carcinoma

B Lymphoma

C Pulmonary tuberculosis

D *Pneumocystis jiroveci* pneumonia

E Sarcoidosis

38. A 68-year-old man has had several episodes of central abdominal pain, loose stools, and vomiting over the past 5 days. He has severe chronic obstructive pulmonary disease (COPD) and was recently treated with 2 weeks of antibiotics for a chest infection. He also takes aminophylline 450mg PO twice daily and prednisolone 10mg PO once daily. The patient suspects he may have suffered a reaction to the antibiotics. Which is the *single* most likely cause? ★ ★ ★

A Amoxicillin

B Cefalexin

C Co-amoxiclav

D Doxycycline

E Erythromycin

39. A 77-year-old man has had a cough with haemoptysis for over a year. During this time, he has lost 20kg and developed a pain in his upper abdomen. He is frail and has become increasingly dependent in his nursing home. The man's daughter tells the medical team that should they find anything worrying through the course of their investigations they should not tell him as it would 'finish him off'. A subsequent CT scan shows a primary bronchial malignancy with metastatic deposits in the liver. Which would be the *single* most appropriate course of action? ★ ★ ★

A Ask the man how much he would like to know about the ongoing investigations

B Refer the man to the palliative care team and allow them to deal with the information

C Tell the daughter and allow her to do what she likes with the information

D Tell the man that the scan was normal as it would not be in his best interests to know the truth

E Wait until either the man or his daughter asks about the scan before venturing any information

40. A 38-year-old woman has had a productive cough with right-sided chest pain for 4 days. Prior to this episode, she had been fit and well.

```
T 38.4°C, HR 110bpm, BP 110/75mmHg, RR 26/
min, SaO₂ 92% on 8L O₂.
```

There is bronchial breathing up to the mid-zone on the right. After 48h of antibiotic therapy, this has progressed to include the upper zone. Her SaO_2 has dropped to 86% on 8L O_2 and an arterial blood gas shows worsening type 1 respiratory failure. Which would be the *single* most appropriate course of action? ★ ★ ★

A Add a course of IV steroids

B Increase O_2 delivery to 15L/min

C Liaise with the Intensive Therapy Unit for ventilatory support

D Request an ultrasound scan of her chest

E Take blood cultures and switch antibiotics

41. A 45-year-old man has had a chest drain inserted for a large right-sided pneumothorax. The on-call junior doctor is asked to review a chest X-ray checking the placement of the drain: the tip of the drain is pointing towards the apex but a 3cm pneumothorax remains and the underwater drain is not bubbling or swinging. Which is the *single* most appropriate next step? ★ ★ ★

A Advance the drain a few centimetres further and repeat the chest X-ray

B Clamp the drain for 12h

C Flush 20ml of saline through the drain

D Remove the drain and leave air to be reabsorbed

E Remove the drain and replace with one further into the apex

42. An 88-year-old man is brought to the Emergency Department with a high fever, acute shortness of breath, and profuse diarrhoea. He is diagnosed with a chest infection and transferred to a ward but dies before any of the admitting team have seen him. The next morning, the hospital bereavement office asks the team's junior doctor to issue a medical certificate of cause of death. Which would be the *single* most appropriate course of action? ★ ★ ★

A Complete the certificate with 1a: Pneumonia

B Direct the office to the Emergency Department

C Gain permission from the family for a post mortem

D Refer the case to the coroner

E Tell the office that the patient's GP should complete the certificate

43. A 71-year-old man is transferred to the Intensive Therapy Unit following an aortic aneurysm repair. He has a long history of severe chronic obstructive pulmonary disease (COPD) and, as well as needing to use a number of inhalers, he takes prednisolone 20mg PO once daily. He is nil by mouth following his surgery but still requires his daily steroid dose. Which is the *single* most appropriate equivalent IV hydrocortisone dose for this patient? ★ ★ ★

A Hydrocortisone 5mg once daily

B Hydrocortisone 10mg once daily

C Hydrocortisone 10mg twice daily

D Hydrocortisone 20mg three times daily

E Hydrocortisone 20mg four times daily

44. A 48-year-old man has developed a non-productive cough. Previously, he felt as if he had 'flu with aching muscles and general malaise. He is normally fit and well and returned from a trip overseas a week ago. He visited no rural areas and does not remember being bitten by anything.

```
T 37.7°C, HR 100bpm, BP 110/75mmHg, SaO₂ 94%
on air.
```

His chest X-ray is shown in Figure 2.3. Which is the *single* most likely causative organism? ★ ★ ★

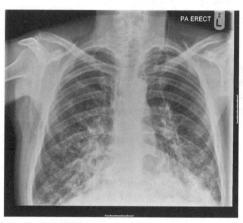

Figure 2.3

A *Chlamydia pneumoniae*

B *Legionella pneumophila*

C *Pneumocystis jiroveci*

D *Staphylococcus aureus*

E *Streptococcus pneumoniae*

45. A 32-year-old woman has been unwell for 3 weeks, initially with a headache and myalgia and latterly with a dry cough. She is a non-smoker and has no past medical history of note. She has reduced air entry bilaterally and symmetrical erythematous skin lesions that blister centrally on her arms and legs. Which is the *single* most likely causative organism? ★ ★ ★

A *Chlamydia pneumoniae*

B *Klebsiella pneumoniae*

C *Legionella pneumophila*

D *Mycoplasma pneumoniae*

E *Streptococcus pneumoniae*

46. A 21-year-old man experiences sudden right-sided chest pain while exercising. The pain persists in the Emergency Department but he is not short of breath. He has no other medical problems.

```
T 36.6°C, HR 90bpm, BP 115/80mmHg, RR 18/
min, SaO₂ 99% on air.
```

An X-ray reveals a 1.5cm sliver of air in the pleural space of the right lung. Which would be the *single* most appropriate course of action? ★ ★ ★

A Admit for observation

B Aspirate the air with a needle and syringe

C Chest drain

D Discharge the man home

E Insert a 16G cannula into the second intercostal space

$47.$ A 55-year-old woman has been increasingly short of breath for 2 weeks. She has felt feverish and has been coughing up green-coloured sputum for the past 5 days. She smokes ten cigarettes a day and drinks 20 units of alcohol a week.

```
T 38.8°C, HR 115bpm, BP 110/65mmHg,
RR 22/min, SaO₂ 91% on air.
```

Percussion of the chest reveals stony dullness up to the mid-zone on the right. Her chest X-ray is shown in Figure 2.4. Which *single* pathological process is the most likely cause? ★ ★ ★

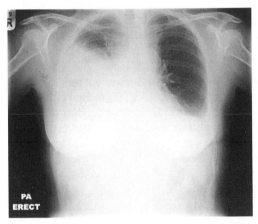

Figure 2.4

A Decreased colloid osmotic pressure

B Elevated hydrostatic pressure

C Impaired lymphatic drainage of the pleural space

D Increased capillary permeability

E Passage of peritoneal fluid through spaces in the diaphragm

48. A 51-year-old man has become increasingly short of breath over a period of 3 years. He worked in ceramics and pottery until recently, but has given up work early because he is unable to exert himself. He is a lifelong non-smoker. He has a chest X-ray performed. Which are the *single* most likely findings on the X-ray? ★ ★ ★

A Bilateral pleural effusions

B Large fibrotic masses in the upper zones

C Multiple bullae in the upper zones

D Nodular pattern in the upper and mid-zones

E Reticulo-nodular shadowing in the lower zones

49. A 42-year-old man is being ventilated in intensive care. He is quadriplegic having contracted tuberculosis of the spine and has been told that he could not survive without respiratory support via his tracheostomy. His mental capacity has not been affected. He has told the doctors that he wants the ventilator to be switched off. Which is the *single* most appropriate course of action for the intensive care team? ★ ★ ★

A Continue ventilatory support as euthanasia is illegal

B Continue ventilatory support as his decision is irrational

C Stop ventilatory support only if the man has an advance directive

D Stop ventilatory support as his condition is terminal

E Stop ventilatory support if he is shown to have capacity

50. A 77-year-old man with metastatic prostate cancer dies on Sunday afternoon on a general medical ward. The junior doctor – part of the medical team looking after him – returns to work on Monday morning and is asked to fill out the required certificates. He completes the death certificate and the cremation form, thus confirming that he has seen the body after death: he plans to do this later on in the day. Unfortunately, he only remembers 3 days later. By the time he contacts the hospital mortuary, he is told the body has already been moved to the funeral directors'. Which is the *single* most appropriate course of action? ★ ★ ★ ★

A Attend the hospital mortuary and ask to see the documents relating to the man's death to confirm his identity

B Confirm date and time of cremation with the crematorium, using that as proof of identity

C Confirm the identity of the patient with the doctor on call at the weekend who certified the death on the ward

D Contact the patient's family and confirm that it was their relative that died at the weekend

E Go to the funeral directors' and view the body before the cremation takes place

51. A 54-year-old man has felt increasingly irritable and tired over the last 6 months and on a number of occasions recently has briefly fallen asleep while driving. He has started to complain of regular headaches in the morning and last week, quite out of character, he forgot his wife's birthday.

```
HR 80 bpm, BP 150/70mmHg.

His BMI is 32kg/m².
```

Which is the *single* most appropriate next step? ★ ★ ★ ★

A Course of antidepressants

B CT scan of the head and neck

C Early morning arterial blood gases

D Sleep studies

E Thyroid function tests

ANSWERS

Single Best Answers

1. E ★

If treatment for a pneumonia is not proving adequate, it is important to re-image the chest. There may be an effusion amenable to drainage ('para-pneumonic'), pus in the pleural space (empyema), or, as here, an actual cavity of pus that will need a longer course of antibiotics (4–6 weeks) and maybe postural drainage.

A This indicates a pneumothorax.

B This indicates focal consolidation.

C This indicates a bronchial tumour.

D This indicates bronchiectasis.

2. E ★

As per the British Thoracic Society (BTS) guidelines, any acute admission to hospital should be seen as a '*window of opportunity to review self-management skills*'. Research has shown that the best way to do this is via personalized action plans. The BTS goes as far as saying that '*no patient should leave hospital without a written personalized action plan*'. Certainly in cases such as this where there has been a long gap since the last episode and where there is doubt as to what therapies have actually been taken, the best place to start is in formalizing a regimen and asking the patient to take ownership of it. The clearer the instructions, the more likely they are to be followed.

N.B. As a note to option D, guidelines state that any admission should be followed up by an asthma specialist within 30 days.

3. E ★

This woman is short of breath, wheezy, and tachycardic. The most likely diagnosis is acute asthma, although anaphylaxis and a pneumothorax should be kept in mind. She is clearly compromised – unable to talk, confused, and cyanosed. This is at least a severe attack and would warrant an early call to the Intensive Therapy Unit while initial treatments are instigated. If her arrival had been telephoned through as a blue call by the paramedics, it would have been sensible to ensure that there was an anaesthetist on the scene to make a preliminary assessment.

However severe the case, BTS guidelines are to use high-dose inhaled β_2 agonists as first-line agents and to administer as early as possible.

A Aminophylline infusions can be used if there has not been sufficient improvement with bronchodilators after 15–30min. By this stage, however, it is likely that the ITU will have been called to make an assessment.

B Epinephrine has a bigger role to play in anaphylaxis.

C Give steroids in all cases of acute asthma.

D Consider a one-off dose of magnesium sulphate in those who do not show a good initial response to bronchodilatators or in life-threatening or near-fatal asthma.

→ http://www.sign.ac.uk/pdf/qrg101.pdf

(*British Guideline on the Management of Asthma.* The British Thoracic Society, Scottish Intercollegiate Guidelines Network, May 2008.)

4. B ★

This is an acute severe asthma attack, but the woman's PEFR recovers to more than 75% of predicted within an hour after initial treatment so she can be discharged unless there are other reasons to prompt an admission. These would include: (i) she still has significant symptoms; (ii) there are concerns about compliance; (iii) she lives alone or is socially isolated; (iv) she has psychological problems, a physical disability, or learning difficulties; (v) she has a previous history of near-fatal or brittle asthma; (vi) exacerbation despite adequate-dose steroid tablets pre-presentation; (vii) she presented at night; or (viii) she is pregnant.

→ http://www.brit-thoracic.org.uk/ClinicalInformation/Asthma/AsthmaGuidelines/tabid/83/Default.aspx

5. B ★   OHCM 8th edn → p820

Running out of breath before the end of a sentence together with a PEFR 33–50% of predicted and HR >110/min is consistent with a severe attack.

A AND C These indicate hypotension and a 'silent chest'.

D AND E All options suggest a life-threatening attack of asthma, largely due to poor respiratory effort due to exhaustion leading to a hypercarbic state, which should prompt immediate referral to the High-Dependency Unit/Intensive Therapy Unit.

6. D ⋆

If a patient thinks their control is slipping, then it probably is. Objective signs of losing control include:

- A history of waking at night with wheeze, cough, or chest pain
- Increased use of bronchodilator therapy
- Decreased effectiveness of bronchodilator therapy
- Work days missed through asthma
- Any change in exercise tolerance.

Only D suggests that current therapy is not sufficient – all the others are expected features of asthma.

7. C ⋆

Patients should be 'stable' on their regular asthma therapy for 24h prior to discharge home. Their peak flow readings should be up to >75% of predicted or best. The prelude to discharge is also a good time to check inhaler technique and that the patient has a firm management plan in place to prevent any further admissions.

→ http://www.brit-thoracic.org.uk/ClinicalInformation/Asthma/ AsthmaGuidelines/tabid/83/Default.aspx

8. A ⋆

The key in the management of asthma is to follow the step-up/ step-down guidelines (as given in the *British Guideline on the Management of Asthma*). This woman is requiring more than one puff of her 'reliever' every day and so needs to move up to step 2 treatment, which is the addition of a regular 'preventer'. Note that Seretide® is an example of a combined preparation of a long-acting β2 agonist and an inhaled steroid (in this case salmeterol and fluticasone). It always contains 50mcg of salmeterol but can contain 100, 250 or 500mcg of steroid. The higher doses tend to be used in the treatment of chronic obstructive pulmonary disease (COPD).

→ http://www.brit-thoracic.org.uk/Portals/0/Clinical%20Information/ Asthma/Guidelines/asthma_final2008.pdf

(*British Guideline on the Management of Asthma*. The British Thoracic Society, Scottish Intercollegiate Guidelines Network, May 2008.)

9. B ⋆

The definition of an asthma attack is: worsening cough, chest pain, breathlessness, or wheeze *not* relieved by a β_2 agonist resulting in breathlessness impairing speech, eating, or sleep.

→ http://www.asthma.org.uk/all_about_asthma/what_to_do_in_an_ asthma_attack/index.html

10. D ★

The guidance from Asthma UK is as follows:

1) Take the 'reliever' inhaler immediately.

2) Sit down and ensure that any tight clothing is loosened. Do not lie down.

3) If there is no immediate improvement during an attack, continue to take one puff of the reliever inhaler every minute for 5min or until symptoms improve.

4) If symptoms do not improve in 5min, call 999 or a doctor urgently.

5) Continue to take one puff of the reliever inhaler every minute until help arrives.

→ http://www.asthma.org.uk/all_about_asthma/what_to_do_in_an_asthma_attack/index.html

11. C ★   OHCM 8th edn → p166

The repeated lung infections that cystic fibrosis sufferers contract lead to the terminal airways remaining permanently open: the result is copious sputum production and the vicious circle of increasingly recurrent infections. Pancreatic insufficiency has led to the development of diabetes.

A This indicates interstitial lung disease.

B AND E These indicate asthma.

D This indicates idiopathic pulmonary fibrosis.

12. B ★

This man has the symptoms of an acute infection with focal signs on his chest. As a smoker, he is at risk of community-acquired bacterial infections, the most common being *Streptococcus pneumoniae*. Although he is systemically unwell (rigors and a tachycardia), he has no core adverse prognostic features: new mental confusion, RR >30/min, systolic BP<90mmHg, or diastolic BP<60mmHg. As he is less than 50 and has no co-existing chronic illness, British Thoracic Society guidelines are that he can be managed safely at home.

A Although this man has a significant smoking history, early 40s would be young to develop a lung cancer. This is an acute illness with no suggestion of the kind of gradual decline that might be expected in a malignant process.

C Sarcoidosis rarely presents with acute breathlessness.

D The combination of haemoptysis and sweats means that tuberculosis is a reasonable differential diagnosis.

A comprehensive travel and contact history should be taken from this man and sputum should be sent for acid-fast bacilli as well as microscopy, culture, and sensitivity. However, with such a short history, and with basal chest sounds and no history of weight loss, a pneumonia is more likely.

E Wegener's granulomatosis is a vasculitis that can present with cough and haemoptysis but usually against a background of chronic symptoms (sinusitis, nasal ulceration, or other upper respiratory tract symptoms) rather than with an acute infection.

British Thoracic Society Standards of Care Committee (2001). BTS Guidelines for the management of community acquired pneumonia in adults. *Thorax* (Suppl. 4) **56**: iv1–iv64.

→ http://thorax.bmj.com/cgi/content/full/56/suppl_4/iv1

13.E ★

Prescriptions for controlled drugs cause confusion among doctors at all levels. They can now be computer-generated (including the date) but require the signature to be handwritten and the patient's address to be included as well as the name and form of the medication to be supplied. The total quantity to be supplied must be written in words and figures, not the dose. The date of birth and GMC number are not necessary.

→ http://www.dh.gov.uk/en/Healthcare/Medicinespharmacyandindustry/Prescriptions/ControlledDrugs/index.htm

14.B ★   OHCM 8th edn → p166

This is suggestive of an infective exacerbation of cystic fibrosis with a bronchiectatic picture. Chronic infection of the bronchi and bronchioles leads to permanent dilatation of these airways.

A This indicates lung carcinoma.

C This indicates systemic lupus erythematosus (SLE).

D This indicates a pulmonary embolism.

E This indicates a Pancoast tumour.

15.D ★

This man is showing signs and symptoms of hypercapnoea. An increase in oxygen administration with non-rebreather masks or nasal oxygen will further increase his carbon dioxide. CPAP is delivered throughout the respiratory cycle but does not change during inspiration or expiration. NIV (also known as bi-level positive airway pressure or BiPAP) aids the inspiratory phase by delivering higher pressures during inspiration and dropping to a CPAP during expiration. This allows retained carbon dioxide to be expired as a result of the positive end-expiratory pressure 'stenting' the airways open.

→ http://thorax.bmj.com/content/vol59/suppl_1/

(Chronic Obstructive Pulmonary Disease. National clinical guideline on management of chronic obstructive pulmonary disease in adults in primary and secondary care. *Thorax* 59, Supplement 1.)

16. B ★

Pneumothoraces do not only afflict fit young men; they also occur as secondary phenomena in those with established lung disease. If the volume of air in the pleural space is large enough, then classic signs elicited are: decreased air entry, reduced expansion, and hyper-resonant percussion note. These cases always require admission to hospital for either aspiration or insertion of a chest drain.

A, D, AND C These suggest consolidation, which would cause a more gradual decline in a COPD sufferer with an increasingly productive cough with or without fever.

E This suggests fluid in the pleural space, which is unlikely to cause such sudden symptoms in someone with lung disease; indeed, there may be chronic effusions that fluctuate in volume and cause minimal symptoms.

Henry M, Arnold T, and Harvey J, on behalf of the BTS Pleural Disease Group, a subgroup of the BTS Standards of Care Committee (2003). BTS Guidelines for the management of spontaneous pneumothorax. *Thorax* 58 (Suppl. II): ii39–ii52.

→ http://www.brit-thoracic.org.uk/Portals/0/Clinical%20Information/ Pleural%20Disease/Guidelines/PleuralDiseaseSpontaneous.pdf

17. C ★   OHCM 8th edn → p726

Inflammation of the costochondral joints presents insidiously until it causes severe, sharp pain originating from the anterior chest wall often radiating around to the back. It should be on the differential diagnosis list for chest pain and – once more serious causes have been excluded – should be considered likely if there is point tenderness over the medial ribs (typically the 2nd to the 5th).

Although this woman has pleuritic chest pain, her observations are almost entirely normal: this would not be the case in E (tachycardia with or without hypoxia) or B (fever and tachycardia with hypoxia), whilst D would be very unlikely in a young woman without risk factors and would more likely present with sudden exertional pain and breathlessness rather than gradually increasing pleuritic pain.

A may be the next most likely cause as it can present with insidious pleuritic chest pain; however, there is also likely to be at least one additional finding: fever, tachycardia and/or tachypnoea, and not associated with tenderness on palpation.

18.C ★

OHCM 8th edn → p170

The new symptoms are those of hypercalcaemia – either from skeletal metastasis, or, as here, from secretion of parathyroid hormone by a squamous cell tumour. Hypercalcaemia as a result of primary hyperparathyroidism can be remembered using:

- 'stones' – renal stones
- 'bones' – pain and sometimes pathological fractures (classically due to osteitis fibrosa cystica)
- 'groans' – abdominal pain from ulcers, nausea, indigestion, or constipation
- 'psychic moans' – lethargy, fatigue, and depression.

19.B ★

Based on the history, this nodule is likely to be a bronchial carcinoma. The right ptosis suggests that it is a Pancoast tumour, i.e. one that causes Horner's syndrome by compressing the sympathetic plexus. Other features include anhidrosis, ptosis, and as infiltration worsens can involve the brachial plexus or recurrent laryngeal nerve.

A This is cranial nerve (CN) XI, which innervates the trapezius and sternocleidomastoid.

C This is CN III; this would cause a 'down-and-out' dilated pupil.

D This would be expected to produce facial and upper limb oedema and dilated neck veins.

E This would result in sensory loss around the eye.

20.D ★

Hyponatraemia in someone with lung cancer is suggestive of the syndrome of inappropriate antidiuretic hormone secretion (SIADH), caused by ectopic hormone secretion by a small cell tumour. These make up about 20% of lung cancers. The remainder are non-small cell and include squamous cell carcinoma, adenocarcinoma, and large cell carcinoma.

21.E ★

Audible gurgling suggests the presence of liquid material in the upper airways and needs to be removed by a suction device such as the wide-bore rigid Yankauer sucker. Although a crash/peri-arrest call should be put out, suctioning the airway may be enough to allow sufficient ventilation to restore this man's full consciousness.

22. E ★

Although writing in notes may not be an explicit part of the medical undergraduate curriculum, a junior doctor has to do it every day. It is also one of the few things for which he can be clearly held accountable. Even if the junior is not confident in what he is writing and is nervous about making bold pronouncements of diagnosis or management plans, he can help himself by obeying a few very simple rules:

1) Write name, designation and sign with bleep number.

2) Write time and date of review.

3) Write reason for review and who was present.

In cases such as this where clinical events probably happened very quickly, it is vital in the aftermath to be able to follow them in chronological order. Omitting the time makes this very difficult. It also lessens the credibility of the entry and calls into question the professionalism of the doctor. Whilst the legal team – and indeed other doctors – may feel that this entry was also lacking for some of the other options listed, the only feature that will actually impair their dissection of events is the lack of a time.

→ http://archive.student.bmj.com/back_issues/1196/st11ed1.htm

23. B ★

Not for resuscitation means not for resuscitation. Although it is hard as a junior doctor not to react instinctively in situations like this and call the arrest team, all that is needed is careful monitoring of breathing and circulation until it is clear that death can be confirmed.

24. C ★

Sudden shortness of breath in a patient with chronic obstructive pulmonary disease (COPD) on NIV should make you think of a spontaneous pneumothorax. The other findings are to be expected in someone with COPD and would not in isolation prompt an immediate review.

25. D ★

The key to this case is the discrepancy between the oxygen saturations and respiratory rate: in someone who has ventilation problems, why would they be breathing so slowly? Their respiratory muscles are either tiring or they are being prevented from working.

This patient has a reason to be on high-dose analgesia so it would be important to examine her pupils urgently: if they are contracted, it may be that naloxone 200mcg IV will go a long way to reversing her current problems (repeated if necessary as it has a very short half-life and can be better given as an infusion). If opioid overdose is responsible, her ventilation rate will improve, as will her oxygen saturations and her level of consciousness.

26.E ★

Sudden-onset pleuritic chest pain is highly suggestive of a thromboembolic event, as is residual hypoxia. This man will need a CT pulmonary angiogram. He has the wheeze of a chronic smoker and no signs of cardiac ischaemia or failure.

27.D ★

The diagnosis is a pulmonary embolism and, although not universal, it is most likely to cause pleuritic chest pain, which is classically worse on inspiration. In this case, it is also associated with a small effusion.

A This would indicate a neoplastic diagnosis.

B AND C These indicate infection.

E This indicates a lung abscess/empyema.

28.D ★

Sudden pain with breathlessness in a young man should make a primary spontaneous pneumothorax top of the list. The patient may be concerned that there is a cardiac cause and this can lead the junior doctor astray: it is therefore vital that, even with a satisfactory SaO$_2$, if the story is convincing, a chest X-ray is performed. Often, in small pneumothoraces, there are no (or very subtle) clinical signs: indeed, tachycardia and tachypnoea may be the only findings.

A This is a reasonable differential in a young man but is unlikely to announce itself so suddenly and does not fit with the clinical sign elicited.

B Sudden pain is unlikely to be the presenting complaint of a chest infection. A young man is more likely to feel gradually short of breath with an increasingly troublesome cough.

C This is a differential not to forget but is more likely to present gradually. It should be considered once other diagnoses have been excluded and is suggested by tenderness on palpation of the costochondral joints.

E This would also present this suddenly and possibly with the same symptoms. However, it is extremely unlikely in a young man with no risk factors and typically there are no signs on examination of the chest.

Mackenzie S and Grey A (2007). Primary spontaneous pneumothorax: why all the confusion over first-line treatment? J R Coll Physicians *Edinb* **37**:335–338.

→ http://www.rcpe.ac.uk/journal/issue/journal_37_4/MackenzieGrey.pdf

29. D ★   OHCM 8th edn → p182

A hyper-resonant percussion note with decreased air entry on the same side suggests that there is air in the pleural space: a pneumothorax should be top of the list when young men become suddenly breathless with chest pain – particularly when they have risk factors, as in this case (asthma and smoking), when it is classified as a secondary pneumothorax and managed differently from a primary spontaneous pneumothorax.

A, B AND C   These are all suggestive of consolidation, which would present gradually with fever and a cough.

E This implies fluid in the pleural cavity, which again would be unlikely to cause sudden symptoms and is more likely to be the result of another process (such as pneumonia, tuberculosis, or malignancy), which would cause symptoms of its own first.

30. B ★   OHCM 8th edn → p370

Patients who have had a course of steroids shorter than 3 weeks and of doses <40mg do not need gradual weaning, unless they have a history of repeated steroid use or previous adrenal suppression.

31. E ★

The doctor's duty is not to be protective of their own clinical reputation in front of their seniors, but to provide the safest level of patient care possible. Although it may be tempting to 'have a go', one of the most important skills for junior doctors is to recognize the limits of their abilities and not to be afraid of admitting if they are unable to carry out a particular task. To this end: '*In providing care you must recognise and work within the limits of your competence*'. The arterial blood gases will give information on acid–base balance and carbon dioxide as well as oxygen levels and are a better indicator than peripheral saturations. The patient should not be coerced into another attempt and the doctor would not be deemed competent just because another doctor has described the procedure to them.

→ http://www.gmc-uk.org/guidance/good_medical_practice/good_clinical_care/index.asp

(*Good Medical Practice 2006,* paragraph 3(a). General Medical Council.)

32. C ★ OHCM 8th edn → pp170, 218

Abdominal pain with postural hypotension is suggestive of adrenocortical insufficiency. In a patient with a lung cancer, this is most likely to be due to metastasis of the cancer to the adrenal glands, causing secondary Addison's disease.

33. A ★

Snoring occurs when the pharynx is partially occluded by the tongue or palate. It therefore heralds partial airway obstruction. In someone who is requiring assistance with his ventilation because of lower respiratory compromise, it should be reversed before too long. The aim of the manoeuvres is to stretch the anterior neck structures. If these measures succeed in stopping the snoring but the man remains drowsy, then other issues such as opioid or carbon dioxide toxicity would need to be addressed. However, as in the first instance of any emergency situation, the airway needs to be managed to allow adequate ventilation.

34. E ★

Whilst arterial blood gases to monitor current oxygenation and a chest X-ray to exclude other pathologies (most notably a pneumothorax) may be useful in the acute setting, spirometry is the preferred initial test to assess the presence and severity of airflow obstruction.

→ http://www.brit-thoracic.org.uk/Portals/0/Clinical%20Information/Asthma/Guidelines/asthma_final2008.pdf

35. C ★

As the British Thoracic Society guidelines explain, '*Evidence that non-pharmacological management is effective can be difficult to obtain and more well controlled intervention studies are required.*' With regard to symptom control, only the so-called Buteyko breathing techniques have been shown to have any impact. They focus on the control of hyperventilation and have been shown to reduce symptoms and the use of bronchodilators but do not alter lung function. Immunotherapy may be of benefit if a specific allergen can be detected and is then considered unavoidable. There is as yet no supporting evidence for acupuncture or dietary modifications, and air ionizers are not recommended.

→ http://www.brit-thoracic.org.uk/Portals/0/Clinical%20Information/
Asthma/Guidelines/asthma_final2008.pdf

36.D ★

When being handed over the care of a patient by another professional, it is always important to review what has been done so far. In this case, the receiving doctor has been told that a chronic obstructive pulmonary disease (COPD) sufferer has shortness of breath that has improved with bronchodilators and low oxygen saturations that have reached 97% on 5L.

His approach should begin with ABCDE (airway, breathing, circulation, disability, exposure). Having assessed his airway, the next port of call is breathing: does a COPD sufferer need to have oxygen saturations in the high 90s? Could this be why he has become confused? Before considering antibiotics and imaging, it is important to ensure that oxygen delivery is sufficient and appropriate without causing compromise in other ways. The best way to do this in COPD sufferers is by employing controlled oxygen therapy (via a Venturi mask) and by regular blood gas monitoring. Whilst it is important to be vigilant for hypercapnoea, it is also illogical to leave patients hypoxaemic. In cases where it is proving difficult to find a balance between the two, an early call to the Intensive Therapy Unit is a smart move as these are the patients who may benefit from mechanical ventilation of some sort (e.g. non-invasive ventilation or bi-level positive airway pressure).

Cooper N (2004). Acute care: treatment with oxygen. *Student BMJ* 12:45–88.

→ http://archive.student.bmj.com/issues/04/02/education/56.php

37.D ★ ★   OHCM 8th edn → pp162, 411

The history of a dry cough with exertional dyspnoea is typical, as is the X-ray showing bilateral pulmonary infiltrates. Another clue is the patches on the tongue, which may be *Candida*, an opportunistic infection in immunosuppression. In a woman of this age with these two unusual infections, a human immunodeficiency virus (HIV) test is essential.

A This is unlikely in someone of this age and with no obvious mass lesion on X-ray.

B Weight loss and night sweats in a young adult should raise the suspicion of haematological malignancy, but with such an obvious respiratory source, it is unlikely in this case. A more common presentation would be weight loss and night sweats and the finding of a non-tender superficial lymph node.

Chest medicine

C This is probably the best differential as the weight loss, cough, and night sweats fit, but the exertional dyspnoea does not and the chest X-ray is not typical.

E Like tuberculosis, this is a granulomatous disease that affects the lungs, but it does not present in this way: breathlessness is not normally the main feature; indeed, it is often discovered incidentally.

38. E ★★★

The drug reaction referred to is aminophylline toxicity following the prescription of antibiotics. This is a common problem in patients with COPD who are using theophyllines, which have a narrow therapeutic range. The antibiotics most likely to cause toxicity are those that inhibit the cytochrome P450 enzyme system – erythromycin, as in this case, and ciprofloxacin.

39. A ★★★

The key to this scenario is the recognition that it is the man who is the patient and not his daughter. Her opinion has been made clear – she may well be right about how the bad news would affect her father but it is incumbent on every medical professional in such a situation to seek the patient's desires or 'information needs' before proceeding.

C singularly misses this point, whilst B would initiate the untenable situation of a man being palliated before he knows he has palliative disease. D is plain deception, whilst E is cowardice that simply postpones a potentially difficult conversation. If bad news exists, then it needs to be broken: the process should begin by setting out initial goals for delivering it by listening – yes, to the patient's family, but crucially, to the patient.

Rabow M and McPhee S (2000). Beyond breaking bad news: helping patients who suffer. *Student BMJ* 8:45–88.

→ http://archive.student.bmj.com/issues/00/03/education/65.php

40. C ★★★

This woman's worsening clinical findings and blood gas show that her current treatment is not working. Although all options may add value at some stage, given her deterioration after 2 days of treatment, it is likely that she will need some assistance to improve her ventilation, probably in the form of continuous positive airway pressure (CPAP).

The key, however, is recognition of the downward trend. Following national guidelines, there should be appropriate local systems in place to ensure that this happens. Whether it is via MEWS (modified early warning score) or PARS (patient at risk score), the aim is to stratify those patients at risk of clinical deterioration based on their physiological observations. Those that fall into the low-risk group require continued monitoring, those in the medium-risk group need assessment by their medical team, and those in the high-risk group need urgent attention from a critical care team. The woman in this case would probably be in the high-risk group. The challenge for the junior doctor is that the information will not always be presented in this way. When confronted with a set of abnormal observations, it is vital that junior doctors perform their own risk stratification based on local systems; they will then be more able to make the appropriate management decision, i.e. increase the frequency of observations, arrange assessment by the senior doctor from the medical team or – as in this case – call for an urgent critical care review.

→ http://www.nice.org.uk/nicemedia/pdf/CG50QuickRefGuide.pdf

(*Acutely Ill Patients in Hospital: Recognition of and Response to Acute Illness in Adults in Hospital.* NICE Clinical Guidance 50, 2007.)

Baines E and Kanagasundaram N (2008). Early warning scores. *Student BMJ* 16:294–336.

→ http://archive.student.bmj.com/issues/08/09/education/320.php

41. C ★ ★ ★

The drain may not be patent for a number of reasons. The holes may be occluded or in a lung fissure, or it may just not be in the right place to drain the remaining air. The first step is to try and unblock the tube with saline. Putting the drain on a high-volume/low-pressure suction might also be tried before it is removed and another re-sited if needed.

A For infection control reasons, drains should never be advanced.

B This will not help the collection of air that remains and could cause a tension pneumothorax.

D The collection of air is too large for this.

E This is what will be required if efforts to unblock the drain are unsuccessful.

Laws D, Neville E, and Duffy J (2003). BTS guidelines for the insertion of a chest drain. *Thorax* 58 (Suppl. 2):ii53–ii59.

42. B ★ ★ ★

The law requires that the certificate be completed by a doctor who attended to the patient during their last illness: 'attended to' means that they should have seen the patient at least twice. For this reason, both A and E are wrong. As this patient died within 24h of being in hospital, the case will need to be referred to the coroner's office. However, this should not be done by a doctor who has not seen the patient at all prior to death. Discussions about post mortems should also be kept between the coroner and the 'attending' doctor. For these reasons, the most appropriate course of action for the junior doctor would be to direct the bereavement office back to the Emergency Department and to the attending doctor.

Dosani S (2002). Dead cert: a guide to death certificates. *Student BMJ* 10:45–88.

→ http://archivestudent.bmj.com/issues/02/03/education/54.php

Fertleman M (1997). A doctor's life after a patient's death: guide to coroners and certificates. *Student BMJ* 5:12–13.

→ http://archive.student.bmj.com/back_issues/0297/data/0297ed2.htm

43.E ★ ★ ★

Prednisolone is four times the strength of hydrocortisone.

44.B ★ ★ ★   OHCM 8th edn → p162

An atypical pneumonia, *Legionella* colonizes water tanks – classically in hotels – causing a 'flu-like illness followed by a dry cough and breathlessness. X-ray findings vary and often lag behind symptoms but may show bilateral consolidation of the lower zones (as in this case). It should be considered in previously fit patients who present with a cough and hypoxia (particularly if they have had recent trips overseas).

A *Chlamydia* typically begins with a combination of pharyngitis and otitis before progressing to a pneumonia.

C *Pneumocystis jiroveci* causes pneumonia symptoms in the immunosuppressed (classically those with human immunodeficiency virus (HIV)).

D *Staphylococcus* causes a cavitating pneumonia in those at either end of the age spectrum or those with underlying lung disease.

E Although *Streptococcus pneumoniae* is the most common causative organism, it tends to affect the elderly or those with some kind of compromise, such as alcohol users and those with heart failure or underlying lung disease.

45.D ★ ★ ★   OHCM 8th edn → p162

The insidious presentation with 'flu-like symptoms is classical. The skin rash is erythema multiforme.

B *Klebsiella pneumoniae* infection is a rare cause of pneumonia.
It produces cavitations, particularly in the upper lobes, in
compromised populations such as the elderly and alcoholics.

See also answers to 44.

46. D ★ ★ ★

As this is not secondary to other medical causes, this is a primary
pneumothorax. Although the patient has some pain, he is not
breathless and has a small defect: patients with small primary
pneumothoraces and minimal symptoms do not require admission to
hospital but they should return should they become breathless.

A Admission in a primary pneumothorax may only be needed after
repeated attempts to aspirate have been unsuccessful and a chest
drain has been placed. Observation is more useful in secondary
pneumothoraces, for example after a successful aspiration.

B Aspiration can be attempted if the patient is breathless and/or
there is a >2cm rim of air on the chest X-ray. A maximum of two
aspirations can be tried.

C An intercostal chest drain should be inserted if the second
attempt at aspiration of the air is unsuccessful. Once air has
stopped leaking, the drain should be left *in situ* for a further 24h
prior to removal and discharge.

E This is needle decompression and is used for tension
pneumothoraces.

Henry M, Arnold T, and Harvey J, on behalf of the BTS Pleural Disease
Group, a subgroup of the BTS Standards of Care Committee (2003).
BTS Guidelines for the management of spontaneous pneumothorax.
Thorax **58** (Suppl. II): ii39–ii52.

→ http://www.brit-thoracic.org.uk/Portals/0/Clinical%20Information/
Pleural%20Disease/Guidelines/PleuralDiseaseSpontaneous.pdf

47. D ★ ★ ★   OHCM 8th edn → p184

The history is suggestive of an infective process, whilst the
clinical findings are that of a pleural effusion. Fluid accumulation
in the pleural space in the setting of an infection is known as
a 'parapneumonic effusion'. The fluid is an exudate and seeps into
the pleural space following inflammation of the lung and resulting
increased capillary permeability. Following Light's criteria, effusions
are either transudates or exudates (based on ratios of fluid:serum
protein and lactate dehydrogenase). Those that occur due to
systemic disturbance are usually transudates, whilst those that are
a response to local factors are usually exudates.

A This occurs due to hypoproteinaemia as seen in liver cirrhosis and the nephrotic syndrome (transudate).

B This is a consequence of increased venous pressure as in heart failure or constrictive pericarditis (transudate).

C This follows obstruction of the superior vena cava and results in decreased absorption of pleural fluid and hence leaking into pleural spaces (exudate).

E This occurs in liver disease with ascites (transudate).

→ http://www.clevelandclinicmeded.com/medicalpubs/disease management/pulmonary/pleural-disease/

48. D ★ ★ ★   OHCM 8th edn → p184

This man has progressive dyspnoea following his exposure to silica during his work in ceramics. The chest X-ray appearance would show a 'miliary' or nodular pattern in the upper and mid-zones and egg-shell calcification of the hilar nodes.

A This would indicate cardiac failure.

B This would indicate progressive massive fibrosis due to progression of coal workers' pneumoconiosis.

C This would indicate emphysematous changes.

E This would indicate pulmonary fibrosis.

49. E ★ ★ ★

'*A competent patient has the right to refuse treatment and their refusal must be respected, even if it will result in their death.*'

→ http://www.gmc-uk.org/guidance/ethical_guidance/consent_ guidance/common_law.asp

(*Consent: Patients and Doctors Making Decisions Together.* See Re B (Adult, refusal of medical treatment) [2002] 2 All ER 449. Right of a patient who has capacity to refuse life-prolonging treatment. General Medical Council.)

50. E ★ ★ ★ ★

This is a strange scenario but one that many junior doctors find themselves in. The most important point to remember is that the death certification that is completed by the doctor is a legal document and that if he signs to say he has seen the body when he has not, he is breaking the law. The body must be seen after death by the doctor unless he was present at the death or certified the death of the patient. If the body has left the hospital, it can be viewed at the funeral directors' to satisfy this requirement.

51.D ★★★★

This man has obstructive sleep apnoea (OSA) and probably snores very badly too if you asked his wife! It would be useful for this man and his wife to complete an Epworth Sleepiness Scale questionnaire. This will allow a subjective assessment of the degree of pre-treatment sleepiness. Pulse oximetry studies might be considered as a first-line approach, but in a man who has symptoms suggestive of OSA and has been sleepy while driving, he should be referred urgently to a sleep centre.

A This man's problems will not be resolved by antidepressants.

B He has had recurrent headaches and a change in personality, but his obesity and daytime somnolence should be investigated first to rule out OSA. If these investigations prove normal, a CT head scan could be warranted.

C This would not provide useful information as he is unlikely to be desaturating once awake.

E This might be useful to check, considering his irritability and high BMI but is not the first choice.

→ http://www.sign.ac.uk/guidelines/fulltext/73/index.html

CHAPTER 3
ENDOCRINOLOGY

Endocrinology is the study of diabetes and the function of mainly three glands. Whilst some may enjoy the colourful findings caused when these glands malfunction, others find that it is in this area that the subject becomes confusingly academic: the complex feedback loops, the intertwining symptoms, eccentric tests, and treatments for rare syndromes.

Conveniently, therefore, both the 'regulars' and the 'unmissables' of endocrinology revolve almost entirely around diabetes mellitus. Junior doctors are exposed to diabetes in all clinical settings, treating acutely low and high blood sugars, the hydration problems that go with it, the regimen changes this may prompt, and the systemic upset that this may cause. It is therefore vital to go armed with a clear understanding of the condition, from its diagnosis to acute and then chronic management via its impact on lifestyle and the population at large.

This chapter will develop an understanding by providing clarity in a range of clinical areas. As well as gaining confidence in detecting and managing a diabetic emergency, it is important to remember that diabetes mellitus is a condition that requires optimum patient motivation and understanding and therefore excellent communication skills on the part of the doctor. This means possessing a solid grounding in, for example, the patterns of eye disease as well as the ability to be able to communicate this to the patient in clear terms. Empowering a patient by arming them with sensitively delivered information may aid control of blood sugars and reduce end organ damage better than any minor tweak to their insulin regimen.

In terms of clinical frequency, thyroid disease is next in line. Dysfunction of this organ is a useful differential diagnosis for a wide range of clinical presentations, so a firm grasp of the concepts behind diagnosis and management in this area will be beneficial. It is also useful as a prototypical endocrine gland. Whilst the concept of negative feedback may make some shudder as they recall a pile of unread first year medical school physiology notes, it is something to cling on to when approaching the remaining pair of rather mysterious glands that are featured in this chapter.

Although neither adrenal nor pituitary gland disease is very common, they create vivid clinical scenarios that are often very recognizable and instructive with regard to basic physiology.

Whilst the main aim of this chapter is to arrive at a working practical knowledge of diabetes, it will also raise awareness of the other glands so that their dysfunction can be recognized and investigated where appropriate. ∎

1. A 32-year-old woman has lost 3kg over the past 3 months. She has no loss of appetite, but has felt rather irritable and 'stressed'.

T 37.1°C, HR 110bpm, BP 100/65mmHg.

Her thyroid function tests are returned as follows:

Thyroid-stimulating hormone (TSH) 0.21mU/L, thyroxine (T4) 218nmol/L.

There is a fine tremor of both hands. She is started on propranolol 40mg PO once daily. Which is the *single* most appropriate next step in management? ★

A Amiodarone 150mg PO once daily

B Carbimazole 40mg PO once daily

C Carbimazole 40mg PO once daily + thyroxine 125mcg PO once daily

D Radioiodine therapy

E Thyroxine 125mcg PO once daily

2. A 68-year-old man undergoes annual retinal screening. He has type 2 diabetes and uses insulin twice daily. Following the scan, he asks his doctor what causes the presence of 'cotton-wool' spots in his report. Which is the *single* most appropriate response? ★

A Areas of tissue starved of oxygen

B Deposits of fat

C Formation of new blood vessels

D Small bleeds

E Small swollen vessels

3. A 40-year-old man is confused. He has an uncontrollable thirst along with the regular passage of large volumes of dilute urine.

```
Urine osmolality 280mOsmol/kg; increases
to 620mOsmol/kg after desmopressin 20µg
nasally.
```

Which is the *single* most appropriate explanation for his symptoms? ★

A Decreased secretion of antidiuretic hormone (ADH) by the pituitary

B Impaired response of the kidney to ADH

C Inappropriately high secretion of ADH by the pituitary

D Primary polydipsia

E Renal hypersensitivity to ADH

4. An 18-year-old man has had abdominal pain for the past 24h. He has been unwell for the last few weeks. He has lost 10kg and has been taking a large bottle of water to bed every night.

```
T 37.5°C, HR 115bpm, BP 110/70mmHg,
RR 30/min.
```

He is clammy, aggressive, and confused. Which is the *single* most likely diagnosis? ★

A Addisonian crisis

B Diabetes insipidus

C Diabetic ketoacidosis (DKA)

D Hyperaldosteronism

E Syndrome of inappropriate antidiuretic hormone secretion (SIADH)

5. A 22-year-old woman is overwhelmingly drowsy and intermittently agitated. She is able to communicate that she has been excessively thirsty for the last 48h and has also been passing increased volumes of urine.

```
T 36.2°C, HR 120bpm, BP 100/75mmHg.
```

She is pale, sweaty, and struggling to stay awake. Which is the *single* most appropriate course of action? ★

A Dextrose 10% 200mL IV

B Glucagon 4mg IV STAT

C Insulin 4U IV STAT

D NaHCO₃ 500mL IV

E Saline 0.9% 1L IV

6. A 24-year-old man has suffered a headache with blurred vision for the past year or more. He has felt continually tired and also reports having to pass urine much more regularly than before. A range of preliminary tests are run:

```
Random venous blood glucose 10.7mmol/L,
fasting venous blood glucose 8.9mmol/L,
glycosylated haemoglobin (HbA1C) 7.8%,
random capillary glucose 14.4mmol/L.

Urine dipstick: glucose 2+.
```

Which *single* result should be given the most consideration in making a diagnosis? ★

A Fasting venous blood glucose

B HbA1C

C Random capillary blood glucose

D Random venous blood glucose

E Urine dipstick

7. A 17-year-old man has lost 6kg over the past 2 months. He has also been excessively thirsty and not his usual self. A venous blood sample is taken.

`Random venous blood glucose 16mmol/L.`

Which is the *single* most appropriate next step in management? ★

A 24h capillary glucose diary

B Fasting venous blood glucose

C Oral glucose tolerance test (OGTT)

D Repeat random venous blood glucose

E Start treatment for diabetes

8. A 78-year-old woman is admitted for the repair of a femoral hernia. She is assessed the night before her scheduled surgery at which time examination reveals a previously undocumented finding (Figure 3.1). The patient has not noticed it before and seems untroubled by it. Which *single* further feature from the history is most likely to support the diagnosis? ★

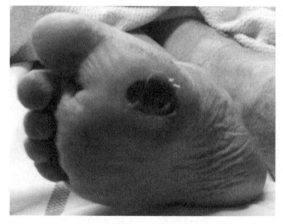

Figure 3.1

A Aching calves after long periods of standing

B Impaired sensation in feet

C Pain in feet when walking

D Persistent swelling resistant to treatment

E Recent history of trauma

9. A 57-year-old man is started on a tablet to reduce his blood glucose. His brother also has type 2 diabetes and has had multiple hypoglycaemic attacks. He returns to see his doctor a week later, angry that he has not been warned about the possibility of these. His doctor tells him that the medication he is taking does not cause this side effect. Which is the *single* most likely medication he is taking? ★

A Glibenclamide

B Gliclazide

C Pioglitazone

D Repaglinide

E Tolbutamide

10. A 28-year-old man has noticed that the tissue around his breasts has become increasingly swollen. They are non-tender. He has recently started chemotherapy for testicular cancer. Which is the *single* most likely biochemical cause for this change? ★

A ↓ Androgen

B ↓ Dopamine

C ↑ Growth hormone

D ↑ Oestrogen:androgen ratio

E ↑ Prolactin

11. A 70-year-old man has been feeling progressively more tired for 2 weeks. He has been drinking increasingly large volumes of fluid each day and passing more urine than normal.

```
Random capillary blood glucose 42mmol/L.

Arterial blood gases: pH 7.37, pO₂ 10.9kPa,
pCO₂ 4.8kPa, HCO₃⁻ 20mmol/L.
```

Which is the *single* most likely precipitant for these symptoms? ★

A Diabetes insipidus

B First-presentation type 1 diabetes

C First-presentation type 2 diabetes

D Pancreatic cancer

E Poorly controlled type 1 diabetes

12. A 28-year-old woman has felt increasingly irritable over the last few months. She describes herself as 'hot and bothered' – she is always trying to cool herself down and is always sweating. She has lost 5kg in this time. She smokes 20 cigarettes a day and drinks 30 units of alcohol a week. Which *single* examination finding is most likely to support the diagnosis? ★

A Dry skin and hair

B Exophthalmos

C Hyperpigmented skin folds

D Lymphadenopathy

E Malar rash

13. An 82-year-old man has become unresponsive. Earlier that morning, he had been talking with the nursing staff, although he declined breakfast. He has atrial fibrillation, insulin-dependent diabetes, and uses high-dose analgesia for severe osteoarthritis.

```
T 35.2°C, HR 120bpm, BP 175/100mmHg,
RR 22/min, SaO₂ 95% on air.

Glasgow Coma Scale (GCS) score: 10/15
(E2, V3, M5).
```

He is noted to be pale and shaking. There is weakness in all four limbs. Which is the *single* most likely cause of his sudden deterioration? ★

A Gastrointestinal haemorrhage

B Hypoglycaemia

C Hypothermia

D Opioid overdose

E Stroke

14. A 58-year-old man has been attempting to control his blood sugars using dietary measures alone for the past 9 months. At the start of this period, his fasting blood glucose was 6.8mmol/L. It is now 8.4mmol/L. His BMI is 32kg/m². Which would be the *single* most appropriate course of action? ★

A Gliclazide

B Glibenclamide

C Metformin

D No drug treatment indicated

E Rosiglitazone

15. A 78-year-old woman has a lump in her neck, which was first noticed by her daughter 3 months ago. There is an obvious midline swelling. It is hard but non-tender and contains several discrete lumps. It moves on swallowing but not on protrusion of the tongue. There are no associated lymph nodes and no dullness to percussion over the sternum. Which is the *single* most likely cause of the swelling? ★

A Graves' disease

B Hashimoto's thyroiditis

C Multinodular goitre

D Physiological goitre

E Subacute thyroiditis

16. A 60-year-old woman has felt generally weak and unwell with a headache for the past year or so. Apart from mild central obesity, the only point of note on examination is the loss of lateral gaze in the right eye. An MRI scan reveals a tumour originating from the pituitary fossa. Which *single* structure is the tumour most likely to have impinged? ★

A Cavernous sinus

B Internal carotid artery

C Optic chiasm

D Sphenoid sinus

E Suprasellar cistern

17. A 68-year-old man undergoes retinal screening. He has type 2 diabetes and uses insulin twice daily. He is told that there is evidence of new vessel formation and asks his doctor for the significance of this finding. Which is the *single* most appropriate response? ★

A Areas of the eye that had previously been damaged have regenerated

B He is likely to lose his sight in this eye within 3 months

C His diabetic control is good and his vision is improving

D His disease is progressing and getting harder to control

E This is a normal finding in someone with type 2 diabetes

18. A 40-year-old woman is on a self-imposed fast that precludes her from taking anything into her system. She has insulin-dependent diabetes, a transplanted kidney, and paranoid schizophrenia.

Urine dipstick: ketones 3+.

Random capillary blood glucose 28mmol/L.

She is refusing all medical help. Which is the *single* most appropriate course of action? ★

A Assess her capacity to make such a decision

B Gain consent for treatment from her next of kin

C Respect her wishes and withhold treatment

D Treat her under 'common law'

E Treat her under a section of the Mental Health Act 2007

19. A 72-year-old man has had progressively severe pain, tingling, and tightness in both feet, especially at night over the past year. He has type 2 diabetes and takes metformin 850mg twice daily. Which *single* examination finding would be most likely to confirm the cause? ★

A Decreased distal vibration sense

B Excessive haemosiderin deposition

C Increased ankle reflexes

D Tenderness over the short saphenous veins

E Wasted quadriceps muscles

20. A 33-year-old woman has not had a period for the last 3 months. She has also noticed frequent milky discharge from her breasts. She is currently being treated for type 1 diabetes, depression, benign positional vertigo, and back pain.

Serum β-human chorionic gonadotropin (β-hCG): negative.

Which *single* drug is most likely to have caused these new symptoms? ★

A Codeine phosphate

B Gabapentin

C Insulin

D Prochlorperazine

E Venlafaxine

21. A 49-year-old woman has felt tired over the last few months and her thyroid function tests are returned as follows:

```
Thyroid-stimulating hormone (TSH) 6.8mU/L,
free thyroxine (fT4) 19pmol/L.
```

She has no detectable goitre. Which is the *single* most likely explanation for the blood results? ★

A Sick euthyroidism

B Subclinical hypothyroidism

C Iodine deficiency

D Hashimoto's thyroiditis

E Unknown use of levothyroxine

22. A 50-year-old woman has had 3 days of tingling fingers followed by an intense 4h period where her jaw and right hand locked up. She recalls a similar episode 20 years ago that required hospital admission. She is housebound due to bad osteoarthritis, has hypertension, and has been treated for depression in the past. Her BMI is 40kg/m². Which *single* investigation would be most useful in the immediate management of symptoms? ★

A Calcium

B Cortisol

C Random venous blood glucose

D Thyroid-stimulating hormone (TSH)

E Urea and electrolytes

23. A 44-year-old man has had a hoarse voice for the past year or so. He has otherwise been well, but in passing he mentions that his shoe size has increased over the past 3 or 4 years. He has a protruding jaw and a large tongue. Which is the *single* most appropriate definitive test to support the likely diagnosis? ★

A Insulin growth factor 1 (IGF-1)

B Oral glucose tolerance test (OGTT) with growth hormone

C Random capillary blood glucose

D Random growth hormone

E Somatostatin

24. A 64-year-old woman has had some blood tests taken for an insurance medical. Her results are all normal except for her thyroid function tests, which are as follows:

```
Thyroid-stimulating hormone (TSH) 8.7mU/L,
free thyroxine (fT4) 11pmol/L.
```

She has no symptoms or detectable goitre.
Which is the *single* most appropriate initial management? ★

A Measure serum thyroid peroxidase antibodies

B Refer for radioiodine therapy

C Review thyroid function in 1 year

D Start a 'block and replace' regimen

E Start levothyroxine

25. A 36-year-old man has had intermittent abdominal pain associated with nausea for several years. He has never sought an explanation for it but has recently started to feel faint, particularly on standing. He has areas of dark skin, most notably in the creases of his palms. Which is the *single* most appropriate explanation for these skin changes? ★

A High circulating levels of adrenocorticotropic hormone (ACTH)

B High circulating levels of aldosterone

C High circulating levels of caeruloplasmin

D High circulating levels of growth hormone

E High circulating levels of iron

26. A 44-year-old woman has had intermittent palpitations increasingly often over the past 6 months. They are associated with anxiety and make it difficult for her to breathe normally. She also feels hot during these episodes and sweats.

```
T 36.6°C, HR 120bpm, BP 115/85mmHg.

Thyroid stimulating hormone (TSH) 0.33mU/L,
thyroxine (T4) 198nmol/L.
```

Which is the *single* most appropriate initial treatment for this woman's symptomatic relief? ★

A Carbimazole 40mg PO once daily

B Digoxin 125mcg PO once daily

C Propranolol 40mg PO four times daily

D Propylthiouracil 30mg PO once daily

E Thyroxine 125mcg PO once daily

27. A 45-year-old man has felt unwell for a year. He has a loss of interest in sex that coincides with the inability to sustain an erection. He has a loss of facial hair as well as intermittent discharge from his nipples. After extensive investigations, an MRI scan shows an 8mm tumour originating from the pituitary fossa. It is decided to postpone surgery in favour of a course of drug therapy. Which is the *single* most appropriate aim of his drug therapy? ★

A Increase dopamine

B Increase growth hormone

C Increase oestrogen

D Increase prolactin

E Increase testosterone

28. A 52-year-old woman has felt more tired than usual over the last 6 months and her thyroid function tests are returned as follows:

Thyroid-stimulating hormone (TSH) 7.9mU/L, free thyroxine (fT4) 14pmol/L.

She has no detectable goitre.
Which is the *single* most appropriate initial management? ★

A Measure anti-TSH antibodies

B Measure total tri-iodothyronine (T3) levels

C Refer for radioiodine therapy

D Start a 'block and replace' regimen

E Start levothyroxine

29. A 52-year-old man has gained 10kg in the past year. He feels as though he has lost all his energy and is low in mood.

`8am cortisol: 36μg/dL.`

His abdomen is distended and is shown in (Figure 3.2).

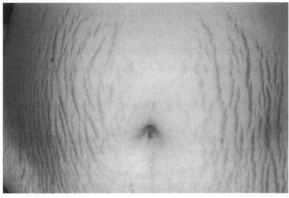

Figure 3.2

Which is the *single* most appropriate subsequent investigation? ★ ★

A CT adrenal glands

B Dexamethasone suppression test

C Midnight cortisol levels

D MRI of the pituitary gland

E Plasma adrenocorticotrophic hormone (ACTH) levels

30. A 40-year-old woman has had recurrent faints. Most recently, she had been sitting on a bus and as she stood, she felt instantly light-headed and could not stop herself from falling.

```
T 36.6°C, HR 90bpm, BP (lying) 125/80mmHg,
BP (standing) 85/55mmHg. Sodium 128mmol/L,
potassium 5.8mmol/L, urea 4.4mmol/L,
creatinine 88µmol/L.
```

Which is the *single* most appropriate medical management? ★ ★

A Doxazosin 4mg PO once daily

B Enalapril 2.5mg PO once daily

C Fludrocortisone 100mg PO once daily

D Furosemide 40mg PO once daily

E Midodrine 10mg PO once daily

31. A 33-year-old woman has fainted twice in the past month. She has recently finished a long course of steroids having been diagnosed with ulcerative colitis 1 year ago. Which *single* investigation is most likely to support the diagnosis? ★ ★

A Calculate the aldosterone:renin ratio

B Collect urine for 24h free catecholamines

C Collect urine for 24h free cortisol

D Give dexamethasone, checking cortisol before and after

E Give tetracosactide, checking cortisol before and after

32. A 66-year-old woman is leaving hospital having been treated for a broad-complex tachycardia. She received two doses of amiodarone 300mg IV and then an oral loading dose before being discharged on 100mg PO once daily. Which is the *single* most appropriate management of potential side effects? ★ ★ ★

A Check thyroid function tests in 6 months

B Only treat if symptoms develop

C Prophylactic carbimazole 20mg PO once daily

D Prophylactic thyroxine 50mcg PO once daily

E Ultrasound scan of thyroid gland in 3 months

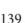

33. A 72-year-old woman attends a routine diabetes outpatient clinic. At her previous check-up 1 year ago, she was told that her eyes were 'normal'. She takes metformin 500mg PO twice daily. Fundoscopy is performed (Figure 3.3). Which is the *single* most likely mechanism behind the appearance seen on fundoscopy? ★ ★ ★

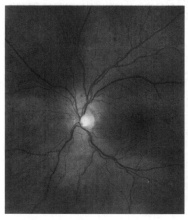

Figure 3.3

A Capillary endothelial change

B Fibrosis of vessels

C Microvascular haemorrhage

D Neovascularization

E Retinal ischaemia

34. A 55-year-old man has suffered intermittent bouts of extreme anxiety over the last 6 months. He has also experienced recurrent headaches, occasional palpitations and lost 5kg. He has recently started taking lisinopril, bendroflumethiazide, and atenolol.

```
HR 60bpm, BP 190/105 mmHg.
```

Which *single* hormone or hormone group is most likely to be the cause? ★ ★ ★

A Aldosterone

B Catecholamines

C Glucocorticoids

D Growth hormone

E Parathyroid hormone

35. A 33-year-old man has been vomiting for 24h. He is unable to keep any food down and is starting to feel weak and very lethargic. He takes hydrocortisone 20mg PO once daily for Addison's disease.

```
T 38.1°C, HR 100bpm, BP 105/70mmHg.
```

Which is the *single* most appropriate management? ★ ★ ★

A Double the daily dose to hydrocortisone 40mg

B Give hydrocortisone 100mg IM STAT

C Halve the daily dose to hydrocortisone 10mg

D Increase the daily dose to hydrocortisone 25mg

E Stop steroids immediately

36. A 75-year-old man has been increasingly irritable, lethargic, and low in mood for 6 months. He has hypertension, chronic kidney disease, type 2 diabetes, and had a partial anterior circulation stroke last year. He takes metformin, phenytoin, and bendroflumethiazide. His 8am cortisol is marginally raised and remains so, even after suppression with dexamethasone 1mg PO. Which *single* factor from the history might explain a false-positive result? ★ ★ ★

A Decreased glomerular filtration rate (GFR)

B Diuretic use

C Phenytoin use

D Presence of diabetes

E Presence of peripheral vascular disease

37. A 66-year-old man has been referred to an ophthalmologist. He was seen nine months ago in a diabetes clinic with what the registrar described at the time as 'pre-proliferative' changes. He is currently controlling his blood sugar with metformin 850mg PO twice daily and gliclazide 160mg PO twice daily. Fundoscopy is performed and reveals new vessel formation (Figure 3.4). Which *single* mechanism is most likely to be responsible for the changes seen on fundoscopy? ★ ★ ★

A Excessive deposition of lipids

B Fibrosis of vessels

C Neovascularization

D Osmotic change in the lens

E Retinal ischaemia

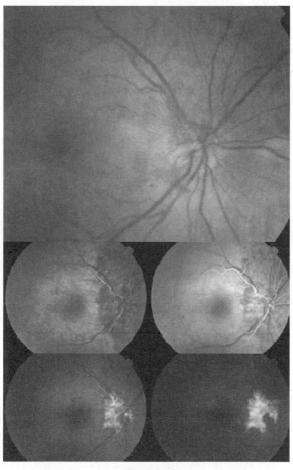

Figure 3.4

38. A 66-year-old man is admitted with abdominal pain and distension, vomiting and his bowels have not opened for 3 days. He is rehydrated with IV fluids and his abdominal X-ray shows multiple distended loops of small bowel. He has recently been diagnosed with type 2 diabetes and takes metformin 500mg PO three times daily. A CT abdomen with IV contrast is booked for the following day, but the nursing staff asks whether the metformin should be continued.

```
Sodium 137mmol/L, potassium 4.3mmol/L,
creatinine 67µmol/L.
```

Which is the *single* most appropriate course of action? ★ ★ ★ ★

A Continue the metformin and give IV fluids for 24h after the scan

B Continue the metformin but do not give IV contrast with the scan

C No additional precautions are required

D Stop the metformin before the scan and restart 48h after

E Stop the metformin before the scan and restart the morning after

EXTENDED MATCHING QUESTIONS

Treatment of type 2 diabetes

For each patient with type 2 diabetes, choose the single most appropriate management decision from the list of options below. Each option may be used once, more than once, or not at all. ★ ★ ★

A Acarbose

B Amlodipine

C Aspirin

D Bezafibrate

E Ezetimibe

F Furosemide

G Gliclazide

H Insulin (IV)

I Insulin (SC)

J Lifestyle advice

K Losartan

L Metformin

M Pioglitazone

N Ramipril

O Simvastatin

1. A 56-year-old man has been trying a low-fat, high-fibre diet over the last 3 months. He has lost 3kg and his BMI is 28.8kg/m². He takes no regular medications. BP 130/80mmHg, HR 75bpm.
Glycosylated haemoglobin (HbA1C) 8.1%.

2. A 78-year-old woman has been taking metformin and glipizide for the last 2 years. She had a myocardial infarction 8 years ago and a recent echocardiogram indicated a left ventricular ejection fraction of 30–40%. She takes aspirin, simvastatin, furosemide, lisinopril, digoxin, and spironolactone.
BP 125/70mmHg, HR 65bpm.
HbA1C 8.8%.

3. A 48-year-old woman has been trying to lose weight over the last few months but returns to her family doctor 4kg heavier. She has no previous medical history. Her BMI is 27.5kg/m².
BP 145/80mmHg, HR 80bpm.
HbA1C 6.2%.

4. A 46-year-old man has been transferred to the Coronary Care Unit following thrombolysis for an acute myocardial infarction (MI). He has type 2 diabetes and usually takes metformin 1g PO three times daily.
Capillary blood glucose 12.2mmol/L.

5. A 42-year-old woman has been taking metformin 1g PO three times daily for the last year. She also takes two antihypertensive medications.
BP 125/80mmHg, HR 78bpm.
HbA1C 8.0%.

ANSWERS

Single Best Answers

1. C ★   OHCM 8th edn → p210

Having addressed symptom control with a β-blocker, the next stage is to reduce circulating levels of thyroid hormones. This can be achieved either by blocking the overactive thyroid gland with carbimazole (and replacing reduced thyroxine to avoid iatrogenic hypothyroidism) or with propylthiouracil, which inhibits thyroid hormone synthesis.

A   Amiodarone is a cause of thyroid disease, rather than a cure.

D   This is used after a period of medical therapy in resistant cases of hyperthyroidism.

E   This is needed to prevent iatrogenic hypothyroidism from anti-thyroid medications but would clearly not work as a sole agent in this case.

2. A ★   OHCM 8th edn → p202

Cotton wool spots are also known as 'soft exudates' and are yellowish-white discolorations of the retina. They are local infarcts of the surface of the retina that occur due to impairment of blood supply.

Along with haemorrhages (D) and venous beading, they are signs of retinal ischaemia. The patient should be told, therefore, that the spots themselves will not cause visual difficulties, but the condition of which they are symptomatic will continue to cause blood-flow problems and further retinal damage if it is not adequately controlled.

B   Lipid deposits are known as 'hard exudates' and are seen in background retinopathy.

C   Once new vessels start forming, proliferative retinopathy has begun, which requires urgent referral.

E   This refers to microaneurysms or 'dots' that are also seen in background retinopathy.

3. A ★   OHCM 8th edn → p232

This is diabetes insipidus, which can have cranial or nephrogenic origins. In this case, the fact that the urine becomes concentrated after administration of synthetic ADH shows that the problem lies in the pituitary (production) rather than the kidneys (site of action). The level of dilution of the urine is too great for primary polydipsia.

4. C ★   OHCM 8th edn → p842

This is a typical first presentation of type 1 diabetes: weight loss, lethargy, and polydipsia leading to acute dehydration. The patient's inability to use his glucose means it leaks out into the urine, pulling excess fluid with it. Untreated, this will result in increasing confusion, coma, and death.

A This is a reasonable differential for a young man presenting with increasing lethargy culminating in shock, but is much less likely than DKA. It is more likely to present with hypoglycaemia and in those known to have the disease or on long-term steroids but who have forgotten to take their tablets.

B This is a good thought in cases of polydipsia but is a much less common cause than DKA. It is less likely to result in profound dehydration and shock.

D This is usually asymptomatic although it can present with polydipsia (more as a result of hypokalaemia rather than dehydration).

E This causes hyponatraemia and therefore confusion, but without the other features of this case – especially thirst. It is unlikely to develop without a precipitant such as a head injury, malignancy, or specific drug use.

5. E ★   OHCM 8th edn → p842

Confusion and drowsiness on a background of polyuria and polydipsia in a young, shocked patient should be treated as diabetic ketoacidosis (DKA) until proven otherwise. Patients with DKA need four things: fluid, insulin, potassium, and education. The fluid normally used in the emergency situation is 0.9% saline.

A Dextrose can be used as the infusion fluid once the blood glucose levels have fallen below 14mmol/L.

B Glucagon is used in the emergency treatment of hypoglycaemia.

C Insulin will be needed soon in this woman's treatment (once her plasma glucose has been confirmed and if it is >20mmol/L), usually in the form of a bolus dose of 6U followed by an infusion running at 6U/h.

D There is conflicting evidence regarding the worth of sodium bicarbonate in DKA. It is certainly not the first-line treatment and should not even be considered without discussion with the diabetic or intensive care teams.

Hardern R and Quinn N (2003). Emergency management of diabetic ketoacidosis in adults. *Emerg Med J* **20**:210–213.

6. A ★

The symptoms of hyperglycaemia along with one fasting glucose >7.1 or one random glucose (D) >11.1 are enough to diagnose diabetes. Neither HbA1C levels (B), nor capillary glucose readings (C) should be used for diagnosis purposes, and glycosuria (E) can be a normal finding.

→ http://www.who.int/diabetes/publications/Definition%20and%20 diagnosis%20of%20diabetes_new.pdf

(*Definition and Diagnosis of Diabetes Mellitus and Intermediate Hyperglycaemia*. World Health Organization, 2006.)

7. E ★

Following the World Health Organization criteria, one random glucose reading of >11.1mmol/L accompanied by the symptoms of hyperglycaemia is enough to diagnose diabetes.

A This is useful once treatment has started.

B A fasting venous reading >7mmol/L is also diagnostic if accompanied by symptoms or if it remains high once repeated.

C An OGTT should be used for people with a fasting reading of 6.1–6.9mmol/L. It is the only means of identifying people with impaired glucose tolerance.

D This would be the right idea if the patient was totally asymptomatic.

→ http://www.who.int/diabetes/publications/Definition%20and%20 diagnosis%20of%20diabetes_new.pdf

(*Definition and Diagnosis of Diabetes Mellitus and Intermediate Hyperglycaemia*. World Health Organization, 2006)

8. B ★   OHCM 8th edn → p206

This is the classical image of a diabetic ulcer induced by peripheral neuropathy: 'punched out' and over an area of hard callus. Patients are usually pain free and suffering from reduced sensation in a 'glove and stocking' distribution.

A This is suggestive of venous disease.

C This occurs in arterial disease.

D This is lymphoedoema.

E This is unlikely.

Edmonds ME and Foster AVM (2006). ABC of wound healing: diabetic foot ulcers. *Student BMJ* 14:177–220.

→ http://archive.student.bmj.com/issues/06/05/education/190.php

9. C ★   OHCM 8th edn → p200

This is from a relatively new class of diabetic medications that work via activation of specific nuclear receptors called peroxisome proliferator-activated receptor-γ, increasing insulin sensitivity of liver, fat, and skeletal muscle cells. They are only associated with hypoglycaemia when combined with insulin/sulphonylureas. Another drug, metformin (a biguanide), works by suppressing hepatic gluconeogenesis and increasing insulin sensitivity; therefore, hypoglycaemia is not a known side effect.

A, B, AND E   These are sulphonylureas and are capable of causing hypoglycaemic attacks. Glibenclamide is a longer-acting agent and is more likely to do this.

D This belongs to the meglitinides and stimulates insulin release from the pancreas by its effects on ATP-dependent potassium channels.

10. D ★   OHCM 8th edn → p222

Increased breast tissue (gynaecomastia) should not be confused with galactorrhoea (spontaneous flow of milk from the nipples), which is caused by high levels of prolactin (E and by association B). A range of drugs and some oestrogen-secreting tumours – such as testicular – alter the oestrogen:androgen ratio. Low androgen levels (A) on their own do not cause breast tissue growth – it is how they relate to oestrogen levels that is crucial. High levels of growth hormone (C) does cause excessive soft-tissue growth but does not commonly affect breast tissue and is not implicated in this scenario.

11. C ★   OHCM 8th edn → p844

The very high blood glucose coupled with a normal pH point away from diabetic ketoacidosis. The symptoms are typical of a hyperosmolar non-ketotic state (HONK), which is the most common way in which type 2 diabetes unmasks itself.

A The history of polyuria and polydipsia would fit, but the very high blood sugar and the lethargy would not.

B It would be unlikely for type 1 diabetes to present at this age. It does not usually present with sugars quite this high – if sugars are very high, then the pH would be likely to show an acidosis.

D Although diabetes can (rarely) be an early sign of pancreatic cancer (particularly in the elderly), such a short history on a background of no other suspicious symptoms make this unlikely in this case.

E This is possible in theory, but someone with type 1 diabetes is unlikely to allow sugars to creep this high without adjusting their insulin regimen. The protracted history is unlikely in someone with known disease, as they are more attuned to the fluctuation of their sugars and better equipped to take appropriate action more quickly.

12.B ★   OHCM 8th edn → p210

The features described (overheating, sweating, weight loss) are those of a hypermetabolic state. Tachycardia and exophthalmos are suggestive of hyperthyroidism, specifically Graves' disease of which this woman is at risk due to her smoking.

A This is a feature of hypothyroidism in which the metabolism is slowed down leading to an almost opposite presentation.

C These are found in Addison's disease (adrenocortical insufficiency), which is more likely to present with lethargy, dizziness, and aches and pains.

D Whilst thyroid dysfunction is more common than lymphoma and should be top of the diagnosis list in such a case, it would be important to examine this woman carefully for any enlarged lymph nodes and to perform a thorough abdominal examination.

E This is suggestive of systemic lupus erythematosus (SLE) – a reasonable differential in a young woman with vague systemic symptoms but more likely to present alongside more concrete findings such as arthritis, serositis, or a rash.

13.B ★

All in-patients with diabetes need to have their sugars closely monitored. They have been taken out of their usual regimen, are eating irregularly, and are unwell. As a result, episodes such as this are a common reason for a drop in GCS score.

A This is possible if he was on high-dose non-steroidal anti-inflammatory drugs (NSAIDs) but there are no suggestive symptoms.

C Hypothermia is <35°C but is unlikely to cause such severe symptoms until <32°C.

D This can suppress the GCS score but would also reduce the respiratory rate and constrict his pupils.

E This would present with focal rather than global weakness.

14. C ★

This man has progressed from a phase of impaired fasting glucose to confirmed type 2 diabetes and cannot continue on dietary control alone (D). Metformin is the first-line oral hypoglycaemic of choice for those with a BMI >25kg/m². (It should also be considered as a potential first-line treatment for those who are not overweight.)

A AND B Sulphonylureas should be considered as a first-line treatment if:

- The patient is not overweight
- The patient does not tolerate metformin (or it is contraindicated)
- A quick response to treatment is needed due to hyperglycaemic symptoms.

They can be added as a second treatment if sugar control remains suboptimal on metformin alone.

E Thiazolidinediones can be added as a third-line treatment if control still needs improvement while on metformin and a sulphonylurea. It can also be considered as a second-line agent in place of a sulphonylurea if the patient has particular concerns over hypoglycaemic episodes.

→ http://www.nice.org.uk/nicemedia/pdf/CG66FullGuideline0509.pdf

(*Type 2 Diabetes: National Clinical Guideline for Management in Primary and Secondary Care (update).* NICE guidelines, May 2008.)

15. C ★   OHCM 8th edn → p210

It may seem obvious but if there are discrete lumps in a thyroid swelling, then it is a nodular goitre. In this case, all options apart from C cause a diffuse 'smooth' goitre. Multinodular goitres cause thyrotoxicosis, whilst single nodule goitres can represent cysts, adenomas, or – very rarely – cancers.

16.A ★ OHCM 8th edn → p218

Lateral gaze is controlled by the abducens nerve (CN VI). It courses through the cavernous sinus, lateral and beneath the pituitary fossa, where it has been affected by invasion or pressure from the tumour.

17.D ★ OHCM 8th edn → p202

New vessel formation or 'neovascularization' is the growth of new fragile blood vessels from the retina. As they tend to form on ischaemic areas, they represent worsening diabetic retinopathy and imply suboptimal blood glucose control. The vessels are dangerous and can leak fluid, bleed, cause scarring, and even detach the retina. Despite this, it would be wrong to tell the patient that his sight will be non-existent in <3 months (B) as variable courses are run. It would be right, however, to tell him that he will need to be seen by an eye specialist for consideration of laser treatment of the new vessels, whilst stressing the need to strive for optimal blood glucose control.

18.A ★

The fact that she has schizophrenia does not automatically mean she lacks capacity to make a decision about medical treatment. Patients who have capacity (that is, who can understand, believe, retain, and weigh up the necessary information) can make their own decisions to refuse treatment, even if those decisions appear irrational to the doctor or may place the patient's health or their life at risk.

B No other adult can consent on her behalf.

C If she has capacity to make the decision and this is entirely voluntary and her own thoughts, then this is correct.

D To treat under 'common law' without the patient's consent, the doctor would first have to prove that the patient lacked capacity to make the decision (which needs to be assessed) and then that it was in their best interests. The only other exception is in an emergency where the doctor feels the patient is at immediate harm, at risk of harming others, or to prevent a crime.

E The Mental Health Act 2007 provides a statutory framework, which sets out when patients can be compulsorily treated for a mental disorder without consent, to protect them or others from harm. Again this would require an assessment of her capacity.

→ http://www.gmc-uk.org/news/articles/Consent_guidance.pdf

(*Consent: Patients and Doctors Making Decisions Together.* General Medical Council.)

19. A ★   OHCM 8th edn → p204

The symptoms are typical of a diabetic sensory neuropathy. Classical examination findings are decreased sensation (especially vibration) in a 'glove and stocking' distribution, with reduced ankle reflexes and resulting deformities of the feet (calluses that can lead to ulcers and Charcot's joints).

B Haemosiderin is an iron storage complex that is released from erythrocytes as they extravasate into the skin in venous ulcer disease. It stimulates melanin production, thus turning the skin brown.

C These are seen in an upper motor neurone lesion.

D Tenderness over the veins at the back of the calf (short saphenous system) is indicative of phlebitis and is common in venous disease.

E This is not suggestive of a sensory neuropathy but rather of amyotrophy, which is painful wasting of muscles, chiefly of the pelvifemoral group.

20. D ★   OHCM 8th edn → p228

This woman is suffering with hyperprolactinaemia and galactorrhoea. The most common cause for this is drugs that reduce the levels of dopamine (which would normally inhibit release of prolactin from the anterior pituitary). A regular offender in this respect is the often-prescribed anti-emetic prochlorperazine. Other examples include metoclopramide and the antipsychotic haloperidol.

21. B ★   OHCM 8th edn → p213

This is subclinical hypothyroidism, but the woman is symptomatic and she should be commenced on a trial of levothyroxine to see whether there is any improvement in her symptoms.

A This is usual in acute illness, with low-to-normal TSH and low/high T4/tri-iodothyronine (T3).

C This would give rise to a goitre.

D This is an autoimmune destruction of the thyroid gland resulting in hypothyroidism.

E This would result in high/normal fT4 with low/normal TSH.

22.A ★

The symptoms described are that of hypocalcaemia. Despite the distracting elements – overweight, hypertension, and depression – they are very typical, especially in someone whose social history suggests likely vitamin D deficiency. The fact that she suffered this many years previously raises the possibility of a genetic abnormality. A subsequent check of parathyroid hormone (PTH) levels would help decide this, but in the acute setting, the focus should be on the calcium levels and correcting them appropriately. Failure to do so can induce cardiac arrhythmias (prolonged QT interval and subsequent collapse).

23.B ★ OHCM 8th edn → p230

This man has the features of acromegaly: growth of feet, prognathism, macroglossia, and hoarseness due to soft-tissue swelling in the larynx. In this condition, there is failure of the feedback loop that should normally see a rise in glucose suppress release of growth hormone. Whilst the other tests may be suggestive and can be employed to monitor disease activity, they offer only isolated data rather than the snapshot of the feedback loop shown by the OGTT.

24.A ★ OHCM 8th edn → p213

This is subclinical hypothyroidism with no signs or symptoms of thyroid dysfunction. It is common, with 10% of those >55 years having a raised TSH. It does not require replacement treatment. If thyroid peroxidase antibodies are present, this suggests that the patient is at risk of an autoimmune thyroiditis and they should be monitored with an annual TSH test (C) or earlier if symptoms are present. If there are no antibodies, they can have 3-yearly follow-up blood tests.

B AND D These are indicated for hyperthyroidism.

25.A ★ OHCM 8th edn → pp218, 220

The symptoms described suggest Addison's disease in which high levels of ACTH cross-react with melanin receptors causing hyperpigmentation, most evident in the buccal mucosa and palmar creases.

B This is tested for via the aldosterone:rennin ratio in patients with resistant hypertension, in young patients with hypertension, or those with hypertension associated with hypokalaemia.

C Serum levels of caeruloplasmin and copper are actually decreased in Wilson's disease, which presents with hepatitis in children and neuropsychiatric symptoms in young adults.

D High levels of growth hormone also occur in acromegaly (which affects the soft tissues rather than skin colour), although the definitive test is an oral glucose tolerance test (OGTT).

E This is found in haemochromatosis due to increased intestinal iron absorption and deposition in organs, including the skin, causing generalized slate-grey skin pigmentation.

26. C ★

β-Blockers are used in the immediate management of the symptoms of hyperthyroidism. β-Blockers such as propranolol and nadolol can provide symptomatic improvement until the euthyroid state has been achieved. Patients who cannot tolerate β-blockers may be treated with calcium channel blockers such as diltiazem. An antithyroid drug such as propylthiouracil or carbimazole is then used to lower thyroid hormone levels with the option for radioiodine therapy or surgery in the future.

Singer P, Cooper DS, Levy EG, et al. (1995). Treatment guidelines for patients with hyperthyroidism. *JAMA* **273**:808–812.

→ http://www.thyroid.org/professionals/publications/documents/GuidelinesHyperHypo_1995.pdf

27. A ★   OHCM 8th edn → p228

This man is displaying hyperprolactinaemia. Tumours less than 10mm are usually treated initially with drugs: the aim is to reduce circulating levels of prolactin by increasing levels of dopamine, hence the use of dopamine agonists such as bromocriptine and cabergoline. If these are poorly tolerated, trans-sphenoidal surgery is the second-line treatment.

28. E ★

This is subclinical hypothyroidism in combination with symptoms of thyroid dysfunction. A trial of T4 replacement should only continue if her symptoms continue to improve.

A This is useful in predicting future hypothyroidism, for example in those who are asymptomatic but with a raised TSH.

B This is not an accurate measure of thyroid activity.

C AND D These are indicated for hyperthyroidism.

29.B ★★

All of these tests are useful in the analysis of the adrenal cortex. However, only if the dexamethasone suppression test reveals abnormal results (i.e. the 8am cortisol level remained high despite attempts to suppress it with an exogenous steroid) would further blood tests (C and E) be required and, depending on results, imaging may be required further down the line (A and D).

30.C ★★   OHCM 8th edn → p218

Postural hypotension associated with hyponatraemia and hyperkalaemia is suggestive of adrenocortical insufficiency. It is the lack of mineralocorticoids that causes the postural drop – to assess their true status, it is useful to check renin and aldosterone levels. If deficient and symptomatic, they need to be replaced by an exogenous steroid i.e. fludrocortisone.

As a general point, measurement of postural blood pressure is an easily performed bedside test that should not be forgotten in the assessment of a patient who has collapsed.

A This is an α-blocker used in the treatment of hypertension and prostatic hypertrophy that is more likely to cause postural hypotension than prevent it.

B This is an angiotensin-converting enzyme (ACE) inhibitor that is used as a first-line treatment for hypertension.

D This is a loop diuretic used to relieve the symptoms of heart failure.

E This is an α_1 sympathomimetic that causes vasoconstriction and is therefore useful in the treatment of orthostatic hypotension. This is the second best answer here as it would help treat the symptoms without actually getting to the source of the problem in the way that fludrocortisone would.

31.E ★★   OHCM 8th edn → pp216–221

The concern is that this woman's adrenal gland has been suppressed by long-term steroid use, which has now come to an end. The initial investigation for this would be E, in other words the short synacthen test, which uses exogenous synthetic adrenocorticotrophic hormone (ACTH) (synacthen) to try and stimulate the adrenal gland into releasing cortisol.

A The aldosterone:renin ratio is a good initial screening test for hyperaldosteronism.

B Three 24h urinary collections are performed as a screening test to look for free catecholamines that would signify a phaeochromocytoma.

C AND D These are both used as screening tests to investigate suspected Cushing's syndrome (D is the dexamethasone suppression test).

32. A ★ ★ ★

Despite the range of potential side effects of amiodarone (partly due to its very long half-life of ~2 months), thyroid toxicity is the most common complication that requires intervention. Indeed, it has been described in up to 10% of patients on long-term amiodarone therapy. Both hyper- and hypothyroidism are possible, although hypothyroidism is more than twice as common. Whilst C and D may be indicated if toxicity develops there is no place for E in the early stages of routine follow-up.

Siddoway L (2003). Amiodarone: guidelines for use and monitoring. *Am Fam Physician* **68**:2189–2196.

→ http://www.aafp.org/afp/20031201/2189.html

33. A ★ ★ ★ OHCM 8th edn → p202

The image shows background diabetic retinopathy with microaneurysms and hard exudates. At the root of this is hyperglycaemia-induced high retinal blood flow, which disturbs the endothelium of the capillaries: all subsequent changes stem from this.

Retinal ischaemia (E) is responsible for neovascularization (D), which then opens up the possibility of these new vessels fibrosing (B). Microvascular haemorrhages (C) are the blots seen in background and pre-proliferative retinopathy; they are features rather than the cause.

34. B ★ ★ ★ OHCM 8th edn → p220

Hypertension in a young person demands that consideration be given to a possible endocrine cause. All of the hormones listed can cause hypertension, but it is the catecholamines – as would be released by an adrenal medulla tumour or phaeochromocytoma – that cause the symptoms seen in this man: the vague general feature of anxiety, the neurological feature of headache, and the cardiovascular features of palpitations and hypertension.

A This is a good differential in cases of hypertension that are resistant to treatment or that occur in people of <40 years, especially if hypokalaemic. However, patients usually remain asymptomatic apart from the raised blood pressure.

C High circulating levels of cortisol occur in Cushing's syndrome and would be more likely to produce a range of physical and psychiatric findings.

D Acromegaly does cause hypertension but presents with very striking soft-tissue findings.

E Hyperparathyroidism can cause hypertension if left untreated for a long time. It is usually asymptomatic or presents with features of hypercalcaemia: lethargy, weakness, depression, and abdominal pain.

35. B ★ ★ ★

As this man cannot take anything orally and does not produce his own cortisol, he is at risk of becoming profoundly hypoglycaemic (lack of cortisol means decreased gluconeogenesis and unopposed insulin activity). He will probably need admission for IV fluids but in the meantime should take a supplementary steroid injection (which all Addison's sufferers should be armed with in case they become unwell).

36. C ★ ★ ★ OHCM 8th edn → p217

This is an example of pseudo-Cushing's syndrome in which cortisol is falsely high due to increased metabolism of dexamethasone, in this case due to a liver enzyme inducer. In other words, this man's symptoms cannot be explained by adrenal gland dysfunction. Whilst this is not a common clinical problem, it serves as a reminder to be careful when interpreting results in patients who are on multiple medications. Some advice from the British National Formulary (BNF), a pharmacist, or a senior medical colleague is a good idea before jumping to a diagnosis on the basis of a one-off result.

37. E ★ ★ ★ OHCM 8th edn → p202

The image indicates new vessels have been formed (thus, C describes what is happening but not the mechanism behind it). This happens in the diabetic eye as a result of occlusion of the microvasculature leading to local hypoxia and areas of the retina becoming ischaemic. This is a serious development, as these new vessels have the potential to bleed and fibrose and can detach the retina.

A This refers to hard exudates that are seen in background retinopathy, i.e. a stage that this man has already been through.

B This is not seen on the image but is the concern once neovascularization has taken place.

D Acute hyperglycaemia can induce a cataract-like state that reverses once normal blood sugar levels are regained.

38.D ★ ★ ★ ★

This is a common situation. This man has small bowel obstruction and type 2 diabetes but normal renal function, and will need the contrast to visualize the bowel properly.

Worldwide, 110 cases of metformin-induced lactic acidosis were reported between 1968 and 1991, with seven developing it following iodinated IV contrast. Metformin is renally cleared and the greatest concern is in those with known renal impairment. Hydration and limiting the dose of contrast can reduce the risk.

The American College of Radiologists' committee on drugs and contrast media state that metformin can be continued in patients with normal renal function and no known co-morbidities associated with lactic acidosis until the time of the scan but should then be withheld for 48h. In those with normal renal function but with co-morbidities, a reassessment of renal function prior to restarting the metformin is advised. In those with pre-exisiting renal dysfunction, much more cautious reinstitution of the metformin is advised.

→ http://www.scribd.com/doc/2952016/Contrast-Media-Administration-Guidelines-by-the-ACR-American-College-of-Radiology-Version-6-2008

(*Manual on Contrast Media, Version 6*. American College of Radiologists, 2008.)

Extended Matching Questions

1. L ★ ★ ★

High-fibre, low-glycaemic-index sources of carbohydrate, low-fat dairy products, and oily fish and limited intake of saturated fats and *trans*-fatty acids should be promoted. The initial body weight loss in an overweight person should be 5–10% but less than this is still beneficial. Following lifestyle interventions but with an HbA1C above 6.5% (or a level agreed with the patient), treatment with metformin should be initiated unless the patient is not overweight or it is contraindicated. HbA1C can be repeated over the next 2–6 months.

2. I ★★★

This woman's blood glucose control is clearly still poor, despite metformin and a sulphonylurea. Thiazolidinediones are well known to cause fluid retention and are contraindicated in this woman due to the increased risk of her developing congestive heart failure. Therefore, the next step has to be SC insulin.

3. N ★★★

After lifestyle interventions, angiotensin-converting enzyme (ACE) inhibitors are the first-line antihypertensives in Caucasians of <55 years. Close blood pressure and blood glucose control are the most important factors in preventing the progression of renal damage in diabetes.

4. H ★★★

The DIGAMI (Diabetes Mellitus, Insulin Glucose Infusion in Acute Myocardial Infarction) study carried out in 1997 suggested that treatment with insulin would be the treatment of choice immediately after acute MI. However, following the acute period there is no reason why metformin cannot be restarted.

Malmberg K (1997). Prospective randomised study of intensive insulin treatment on long term survival after acute myocardial infarction in patients with diabetes mellitus. *BMJ* **314**:1512–1515.

→ http://www.bmj.com/cgi/content/full/314/7093/1512

5. G ★★★

Her blood pressure is well controlled but her blood glucose control is still suboptimal and a sulphonylurea should be added to the therapy if metformin alone cannot control the diabetes sufficiently.

CHAPTER 4

GASTROENTEROLOGY

W hilst the function of the heart and lungs can readily be assessed after a basic examination, the gastrointestinal tract can seem rather less forthcoming. Indeed, whilst a junior doctor can get to grips with the cardiorespiratory system via their stethoscope, they may feel that it is not until they have mastered the specialized skills of endoscopy that they can acquire equivalent knowledge of the gastrointestinal tract.

This is far from the truth: whilst it is relatively inaccessible, the gastrointestinal tract malfunctions in colourful ways: jaundice, haematemesis, and melaena are arguably easier to interpret than the waveform of the jugular venous pulse. Even the 'vague' symptoms such as weight loss, vomiting, constipation, and nausea can be very telling once analysed in detail. Screening for risk factors by taking alcohol, smoking, diet, and drug histories provides a useful backdrop for the acute presentation.

Beyond the history, an initial inspection can tell us more about how well the gastrointestinal tract is functioning.

- What is the patient's BMI?

- Are they gaunt and drawn?

- Is there any evidence of pallor or yellowing around the eyes?

- Is there any venous distension or obvious bulky swellings tenting the thin overlying skin?

Although we only get short glimpses of the beginning and end of the gastrointestinal tract, much can be learned about the problems that lie deeper within. The mucosa in and around the oral cavity tells us much more than just the hydration status and level of oral hygiene. It can also hint at nutrition (sore corners of the patient's mouth and tongue), immune dysfunction (presence of fungal overgrowth), and inflammatory disease (multiple aphthous ulcers).

The bowel lumen is designed to be able to cope with different consistencies of solids and liquids, but there are a number of ways in which the journey can be interrupted. Narrowing (carcinoma), twisting (volvulus), absence of propulsive forces (achalasia), and trapped bowel (hernias) can prolong or prevent downstream passage throughout the stomach and small and large bowel. Each of these present in typical ways, and because of the mixed medical and surgical approach, these teams often work closely together: as a result, there is a natural overlap between these two chapters.

Consequences of an excessive alcohol intake dominate both the gastro wards and the pages of this chapter: gastritis, peptic ulceration, diarrhoea, jaundice, varices, and upper gastrointestinal haemorrhage can all lead to fulminant liver failure. As well as developing a confident approach to assessment (that does not rely on the oesophagogastroduodenoscopy report), it is the ability to manage these 'bread-and-butter' situations that is at stake here. As befits a surgical–medical specialty, these skills need to be supplemented by basic practical nous and an awareness of urgent referral criteria and procedures. ■

SINGLE BEST ANSWERS

1. A 42-year-old woman has had dysphagia of all liquids and solids for 3 months. She has regular central chest pain and regurgitates undigested food on most occasions but does not suffer from acid reflux. She has lost nearly half a stone over 6 months. Which is the *single* most likely diagnosis? ★

A Achalasia

B Benign oesophageal stricture

C Bulbar palsy

D Diffuse oesophageal spasm

E Pharyngeal pouch

2. A 74-year-old man has had a retrosternal pain and bloating for 8 weeks. He has had no loss of appetite or weight loss. He has recently been started on some new medication and feels that this may be the cause of his symptoms. Which is the *single* most likely cause of his symptoms? ★

A Alendronate

B Bisoprolol

C Codeine phosphate

D Digoxin

E Quinine sulphate

3. A 63-year-old man has lost 2 stone in weight and become increasingly jaundiced over the last 4 weeks. He has no abdominal discomfort but his urine has become very dark and his stools pale in colour. He drinks 15 units of alcohol per week. An ultrasound scan of the liver shows a dilated common bile duct. Which *single* liver function test results would confirm the most likely diagnosis? ★

A Bilirubin 30µmol/L, ALP 240IU/L, AST 30IU/L, GGT 55IU/L

B Bilirubin 35µmol/L, ALP 30IU/L, AST 28IU/L, GGT 35IU/L

C Bilirubin 55µmol/L, ALP 470IU/L, AST 60IU/L, GGT 415IU/L

D Bilirubin 58µmol/L, ALP 210IU/L, AST 205IU/L, GGT 145IU/L

E Bilirubin 120µmol/L, ALP 130IU/L, AST 1020IU/L, GGT 630IU/L

4. A 72-year-old man has vomited more than five times over the past 24h. He has also begun passing very frequent loose stools. He feels weak, dizzy, and slightly confused. He is on a disease-modifying agent for rheumatoid arthritis and has type 2 diabetes. He does not smoke, drinks 20–30 units of alcohol a week and has not travelled abroad recently.

```
T 37.1°C, HR 100bpm, BP 95/50mmHg.
```

His abdomen is soft with tenderness at the epigastrium. A digital rectal examination reveals an empty rectum. Which is the *single* most appropriate course of action? ★

A Colonoscopy

B CT scan of the abdomen

C Insertion of nasogastric tube

D IV fluids

E Loperamide PO

5. A 53-year-old man has been troubled by recurrent bouts of epigastric pain associated with nausea and sweating. He has recently moved house and feels the pain has been worse as he has needed to carry lots of heavy boxes up and down stairs. He has tried omeprazole 20mg PO once daily with no improvement over the last 3 weeks. His BMI is 33kg/m^2.

```
HR 82bpm, BP 155/85mmHg.
```

Which is the *single* most appropriate initial management? ★

A Barium meal

B Chest X-ray

C CT scan of the abdomen

D Exercise ECG

E Oesophagogastroduodenoscopy (OGD)

6. A 62-year-old man has had worsening acid reflux over the last 4 months. He has been eating large amounts of rich fatty foods over this period and attributed his symptoms to this. He uses a salbutamol inhaler for asthma when required but otherwise has no medical problems. Which *single* additional factor in his history would warrant urgent referral for endoscopy? ★

ALARMS

A Family history of oesophageal cancer

B Progressively worsening shortness of breath

C Smoker of 20 cigarettes per day

D The recent onset of reflux-like symptoms

E Weight gain of half a stone

7. A 37-year-old man has had upper abdominal pain and belching for the last 2 weeks. Over the last month, he has been taking regular diclofenac since dislocating his shoulder playing rugby. His bowels are opening normally and his stools are normal in colour. He smokes ten cigarettes per day and drinks 25 units of alcohol per week. Which is the *single* most appropriate next step? ★

A Advise to reduce alcohol intake and stop smoking

B Advise to stop taking diclofenac tablets

C Empirical *Helicobacter pylori* treatment

D Stool antigen test for *Helicobacter pylori*

E Urgent referral for oesophagogastroduodenoscopy (OGD) within 2 weeks

8. A 60-year-old man is experiencing pain on swallowing. Over the last 3 months, it has been worsening such that he can no longer tolerate food unless it is pureed. He has had chronic reflux symptoms but no other medical problems. He has smoked 20 cigarettes a day for 40 years. Which *single* further feature is most likely to support the diagnosis? ★

A Coughs on swallowing

B Neck bulges on drinking

C Pain is intermittent

D Regurgitates oral intake

E Voice is hoarse

9. A 66-year-old man has fallen three times in a day. He is confused and is responding to things that are not there.

```
T 36.5°C, HR 110bpm, BP 85/60mmHg.

Hb 8.5g/dL, MCV 105fL, INR 1.7, albumin
26g/L.
```

His abdomen is distended and tense with shifting dullness. Which is the *single* most appropriate course of action? ★

A Abdominal paracentesis

B Lactulose 45mL

C Packed red cells 2U

D Propranolol 80mg

E Spironolactone 100mg

10. A 62-year-old woman has an increasingly painful and swollen abdomen. She has suffered these problems many times in the past but this time it is impairing her breathing. She consumes 60–80 units of alcohol per week. The palms of her hands are flushed pink and the digits are oedematous with white nails. Her abdomen is markedly distended, with a palpable non-tender liver edge 4cm below the costal margin. Shifting dullness is demonstrated. There is bilateral ankle oedema pitting to the mid-calf. Which *single* factor is most likely to be responsible for this woman's peripheral oedema? ★

A Concurrent renal failure

B Hepatic vein thrombosis

C Low levels of serum albumin

D Portal hypertension

E Right heart failure

11. A 58-year-old woman has felt increasingly lethargic over the past 3 or 4 years and has noticed that her eyes look 'yellow'. She has recently been diagnosed with hypothyroidism for which she takes replacement therapy. She has no previous medical history but occasionally takes chlorphenamine. Which *single* autoantibody is most consistent with the diagnosis? ★

A Anti-centromere

B Anti-double-stranded DNA

C Anti-mitochondrial

D Anti-phospholipid

E Anti-smooth muscle

12. A 54-year-old woman has been dizzy and nauseous for 1 day. Prior to this, she had 3 days of epigastric pain and vomiting. She has type 2 diabetes and had a pituitary tumour excised 20 years previously for which she remains on steroid replacement therapy. She is pale. Her abdomen is soft with epigastric tenderness. Digital rectal examination finds tar-like liquid stool in the rectum. Which is the *single* most likely diagnosis? ★

A Angiodysplasia

B Diverticulitis

C Gastric carcinoma

D Mallory–Weiss tear

E Perforated gastric ulcer

13. A 78-year-old woman has had epigastric pain for 1 week and had one episode of passing tarry stool. She has cognitive impairment with a mini mental state examination (MMSE) score of 12/30. The medical team plan to investigate her symptoms with an oesophagogastroduodenoscopy (OGD). When seeking her consent, it is noted that she does not seem to understand the explanations and cannot retain information or weigh up the risks and benefits. Which is the *single* most appropriate course of action for the medical team? ★

A Gain verbal consent from the woman's next of kin

B Gain written consent from the woman's next of kin

C Get one of the doctors to sign for consent as a proxy

D No consent is needed for such a minor procedure

E Postpone the procedure

14. A 34-year-old woman undergoes an ileal–caecal resection for Crohn's disease. The operation is uneventful and she is discharged 1 week later. The patient asks the junior doctor whether she will need any supplementation as a result of the operation. Which is the *single* most likely supplementation she will need? ★

A Bile salts

B Folic acid

C Intrinsic factor

D Vitamins A and D

E Vitamin B_{12}

15. A 70-year-old woman has had three bouts of haematemesis. She is dizzy, confused, and hallucinating. She is a non-smoker but admits to heavy alcohol use since her husband died 15 years previously.

`T 36.5°C, HR 120bpm, BP 85/55mmHg.`

Her abdomen is distended and tense and demonstrates shifting dullness. Which is the *single* most likely diagnosis? ★

A Erosive oesophagitis

B Mallory–Weiss tear

C Oesophageal carcinoma

D Oesophageal varices

E Perforated gastric ulcer

16. A 47-year-old woman vomits repeatedly with dark red specks visible throughout. She is initially confused but settles while being attended to in the Emergency Department. She has suffered several such episodes in the past 5 years. Pending an endoscopy, it is decided to control the bleeding with some medical therapy. The patient is sceptical and refuses the treatment. Which is the *single* most appropriate explanation of how this treatment works? ★ ★

A Increases the levels of vitamins that encourage clot formation

B Narrows the blood vessels to the small intestines

C Prevents the formation of proteins that break down clots

D Reduces the pressure of the blood coming from the liver

E Replaces the body's lost stores of protein

17. A man consumes between 100 and 150 units of alcohol per week. He has slight ascites but no evidence of encephalopathy.

```
Prothrombin time: 3s > normal.
```

The doctor who sees him uses the Child–Pugh grading system to assess his risk of variceal bleeding. Which *single* pair of additional variables should be used to grade his risk? ★ ★

A Age + urea

B Alanine transferase + amylase

C Bilirubin + albumin

D Creatinine + sodium

E Platelet count + ferritin

18. A 42-year-old woman has had difficulty swallowing for the last 18 months. From the beginning she has been struggling to tolerate both solids and fluids. She often regurgitates her oral intake and has lost over 5kg. She is a non-smoker and has no other medical problems. Which *single* investigation is most likely to support the diagnosis? ★

A Abdominal X-ray

B Barium swallow

C Chest X-ray

D Endoscopic ultrasound scan

E Oesophagogastroduodenoscopy (OGD)

19. A 49-year-old man has had retrosternal burning pain for the last 2 months. He has no ALARM Symptoms (see answer to question 6) and does not take any regular medications. He initially took a proton pump inhibitor (PPI) but returned to his doctor 1 month later with no improvement in symptoms. He subsequently tested positive for *Helicobacter pylori* and was given eradication therapy for 1 week. He has returned 10 days later with persisting symptoms. Which is the *single* most appropriate next step? ★ ★

A 2-week course of *H. pylori* eradication therapy

B Metoclopramide 10mg PO three times daily

C Omeprazole 40mg twice daily

D Retest for *H. pylori* infection

E Urgent endoscopy

20. A 44-year-old man has experienced acid reflux over the last 2 months and describes some difficulty swallowing. Some blood tests are taken and he is awaiting an urgent endoscopy in the next 2 weeks. He smokes 20 cigarettes a day and his BMI is 31kg/m². Which is the *single* most appropriate piece of advice to give before the endoscopy? ★

A Advise him to lose weight and stop smoking

B Start a proton pump inhibitor (PPI)

C Start an alginate antacid

D Start an H₂-receptor antagonist

E Start triple therapy to eradicate *Helicobacter pylori*

21. A 44-year-old woman has had diarrhoea for 2 days. It has progressed such that she has passed 15 liquid motions in the last 12h. Seven days previously, she completed her second cycle of chemotherapy for breast cancer.

```
T 38.4°C, HR 110bpm, BP 105/75mmHg.
```

Which is the *single* most appropriate next step? ★ ★

A Await stool and blood cultures before starting antibiotics

B Do not consider antibiotics so soon after chemotherapy

C Only start antibiotics if T >38°C and HR>90bpm for >12h

D Start blind broad-spectrum antibiotics

E Start loperamide 4mg PO four times daily

22. A 33-year-old woman has a medical assessment prior to a new job. She has been well apart from some mild coryzal symptoms the previous week.

```
Bilirubin 42μmol/L, ALP 60IU/L, AST 28IU/L,
GGT 30IU/L.
```

```
Urine dipstick: no bilirubin detected.
```

Which is the *single* most likely explanation for these results? ★ ★

A Crigler–Najjar syndrome

B Epstein–Barr virus

C Gilbert's syndrome

D Hepatitis B virus infection

E Rotor syndrome

23. A 48-year-old man has an endoscopy for dyspepsia, which shows a duodenal ulcer. He is homeless and drinks more than 100 units of alcohol per week. He has no allergies and takes no regular medications. His *Campylobacter*-like organism (CLO) test is positive and the doctor wants to start *Helicobacter pylori* eradication therapy. Which is the *single* most appropriate next step? ★ ★

A Amoxicillin 1g twice daily, clarithromycin 500mg twice daily, and omeprazole 20mg twice daily for 1 week

B Amoxicillin 1g twice daily, metronidazole 400mg twice daily, and omeprazole 20mg twice daily for 1 week

C Bismuth subcitrate 120mg four times daily, tetracycline 500mg four times daily, omeprazole 20mg twice daily, and amoxicillin 1g twice daily for 2 weeks

D Bismuth subcitrate 120mg four times daily, tetracycline 500mg four times daily, omeprazole 20mg twice daily, and metronidazole 400mg twice daily for 2 weeks

E Clarithromycin 500mg twice daily, metronidazole 400mg twice daily, and omeprazole 20mg twice daily for 1 week

24. A 28-year-old woman has been admitted with abdominal pain and profuse vomiting and diarrhoea. Nursing staff call the on-call junior doctor and report that she has rolled her eyes back and is unable to prevent protrusion of her tongue. She is currently being treated with a number of different medications for a presumed gastroenteritis. Which *single* drug is most likely to have caused these symptoms? ★ ★

A Cyclizine

B Hyoscine butylbromide

C Metoclopramide

D Omeprazole

E Ondansetron

25. An 80-year-old woman has taken 70 paracetamol tablets and is acutely unwell in hospital. She says that she did not want to be found and wants to die. She is refusing any further treatment. Which is the *single* most appropriate course of action? ★ ★

A Assess her capacity to make such a decision

B Gain consent for treatment from her next of kin

C Respect her wishes and aim to keep her comfortable

D Treat her under a section of the Mental Health Act 2007

E Treat her under common law

26. A 40-year-old woman is extremely tired and lethargic. She has been otherwise well, although she has been increasingly itchy over the past few months. She takes thyroxine 50mcg PO once daily.

```
T 36.9°C, HR 85bpm, BP 135/90mmHg.
```

Her sclerae are tinged yellow. Her abdomen is soft and non-tender but diffusely excoriated. Which *single* investigation would be most likely to support the diagnosis? ★ ★

A Anti-mitochondrial antibodies

B Anti-nuclear antibodies

C Caeruloplasmin

D Hepatitis serology

E Paul–Bunnell monospot test

27. A 60-year-old man is weak, lethargic, and confused. He has been deteriorating gradually over many months and has just finished a 3-day alcoholic binge. He has longstanding alcohol misuse and chronic pancreatitis. He is tremulous and cachectic with dry mucous membranes. The attending doctor plans to rehydrate him with 1L of 5% dextrose IV. Which *single* medication should be given beforehand? ★ ★

A Chlordiazepoxide 30mg PO

B Omeprazole 40mg IV

C Pancreatin 10,000U

D Vitamin B + C ampoules I and II

E Vitamin B Compound Strong 2 tablets PO

28. A 55-year-old woman had a stroke 3 days ago. She fails a swallowing assessment carried out by the speech and language therapist. The decision is made to commence her on enteral feeding via a nasogastric feeding tube. The tube is inserted and the junior doctor on call has been asked to confirm the position of the tube prior to commencing feeding. Which is the *single* most reliable way to confirm that the tube is in the correct position? ★ ★ ★

A Aspirate yellow/green-coloured fluid

B Listen over the stomach as air is passed through the tube

C Measure the length of tube left externally

D Percuss over the stomach as air is passed through the tube

E Test the pH of the aspirate with graduated pH paper

29. A 38-year-old man has felt increasingly tired and lethargic over the last 4 weeks. He has not noticed any change in his bowels recently and normally passes a small amount of blood with his motions, which he says has not changed. He was diagnosed with ulcerative colitis 15 years ago and takes mesalazine enteric coated (EC) 800mg PO twice daily. His abdomen is soft and non-tender. On digital rectal examination, no masses are felt and there is a small amount of fresh blood on the finger.

```
Hb 10.6g/dL, MCV 75.6fL, ferritin 10ng/ml.
```

Which is the *single* most appropriate management? ★ ★ ★

A Increase mesalazine EC to 800mg three times daily

B Reassure that this is to be expected in ulcerative colitis

C Start a 5-day course of prednisolone 40mg PO once daily

D Start ferrous sulphate 200mg PO three times daily

E Urgent 2-week referral to surgical outpatient clinic

30. A 57-year-old man has vomited more than 350mls of fresh blood. He is dependent on alcohol and has consumed in excess of 200 units of alcohol over the last 4 days.

```
T 36.2°C, HR 112bpm, BP 105/60mmHg.
```

IV fluids and a dose of vitamin K are given. A request is made for packed red cells and fresh frozen plasma (FFP). As the registrar opens the endoscopy suite, he asks the junior doctor to reduce the portal venous pressure. Which is the *single* most appropriate initial management? ★ ★ ★

A Furosemide

B Glyceryl trinitrate

C Octreotide

D Propranolol

E Terlipressin

31. A 62-year-old man has been passing small amounts of blood with his bowel movements for 2 months. He is not sure whether it is mixed with the stool, but the blood is bright red in colour and he thinks it is getting less. He has always been troubled by constipation, but he has not noticed any change in his bowels recently. He has osteoarthritis and takes regular diclofenac for symptomatic relief. He has no family history of bowel cancer. Which is the *single* most appropriate management? ★ ★ ★

A Add omeprazole 40mg PO once daily

B Commence regular lactulose 20ml PO twice daily

C Routine referral to surgical outpatient clinic

D Send a full blood count and review whether he is anaemic

E Urgent 2-week referral to surgical outpatient clinic

32. A 68-year-old man has passed a large amount of melaena over the last 2 hours and has also vomited some altered blood. He is not currently bleeding and, having been resuscitated by a junior doctor in the Emergency Department, is now being assessed for his predictive risk of rebleeding and death using the Rockall scoring system. Which *single* factor in the history would have the greatest effect on predicting his risk? ★ ★ ★ ★

A 40 units of alcohol per week

B Aged 68 years

C Chronic kidney disease

D Ischaemic heart disease

E Oesophageal carcinoma

33. A 44-year-old homeless man has developed difficulty breathing and has palpitations. He has been recovering in hospital for several days following an alcoholic binge of around 100 units and had been encouraged to eat and drink normally prior to discharge. He is very unkempt. His BMI is 19kg/m².

```
T 36.7°C, HR 95bpm, BP 115/80mmHg, SaO₂ 98%
on 4L oxygen.
```

Which *single* pair of tests is the most appropriate next step? ★ ★ ★ ★

A Chest X-ray + arterial blood gasses

B ECG + troponin level

C Full blood count + sputum sample

D Liver function tests + calcium

E Urea and electrolytes + phosphate

34. A 64-year-old man is jaundiced and confused. Two years ago, he underwent surgery for a colonic carcinoma but refused adjuvant chemotherapy on the basis that he felt well. Imaging shows disseminated metastatic disease with most of the liver parenchyma being replaced by tumour. The intrinsic and extrinsic hepatic ducts are dilated and an attempt to stent the common bile duct fails. His family ask the doctor to do everything possible. Which is the *single* most appropriate next step? ★ ★ ★ ★

A Attempt percutaneous drainage of the obstructed biliary duct

B Debulking of the hepatic tumour to reduce the obstruction

C Focus on symptom relief using a palliative care approach

D Start chemotherapy to reduce the size of the obstructing tumour

E Try to stent the biliary duct again during another endoscopic retrograde cholangiopancreatography (ERCP)

35. A 55-year-old man has just been told he has oesophageal cancer with liver metastases. He currently spends more than 50% of the time in bed or lying down and is capable of only limited self-care. As a result, he has a WHO performance status of 3. He feels very positive about enjoying the time he has got left with his family and asks how much longer he has to live. Which is the *single* most appropriate response? ★ ★ ★ ★

A Less than a week

B 1–3 months

C 6–12 months

D 1–2 years

E More than 2 years

EXTENDED MATCHING QUESTIONS

Changes in bowel habit

For each patient with a change in bowel habit, choose the *single* most likely diagnosis from the list of options below. Each option may be used once, more than once, or not at all. ★

A Autonomic neuropathy

B Carcinoid syndrome

C Chronic pancreatitis

D Coeliac disease

E Colorectal cancer

F Conversion disorder

G Diverticulosis

H Hyperthyroidism

I Inflammatory bowel disease

J Irritable bowel syndrome

K Lymphoma

L Porphyria

M Systemic sclerosis

N Viral gastroenteritis

1. A 60-year-old man has had alternating cycles of diarrhoea and constipation for the last few months. He has noticed that, even when he passes formed stool, it is often covered in mucus. He also reports feeling that he has never completely emptied his rectum, even immediately after opening bowels.

2. A 64-year-old woman feels that for the past couple of years, her bowel motions have either been far too loose or far too infrequent. She also has intermittent left-sided abdominal pain. It feels like a cramp and is relieved temporarily by bending over and more definitely by defaecating. It is associated with nausea and the frequent passage of wind.

3. A 66-year-old man has been passing loose stools for the past 2 weeks. They are light in colour and resistant to being flushed away. He also has generalized abdominal pain that has never really improved since its onset some years ago and has continued to lose weight.

4. A 62-year-old woman has had recurrent cycles of diarrhoea alternating with constipation over many years. She suffers with intermittent lower abdominal pain. It is usually eased by opening her bowels, but has been generally worse since her partner died unexpectedly last month.

5. A 60-year-old man has had profuse watery diarrhoea for the last 72h. He feels generally unwell, with abdominal pain, sore joints, and gritty eyes. He has been prone to similar such episodes in the past. He suspects he has lost weight recently, and he has not travelled abroad.

Causes of dysphagia

For each patient with dysphagia, choose the *single* most likely diagnosis from the list of options below. Each option may be used once, more than once, or not at all. ★ ★ ★

A Achalasia

B Aortic aneurysm

C Bronchial cancer

D Bulbar palsy

E Gastric cancer

F Gastro-oesophageal reflux disease (GORD)

G Mediastinal lymph nodes

H Myaesthenia gravis

I Oesophageal cancer

J Oesophageal spasm

K Oesophagitis

L Retrosternal goitre

M Syringobulbia

N Systemic sclerosis

6. A 65-year-old woman has had difficulty swallowing both solids and liquids for 3 months. She has non-insulin-dependent diabetes, has had two strokes, and has a BMI of 45kg/m^2. A barium swallow diagnoses the cause of her symptoms but she is deemed by a gastroenterologist to be a high-risk surgical candidate and instead is offered therapy with botulinum toxin.

7. A 60-year-old man has sudden severe chest pain while at rest. He reports having had the pain before, always during meals. Rather than being accompanied by shortness of breath, it is associated with difficulty swallowing. After having a normal ECG, the man is discharged with an appointment for a barium swallow as an outpatient.

8. A 75-year-old woman has recently developed difficulty in making the swallowing movement and has weakness in all four limbs. She has spent 4 weeks on a surgical ward recovering after a complicated anterior resection of a rectal tumour. Earlier in the week, she had a severe hyponatraemia, rapidly corrected by the on-call house officer.

9. A 58-year-old woman has had pain on swallowing that has developed over the past few months. Prior to this, she suffered from pain in the centre of her chest, especially when lying down or bending over. She has osteoarthritis but is otherwise fit and well.

10. A 66-year-old man feels pain on trying to swallow solid foods. He can still tolerate fluids without any discomfort. He has lost 5kg since the start of this pain 2 months ago. He attributes the onset of these symptoms to his quitting smoking.

ANSWERS

Single Best Answers

1. A ★   OHCM 8th edn → p240

This is achalasia where loss of the oesophageal myenteric plexus means peristalsis is absent and the lower oesophageal sphincter does not relax.

B There is no history to suggest this.

C This involves lower motor neurones (LMN IX–XI), often slurred speech, nasal regurgitation of food, difficulty chewing, and choking on liquids. Signs include tongue fasciculation and absence of a gag reflex.

D This involves uncoordinated peristaltic contractions such as the 'nut-cracker oesophagus' where the distal contractions are of excessive amplitude and cause retrosternal chest pain and intermittent dysphagia.

E A cough and lump in the neck would be more prominent.

2. A ★

The most common reaction to bisphosphonates is irritation, inflammation, or ulceration of the oesophagus. As a precaution, therefore, it should be taken 30min before food (usually breakfast) and the patient should not lie down for at least 30min after taking the medication.

3. C ★

The scenario suggests a diagnosis of cholestatic jaundice, compatible with biliary obstruction due to a pancreatic mass.

A Raised ALP (normal GGT) suggests a bone source for the ALP.

B This indicates Gilbert's syndrome.

D This is a mixed hepatitic–cholestatic picture.

E This indicates hepatitis.

4. D ★

Whilst the majority of patients with diarrhoea do not attend hospital, if it occurs in the elderly (or immunocompromised), then it is an indication for hospital admission. Although this man is not feverish and has not passed any blood, he is weak, confused, tachycardic, and hypotensive. The most likely cause is a viral gastroenteritis, but he would need admission to an isolation room in the first instance for fluid and electrolyte replacement. Stool cultures should be sent and, as he is >60 years and immunocompromised, he is classified as high risk by the British Infection Society and should be considered for antibiotics on admission (usually ciprofloxacin PO). If there is a recent history of antibiotic use, then *Clostridium difficile*-associated diarrhoea may well be the cause, in which case metronidazole or vancomycin should be used.

A This is rarely indicated except in cases of diarrhoea in inflammatory bowel disease-associated colitis.

B This is only indicated if other pathologies are suspected.

C There is no suggestion of bowel obstruction here and so no need to decompress the stomach.

E Anti-motility agents should be avoided as they are known either to worsen or to prolong symptoms.

→ http://www.rcpe.ac.uk/education/cme/infect-dis/dundas/dundas_2.html

(*Acute Diarrhoea and Fever.* Royal College of Physicians of Edinburgh, General Medical Review, 2007)

5. D ★

Epigastric pain in association with nausea and sweating should not automatically be attributed to a gastrointestinal cause. Instead, cardiac disease needs to be ruled out, especially in a man with risk factors and no response to proton pump inhibitors.

6. D ★   OHCM 8th edn → p242

The recent onset of persistent/unexplained symptoms of dyspepsia in anyone over 55 years should prompt urgent referral for endoscopy. This should happen regardless of whether any ALARM Symptoms are present. **ALARM S**ymptoms are:

Anaemia

Loss of weight

Anorexia

Recent onset of progressive symptoms

Melaena or haematemesis

Swallowing difficulty

→ http://www.nice.org.uk/guidance/CG27

(*Referral Guidelines for Suspected Cancer*. NICE Clinical Guideline 27, 2005.)

7. B ★

This man has symptoms of dyspepsia but there are no 'red flags' present. There is no reason to test for or empirically eradicate *H. pylori*. The offending medication should be stopped. If the pain continues, he could be given a proton pump inhibitor. There is no need for further investigations and he could be reviewed in a month's time.

8. E ★　　　OHCM 8th edn → pp240, 620

Odynophagia is a concerning symptom. In someone with a background of reflux disease (and smoking), it is likely to be progressive and associated with weight loss and signals either a squamous cell or adenocarcinoma of the oesophagus. One in five occurrences is in the upper part of the oesophagus and it is these that are associated with a hoarse voice.

A Coughing mid-swallow indicates difficulty in making the movement as in, for example, a bulbar palsy.

B This is suggestive of a pharyngeal pouch.

C Intermittent pain is likely to be due to abnormal contractions of the oesophagus, as occurs in oesophageal spasm.

D Regurgitation is symptomatic of a motility disorder (e.g. achalasia) as opposed to a mechanical blockage (e.g. a malignant stricture).

9. B ★

The clinical findings and blood results are suggestive of liver failure; with this as the background, the history of repeated falls and strange responses should be interpreted as hepatic encephalopathy (HE). This is defined as a disturbance in brain functioning due to nitrogenous substances derived from the gut that are allowed to build up by a failing liver.

The aims in this situation are therefore:

1) Nutritional management, i.e. reduction in protein intake while still receiving the maximum tolerable (~1.2g/24h).

2) Reduction in the 'nitrogenous load': this can be achieved via bowel cleansing (regular enemas) and non-absorbable disaccharides (lactulose is the first-line pharmacological treatment of HE).

For acute encephalopathy, give lactulose 45mL PO followed by an hourly dose until there is a bowel movement; after this, the target is two to three soft bowel movements a day (usually 15–45mL 8–12h).

A This can be used for symptomatic tense, refractory, or recurrent ascites, but not before attempts are made to increase ammonia excretion.

C This man is anaemic but not critically; transfusing him is not the priority at this stage.

D This is used in the prevention of variceal haemorrhage, as it reduces cardiac output and vasoconstricts.

E This is a first-line treatment of ascites (along with salt restriction) but will not address the problem of HE as directly as lactulose.

Blei A and Córdoba J (2001). Hepatic encephalopathy. *Am J Gastroenterol* **96**: 1968–1976.

→ http://www.acg.gi.org/physicians/guidelines/Hepatic Encephalopathy.pdf

10. C ★

This woman has liver failure with ascites and peripheral oedema. Ascites has developed, in this case most likely as a complication of liver cirrhosis and portal hypertension. Liver failure impairs synthetic function leading to hypoalbuminaemia, the effects of which are seen in increasing peritoneal fluid, peripheral fluid distribution, and leuconychia.

11. C ★   OHCM 8th edn → pp266, 555

This is primary biliary cirrhosis with anti-mitochondrial antibodies detected in up to 98% of cases. Interlobular bile ducts are damaged by chronic granulomatous inflammation, which leads to progressive cholestasis, cirrhosis, and portal hypertension. Often this is diagnosed after finding a raised ALP level during routine blood examination and as in this case lethargy and pruritus can precede the jaundice by a number of years.

A This occurs in up to 30% of limited systemic sclerosis.

B This occurs in 60–75% of systemic lupus erythematosus (SLE).

D This occurs in SLE and anti-phospholipid syndrome.

E This occurs in 70% of auto-immune hepatitis.

12. E ★   OHCM 8th edn → p252

Symptoms of hypotension and melaena in someone on long-term steroid therapy are highly suspicious for a bleeding ulcer. The key, however, is to discover the melaena, because the patient will not always do it themselves. In this case, for example, the presenting complaint was nausea and dizziness – in someone with an endocrine history it would be easy to be distracted by thoughts of an Addisonian crisis. It is vital, however, to keep it simple and work through the common causes of dizziness first; among other things, this means performing a digital rectal examination.

A This is a cause of a lower rather than an upper gastrointestinal bleed, i.e. it causes fresh rectal bleeding, usually in the elderly.

B This also causes fresh bleeding that is usually sudden and painless.

C This is more likely to present with vomiting, dysphagia, and weight loss after several weeks of non-specific symptoms.

D This is probably the next best answer, as 3 days of vomiting could be enough to cause a tear in the oesophagus resulting in altered blood per rectum and symptoms of hypotension. However, as this woman is at high risk because of the steroid use, gastric ulceration would be more likely.

13.C ★

The scenario suggests that the woman does not have capacity. The procedure is important to investigate the gastrointestinal bleeding but her next of kin cannot consent on her behalf. The team need to sign a form stating this, with one of them acting as proxy consent giver, explaining why the procedure is necessary.

14.E ★

Loss of the terminal ileum results in an inability to absorb the intrinsic factor–vitamin B_{12} complex. If there has been extensive surgery to the small bowel, folic acid and fat absorption (and hence fat-soluble vitamins) may be reduced requiring supplementation. Impaired bile salts absorption can be compensated by an increase in their synthesis.

15.D ★   OHCM 8th edn → pp252–256

Given that this woman is hallucinating (encephalopathy) and has fluid in her abdomen (ascites), it is likely that her heavy alcohol use has caused her liver to fail. She is now bleeding from the dilated collateral veins that have developed at sites of portosystemic anastomoses in response to portal hypertension.

A This usually presents with burning retrosternal pain and dysphagia with no features of alcoholic liver disease.

B This does present with haematemesis but usually after some violent vomiting has caused an oesophageal tear in the first place. It is a reasonable differential but is less likely given the background of alcoholic liver disease.

C This causes dysphagia, retrosternal pain, and hoarseness.

E This can cause both coffee-ground haematemesis and melaena but does not fit with the clinical scenario.

16. B ★★

This describes how vasopressin and its analogues (including terlipressin) work in this situation, i.e. an upper gastrointestinal bleed in someone with likely chronic liver disease and thus bleeding oesophageal varices.

A This is the method of action of tranexamic acid.

C This describes the effects of vitamin K.

D This describes how somatostatin works.

E This is the effect of treatment with human albumin solution.

17. C ★★   OHCM 8th edn → p261

The Child–Pugh score is a method of grading cirrhosis and the risk of variceal bleeding. It is calculated using:

- Bilirubin, albumin, and prothrombin time (PT) *and*
- grades for ascites and encephalopathy.

Having established that this man has slight ascites, is not encephalopathic, but has a PT 3s > normal, bloods for albumin and bilirubin need to be sent to give him a Child–Pugh grade and stratify his risk of variceal bleeding. It can also be used to predict mortality and quantify the need for a liver transplant.

18. B ★   OHCM 8th edn → p240

The history of difficulty swallowing solids and liquids from the start is that of a motility disorder. In disorders like achalasia (in which the lower oesophageal sphincter cannot relax due to degeneration of the myenteric plexus), contrast material is seen to pass slowly through a distally tapering oesophagus into the stomach. Oesophageal manometry can then be used to perform more specific diagnostics and show features such as the resting pressure of the sphincter and the exact pattern of oesophageal peristalsis.

A In the setting of dysphagia, this does not offer much extra to an erect chest film.

C This is a useful although non-specific first step in dysphagia, but may clearly show a hiatus hernia.

D AND E These can be used together: an OGD to rule out a tumour at the gastro-oesophageal junction and an endoscopic ultrasound scan for further visualization if a tumour is detected.

19. B ★ ★

The man has tried 1 month of PPI treatment and has been tested for and eradicated of *H. pylori* infection. However, he still has symptoms and if this is the case the guidelines recommend a trial of a prokinetic such as metoclopramide or domperidone or an H_2 antagonist for a month. If symptoms continue to persist after this, he should be referred to secondary care. To retest for *H. pylori* infection, the patient must stop the PPI for 14 days and be 28 days from last taking the antibiotic.

→ http://cks.library.nhs.uk/dyspepsia_proven_gord#-323460

20. C ★

PPIs and H_2 antagonists should not be used for a minimum of 2 weeks before the endoscopy. Lifestyle advice regarding his weight and current smoking is appropriate, but will not affect the result or interpretation of the endoscopy. Triple therapy can be given in situations where there are no ALARM Symptoms (see answer to question 6), but the decision to undertake an endoscopy has already been taken so the treatment should not be started beforehand.

→ http://www.nice.org.uk/nicemedia/pdf/cg027niceguideline.pdf

21. D ★ ★

This woman has a systemic inflammatory response (T >38°C, HR >90bpm) with potentially infective diarrhoea. As she is potentially septic so soon after completing a course of chemotherapy, this is febrile neutropenia. She should therefore be treated following the hospital neutropenia regimen. This may differ from trust to trust but will always stipulate that in the presence of systemic inflammatory response syndrome (SIRS) or sepsis in this situation, broad-spectrum antibiotics need to be instituted, even before any cultures have been received.

22. C ★ ★

Although not serious, Gilbert's syndrome is common, with up to 2% prevalence. It is often detected incidentally, as in this case. It causes an unconjugated hyperbilirubinaemia, thus differentiating itself from

Rotor syndrome (E), which causes a conjugated hyperbilirubinaemia and is therefore urine positive for bilirubin. The enzyme deficit that causes the bilirubin rise in Gilbert's syndrome is heightened in intercurrent illnesses (as suggested here by the recent viral symptoms) and fasting.

A This is a more extreme form of Gilbert's (the enzyme is totally absent) that usually presents in the neonatal period and requires liver transplantation.

23. A ★★

In a man who drinks excessive amounts of alcohol, it would be a bad idea to give him a metronidazole-based eradication therapy (disulphiram-like reaction). First-line eradication therapy should be a proton pump inhibitor (PPI)-based triple therapy for a week and, in general, these should be based around either clarithromycin or metronidazole. This is due to the high levels of resistance that occur with treatment failure and would ultimately leave no other option for treatment. Second-line treatment is a four-drug combination using the other agent, i.e. metronidazole or clarithromycin and bismuth, tetracycline and PPI, this time for 2 weeks.

Romano M and Cuomo A (2004). Eradication of *Helicobacter pylori*: a clinical update. *MedGenMed* 6:19.

→ http://www.pubmedcentral.nih.gov/articlerender.fcgi?artid=1140724

24. C ★★

This is an oculogyric crisis caused by blockade of the D_2 receptor by the centrally acting anti-emetic metoclopramide.

A This is an antihistamine that can cause drowsiness and a dry mouth.

B This is an antispasmodic that largely causes antimuscarinic side effects such as dry mouth and blurred vision.

D This is a proton pump inhibitor (PPI) that can cause headache and gastrointestinal upset.

E This is an anti-emetic that can cause headache and constipation.

25. A ★★

An adult shown to have capacity can refuse treatment. Patients who have capacity (i.e. who can understand, believe, retain, and weigh up the necessary information) can make their own decisions to refuse treatment, even if those decisions appear irrational to the doctor or may place the patient's health or their life at risk.

B No other adult can consent on her behalf.

C If she has capacity to make the decision and this is entirely
   voluntary and her own thoughts, then this is correct.

D The Mental Health Act 2007 provides a statutory framework,
   which sets out when patients can be compulsorily treated for
   a mental disorder without consent, to protect them or others
   from harm. Again, this would require an assessment of her
   capacity.

E To treat under common law without the patient's consent, the
   doctor would first have to prove that the patient lacked capacity
   to make the decision (which needs to be assessed) and then that
   it was in their best interests. The only other exception is in an
   emergency where the doctor feels that the patient is at immediate
   harm, or at risk of harming others, or to prevent a crime.

→ http://www.gmc-uk.org/news/articles/Consent_guidance.pdf

(*Consent: Patients and Doctors Making Decisions Together.* General
Medical Council.)

26. A ★ ★   OHCM 8th edn → p266

When confronted with a history of systemic pruritus, it is important to
look for other clues, as there is a vast range of possible causes. As this
woman also has jaundice, the most likely is an accumulation of bile salts.
This can follow either damage to hepatocytes (hepatitis or cirrhosis) or
obstruction of normal biliary flow, so should prompt a full screen for liver
disease. However, the most likely cause is primary biliary cirrhosis, as the
patient also has thyroid disease and the two autoimmune processes
frequently co-exist. The diagnostic test is therefore anti-mitochondrial
antibodies, which are positive in 98% of cases.

B This is more likely to be positive in primary sclerosing cholangitis
   (which can present with similar symptoms but is more likely to
   fluctuate, is associated with inflammatory bowel disease, and
   is more common in men) and autoimmune hepatitis (which can
   present as an acute hepatitis or as insidious liver failure).

C This woman has no signs of infection and only jaundice, rather
   than progressive liver failure, but it would still be useful to
   establish her hepatitis status.

D This is a test for heterophil antibodies, which develop in 90% of
   patients with infectious mononucleosis. This runs a shorter course,
   usually starting with a sore throat, fever, swollen glands, and
   general malaise.

E Low serum levels of copper and caeruloplasmin are found in
   Wilson's disease: presentation is usually with liver failure in
   children or central nervous system disturbance in adults.

27.D ★★

The key here is to realize that giving dextrose – both for rehydration and for correcting hypoglycaemia – to a potentially thiamine-deficient patient can precipitate Wernicke's encephalopathy. This man has incipient Wernicke's encephalopathy and should be treated initially with two doses of vitamins B + C (i.e. Pabrinex™ ampoules I + II) IV three times daily. All of the other drugs may be given, but not necessarily before the fluids.

A This is a benzodiazepine given for symptoms of alcohol withdrawal.

B This is often used for alcoholic gastritis.

C This is a pancreatic enzyme supplement.

E This is reasonable in the acute setting if the patient is low risk and is a good idea for almost all patients once they are discharged.

→ http://www.rcplondon.ac.uk/pubs/contents/0f0aa30e-8616-4942-ad07-5e5a0af7e91d.pdf

28.E ★★★

A patient with an aspirate with pH between 0 and 5.5 can safely be started on enteral feeding. There are no known reports of pulmonary aspirates at or below this figure. If the pH of the aspirate is >6, the patient should be left for an hour before retesting the aspirate. If the aspirate is still above pH 6, consider replacing the tube or checking the position by X-ray.

→ http://www.npsa.nhs.uk/nrls/alerts-and-directives/alerts/nasogastric-feeding-tubes

(*Reducing the Harm Caused by Misplaced Nasogastric Feeding Tubes*. The National Patient Safety Agency, February 2005; updated February 2007.)

29.E ★★★

A man of any age with unexplained iron deficiency anaemia and an Hb of 11g/dL or below should be urgently referred to rule out a malignant cause. He is at increased risk of bowel cancer with his co-diagnosis of ulcerative colitis

30.E ★★★   OHCM 8th edn → pp254–256

This man is haemodynamically compromised following his variceal bleed and should be given terlipressin to reduce his portal venous pressure. Terlipressin use in variceal bleeding has been shown to produce a 34% relative risk reduction in mortality and is the only vasoactive agent that has been shown to reduce mortality.

A AND B   These are indicated in the acute management of pulmonary oedema and angina.

C Octreotide causes a small reduction in the need for blood transfusions but does not have any effect on mortality.

D Propranolol is used in the prophylaxis of variceal bleeding rather than the acute management.

Ioannou G, Doust J, and Rockey DC (2003). Terlipressin for acute esophageal variceal hemorrhage. *Cochrane Database Syst Rev* Issue 1: CD002147.

→ http://www.cochrane.org/reviews/en/ab002147.html

Gøtzsche PC and Hróbjartsson A (2008). Somatostatin analogues for acute bleeding oesophageal varices. *Cochrane Database Syst Rev* Issue 3: CD000193.

→ http://mrw.interscience.wiley.com/cochrane/clsysrev/articles/CD000193/frame.html

31.E ★★★

In those over the age of 60 years, a history of fresh rectal bleeding of more than 6 weeks' duration should not be attributed to diclofenac or haemorrhoids. Regardless of whether there is any change in bowel habit, an urgent referral should be made to be seen within 2 weeks in a surgical outpatient clinic. Guidance states that when referring, all that is required is an abdominal and rectal examination and a full blood count, so as to not delay specialist assessment.

→ http://www.nice.org.uk/guidance/CG27

(*Referral Guidelines for Suspected Cancer*. NICE Clinical Guideline 27, 2005.)

32.C ★★★★

Rockall defined a number of independent risk factors that predict death using four factors: age, co-morbidities, shock, and endoscopic findings. A score of more than 8 is associated with a high risk of death.

Rockall TA, Logan RF, Devlin HB, and Northfield TC (1996). Risk assessment after acute upper gastrointestinal haemorrhage. *Gut* **38**:316–321.

33.E ★★★★

In prolonged starvation, the lack of dietary carbohydrate means insulin secretion is reduced. As fat and protein stores are preferentially catabolized for energy, there is a loss of intracellular electrolytes, especially phosphate. When food becomes available again, a shift from fat back to carbohydrate metabolism and the resultant rise in insulin stimulate cellular uptake of phosphate. Features of refeeding syndrome can occur if this leads to a profound hypophosphataemia (<0.5mmol/L). Early features are often non-specific but patients can go on to develop cardiorespiratory failure, arrhythmias, rhabdomyolysis, seizures, coma, and sudden death. Magnesium, glucose, and thiamine can also be low.

A AND B These are useful in patients with cardiorespiratory signs/ symptoms but are not the most appropriate here.

C This would be useful if this was a chest infection.

D This might show changes consistent with alcoholic excess.

Hearing SD (2004). Refeeding syndrome. *BMJ* **328**:908–909.

34. C ★★★★

This man has metastatic colonic carcinoma with tumour spread to the adrenals, liver, and lung. The ERCP stenting failed, and considering the degree of not only intrinsic and extrinsic obstruction, this was unlikely to improve symptoms radically. Percutaneous drainage would have similar effects. This man now has end-stage metastatic disease and is encephalopathic; he should be commenced on the Liverpool Care Pathway. This is a nationally recognized pathway for symptom relief and dignity of the dying patient of all causes. Drugs included on this pathway include midazolam, morphine, and glycopyrronium.

→ http://www.mcpcil.org.uk/liverpool_care_pathway

35. B ★★★★

This is not core knowledge but it is useful to understand the concept, which is likely to be discussed in multidisciplinary team meetings you may sit in on as a junior doctor. With metastatic cancer and a performance status of 3 (>50% time in bed/lying down, capable of only limited self-care), the prognosis in this case is less than 3 months. The WHO performance status assesses general health and grades from 0 (fully active) to 4 (almost fully dependent).

→ http://www.cancerhelp.org.uk/help/default.asp?page=5566

→ http://www.goldstandardsframework.nhs.uk/

(Gold Standards Framework Programme, England 2005.)

Extended Matching Questions

1. E ★

A fluctuating bowel habit with the passage of mucus per rectum is highly suspicious of malignancy. The feeling of incomplete emptying is tenesmus, which is common in inflammatory bowel syndrome but can also be caused by a tumour.

2. G ★

This is the presence of outpouchings of the gut wall; it is often asymptomatic but can present with non-specific abdominal pain and the feeling of bloating.

3. C ★

This man has steatorrhoea – indicative of fat malabsorption – and acute on chronic abdominal pain. Continued weight loss is also caused by general malabsorption due to an atrophic pancreas that is caused in more than 70% of cases by alcohol.

4. J ★

She is showing chronic intermittent symptoms that are exacerbated by stress.

5. I ★

Arthritis and conjunctivitis in the setting of abdominal pain and diarrhoea is suggestive of inflammatory bowel disease and would need urgent investigation via a sigmoidoscopy.

6. A ★ ★ ★

This occurs due to failure of relaxation of the lower oesophageal sphincter as a result of degeneration of the myenteric plexus, although the cause is unknown. Dysphagia and regurgitation of undigested food are the commonest symptoms.

7. J ★ ★ ★

Loss of the normal oesophageal propulsive motility is responsible for the chest pain, regurgitation, and dysphagia experienced. It is often treated with calcium channel blockers or nitrates.

8. D ★ ★ ★

Rapid correction of hyponatraemia can lead to bulbar palsy and central pontine myelinolysis. This is severe damage to pontine nerve cell myelin sheaths, leading to limb weakness and difficulty speaking and swallowing. The signs are of a lower motor neurone lesion.

9. K ★★★

It is the pain on swallowing that suggests that this has developed from GORD to actual oesophageal inflammation. However, it may also indicate cancer and this woman will need an oesophagogastroduodenoscopy (OGD).

10. I ★★★

Dysphagia, weight loss, and retrosternal chest pain should prompt immediate referral for investigations to rule out this diagnosis.

Gastroenterology

CHAPTER 5

RENAL MEDICINE

The kidney causes problems for medical students and junior doctors alike: the convoluted journey from plasma to urine, the conundrum of what is reabsorbed and excreted where, and the ever-tangled web of the glomerulonephritides are traditionally learnt rather than actually understood.

As in all clinical medicine, a good place to start is with the fundamentals of the organ in question. The passage from plasma to urine follows the pathway:

Blood
→Nephron
→Glomerulus
→Tubules
→Collecting duct
→Ureter
→Bladder
→Urethra

The primary functions of the kidney are:

- Removal of toxic waste

- Balancing of electrolytes

- Stabilizing pH

- Activating vitamin D

- Stimulating erythropoiesis

- Maintaining the blood volume.

The challenge, then, is to implement these basics by being sensitive to deviations from normal physiology: recognizing the accumulation of any potential toxins (hyperkalaemia, uraemia, and acidosis) or the lack of any synthetic products (hypocalcaemia and anaemia), suggesting triggers for such deviations and pinpointing the specific parts of anatomy that may be malfunctioning in some way so as to cause impairment.

Despite its bad reputation, the kidney reveals more about itself than any other organ and, in theory, should be the easiest to monitor. It achieves this through its *raison d'être*: urine. Its presence, absence, contents, smell, and colour offer a running commentary on the activity of the renal tract at any given point in time: it is the internal, intangible workings of specialized cells made physical, measurable, and dippable. So, far from being those much feared OSCE stations, the dipstick and the catheter are our friends.

Or they should be, for it is our ability to harness the information that they provide, allied to the series of numbers on the oft-requested 'U&E' against a background of wide-ranging symptoms that will make us sensitive to the running of the kidney. This – not just our ability to regurgitate the three types of renal tubular acidosis – is what is at stake in this chapter.

Indeed, as the span of the questions that follow confirms, it is the urinary tract infections, blocked catheters, stones, and hypovolaemic failures that are our bread and butter. Identify and treat these successfully and the interstitial nephritides, Fanconi's syndrome, and even glomerulonephritis will seem less daunting and may even start to make sense. ∎

1. A 70 year old man attends his local general hospital for a blood test having started taking lisinopril 10mg PO once daily 2 weeks previously. His doctor contacts him with the results:

	Pre-lisinopril	2 weeks later
Estimated glomerular filtration rate (eGFR; ml/min)	50	40
Creatinine (μmol/L)	150	180

Which is the *single* most appropriate management? ★

A Admit the man to hospital for investigations

B Halve the dose of lisinopril

C Repeat the test in 10 days' time

D Stop lisinopril immediately

E Switch to bendroflumethiazide 2.5mg PO once daily

2. A 66-year-old man has had a right femoral popliteal bypass. He had 2.5L of IV fluids (a mixture of colloid and crystalloid) during the operation.

```
T 36.5°C, HR 72bpm, BP 105/65mmHg,
RR 14/min.
```

There is a central venous line, a urinary catheter and an epidural *in situ*. The nursing staff call the on-call junior doctor because the patient has not passed urine in the last 4h. Which is the *single* most appropriate course of action? ★

A Abdominal examination

B Change catheter

C Fluid challenge: colloid 500mL IV STAT

D Mixed venous saturation from the CVP line

E Turn off the epidural

3. A 37-year-old man has had 12h of severe abdominal pain. It comes in waves and is associated with nausea. He has had this pain once before but it passed without him having to resort to medical help. His kidneys, ureters and bladder film (KUB) is shown in Figure 5.1. Which *single* finding on the image is most supportive of the likely diagnosis? ★

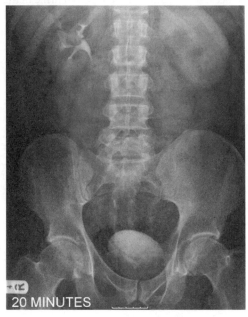

Figure 5.1

A Calculus at the left vesico-ureteric junction

B Calculus at the right vesico-ureteric junction

C Dilated right pelvic calyces

D Distended bladder

E Left delayed nephrogram

4. A 35-year-old woman has severe abdominal pain with vomiting. She reports similar episodes occurring every few hours for the last 3 or 4 days. The pain starts in her right side and moves down into her groin. As the pain intensifies, she becomes more and more nauseous and less able to stay still. Which is the *single* most likely explanation for her pain? ★

A Collection of fluid within a restricted area

B Inflammation of the visceral peritoneum

C Irritation of the parietal peritoneum

D Loss of local blood supply

E Obstruction of a hollow viscus

5. A 30-year-old man has had intermittent abdominal pain for the past 3 days. It begins in his left side and travels down into his groin. He has also felt nauseous and is finding it difficult to lie still. Which is the *single* most appropriate analgesia? ★

A Codeine phosphate 60mg PO

B Diclofenac 100mg PR

C Morphine 10mg PO

D Pethidine 150mg IM

E Tramadol 100mg PO

6. A 66-year-old man has had a sudden onset of right-sided abdominal pain for 2h. The pain comes and goes but is mostly in the right side of his abdomen moving down towards the top of his thigh. He has vomited three times since the pain started. He has ankle oedema, which is treated with furosemide 40mg PO once daily.

```
T 36.5°C, HR 75bpm, BP 140/75mmHg.
```

His abdomen is soft but tender in the right upper quadrant and right loin. Which *single* finding on urinalysis is most likely to support the diagnosis? ★

A Blood 2+

B Ketones 4+

C Leucocytes 3+

D Nitrite positive

E Protein 3+

7. A 48-year-old woman who has type 1 diabetes has felt increasingly lethargic and nauseous over the last few weeks and she undergoes some blood tests.

```
Creatinine 630µmol/L, ALP 45IU/L, calcium
2.6mmol/L, Hb 13.5g/dL, potassium 6.5mmol/L,
phosphate 1.8mmol/L.
```

Which *single* blood test result supports a diagnosis of chronic kidney disease? ★

A ALP

B Calcium

C Hb

D Phosphate

E Potassium

8. A 78-year-old man has a painfully distended lower abdomen that has developed over the past 2 days and he has not passed urine during this time. He has benign prostatic hypertrophy and has had this problem before. A urinary catheter is placed. Which is the *single* most appropriate course of action? ★

A Abdominal X-ray

B Digital rectal examination

C IV antibiotics

D IV fluids

E Ultrasound scan of the kidneys

9. A 69-year-old man has recently started taking lisinopril 10mg PO once daily. Two weeks later he attends a follow-up appointment. The clinical findings are:

```
BP 145/90mmHg.

Urinary albumin:creatinine ratio 50mg/mmol.

Potassium 6.3mmol/L (pre-lisinopril:
4.9mmol/L).
```

Which is the *single* most appropriate next step? ★

A Continue lisinopril at the current dose

B Continue lisinopril with furosemide 40mg PO once daily

C Stop lisinopril

D Switch to losartan 50mg PO once daily

E Switch to ramipril 2.5mg PO once daily

10. A 35-year-old woman has had left-sided abdominal pain for 6h. It started suddenly and is severe. She is nauseous and has vomited twice.

```
T 37.2°C, HR 110bpm, BP 135/90mmHg.
```

Her abdomen is soft with tenderness from the left iliac fossa to the left flank. Her kidneys, ureters and bladder (KUB) film is shown in Figure 5.2. Which *single* arrow indicates the most likely source of her symptoms? ★

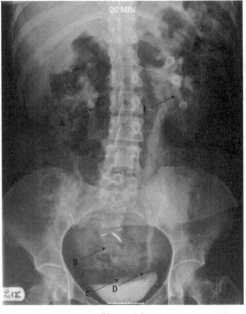

Figure 5.2

11. A 28-year-old man has noticed red specks in his urine for the second time. He recovered quickly after the first occasion but became unwell with a sore throat prior to this episode.

```
Urine dipstick: blood 3+.
```

Which is the *single* most likely explanation for the urine dip results? ★

A Antibodies binding the kidney's basement membrane

B Congenitally enlarged cystic kidneys

C Immune complex deposition within the glomerulus

D Inflammation of the bladder wall

E Necrotizing granulomatous inflammation in Bowman's capsule

12. A 72-year-old African-Caribbean man has a routine check-up. At the end of the consultation, it is suggested that he provide a urine sample and go for an ultrasound scan as screening for possible chronic kidney disease. His BMI is 33kg/m².

```
BP 135/90mmHg.
```

```
Fasting venous blood glucose 6.4mmol/L.
```

Which *single* factor should have prompted the doctor to suggest these tests? ★

A Age

B Ethnicity

C Fasting glucose

D Gender

E None

13. A 30-year-old woman has been passing minimal amounts of concentrated urine for the past 3 days. She is starting to feel tired, but prior to this had been well except for a minor skin infection for which she received a short course of oral antibiotics.

```
BP 140/90mmHg.

Urea 9.2mmol/L, creatinine 105μmol/L,
albumin 38g/L.

Urine dipstick: protein 1+, blood 2+.
```

Which is the *single* most likely diagnosis? ★

A Acute tubular necrosis

B Interstitial nephritis

C Nephritic syndrome

D Nephrotic syndrome

E Renovascular disease

14. A 25-year-old man has had intermittent right-sided abdominal pain for the last 5 days. It has struck several times for short periods, always focused on the right side of the back, before moving towards his groin. When it comes, it is severe – enough to wake him from sleep on one occasion – and causes him to roll around to try and get comfortable.

```
T 36.6°C, HR 90bpm, BP 125/80mmHg.
```

Which *single* pair of investigations would be most likely to support the diagnosis? ★

A Amylase + CT scan of the abdomen

B Digital rectal examination + abdominal X-ray

C Full blood count + laparotomy

D Liver function tests + liver ultrasound scan

E Urine dipstick + kidneys, ureters, and bladder (KUB) X-ray

15. A 76-year-old man has become increasingly confused over the past 3 days. He has also not opened his bowels in the last 48h.

```
T 37.8°C, HR 100bpm, BP 135/80mmHg, SaO₂ 97%
on air.
```

His chest is clear. His abdomen is distended with suprapubic dullness to percussion. Which is the *single* most appropriate immediate management? ★

A Give a phosphate enema

B Pass a urinary catheter

C Request an abdominal X-ray

D Request urinalysis

E Start broad-spectrum antibiotics

16. A 27-year-old man attends a pre-assessment clinic prior to the routine repair of an inguinal hernia. Urinalysis is done as part of the routine work-up:

```
Urine dipstick: blood 1+, protein 2+.
```

The junior doctor assessing him contacts the medical registrar who asks whether there is anything in the man's history that would raise the suspicion of a vasculitis. Which would be the *single* most relevant feature? ★

A Epistaxis

B Exposure to tuberculosis

C Fever

D Skin infection

E Sore throat

17. A 68-year-old woman has an acutely swollen and painful left knee. She is receiving IV fluids and antibiotics and is awaiting a wash-out of the knee joint under general anaesthetic. Through the course of the day prior to the procedure, the woman's urine output tails off such that in 4h she has only produced 10mL of dark urine. There is blood oozing from around the cannula site. Which is the *single* most appropriate step before proceeding with the knee wash-out? ★ ★

A Fresh frozen plasma (FFP) 300mL IV STAT

B Gentamicin 4mg/kg IV STAT

C Haemodialysis

D Insertion of CVP line

E Packed red cells 2U IV

18. An 82-year-old woman has had a laparoscopic repair of a femoral hernia. On the morning after surgery, the consultant notes that she has not received sufficient IV fluid therapy and has remained on metformin throughout, rather than being on a sliding scale of insulin for her diabetes. She is vomiting and taking rapid deep breaths. Which *single* investigation would be most likely to support the diagnosis? ★ ★

A Arterial blood gasses

B Chest X-ray

C Full blood count

D Random capillary blood glucose

E Urea and electrolytes

19. A 22-year-old woman has longstanding intermittent joint pains and mouth ulcers. She has had a renal biopsy and various courses of immunosuppressive therapy.

```
T 37.8°C, HR 90bpm, BP 135/95mmHg.
```
```
Urine dipstick: protein 3+.
```

Which *single* site within the kidney is most likely to be responsible for her proteinuria? ★ ★

A Collecting duct

B Distal tubule

C Glomerulus

D Interstitium

E Proximal tubule

20. A 72-year-old man is recovering from major colorectal surgery. Two days after the operation, his urine output has tailed off. There is no previous history of renal disease. His abdomen is not distended and there is no bladder palpable, but he appears adequately hydrated. There is a catheter *in situ* that remains patent on flushing.

```
Urea 16mmol/L, creatinine 323µmol/L.
```

Which is the *single* most appropriate initial management? ★ ★

A Change the catheter

B Insert a CVP line

C Request an ultrasound scan of the bladder and kidneys

D Start cefuroxime 1.5g IV three times daily

E Start furosemide 40mg PO once daily

21. An 82-year-old man has had a series of heavy epistaxes. These started yesterday and occur whenever he exerts himself or leans forward. Three days ago, he started an antibiotic for a urinary infection. He has atrial fibrillation for which he takes warfarin. His INR is 6.4. Which *single* antibiotic has he been taking? ★ ★

A Amoxicillin

B Cefalexin

C Co-amoxiclav

D Nitrofurantoin

E Trimethoprim

22. A 55-year-old woman is listed for a Nissen's fundoplication. She has type 2 diabetes with nephropathy. She is prescribed a sliding-scale insulin regime and requires thromboprophylaxis. Her creatinine clearance is calculated at 21ml/min. Which is the *single* most appropriate management? ★ ★ ★

A Aspirin 75mg PO once daily

B Enoxaparin 1mg/kg SC once daily

C Heparin 5000U SC twice daily

D Thromboembolic disease stockings

E Thromboprophylaxis is contraindicated in severe renal impairment

23. A 66-year-old man attends his annual check-up at the renal outpatients department. He is currently taking lisinopril 10mg PO twice daily. His results are:

	Last year	This year
Blood pressure (mmHg)	130/85	140/95
Hb (g/dL)	11.1	10.2
Estimated glomerular filtration rate (eGFR; ml/min)	55	50
Creatinine (μmol/L)	130	140

Which *single* additional investigation would be most useful in the planning of further treatment? ★ ★ ★

A 24h urine collection for protein

B Calcium, phosphate, parathyroid hormone and vitamin D

C Ferritin

D Urinary albumin:creatinine ratio

E Ultrasound scan of kidneys, ureters, and bladder

24. A 35-year-old man is worried that his urine has been slightly red in colour over the last few days. He is a keen runner and usually exercises three times a week, but has been off work for the last few days with a cough and sore throat.

```
T 37.1°C, HR 85bpm, BP 125/60mmHg.

Urine dipstick: leucocytes -, nitrites -,
protein 1+, blood 3+.
```

Which is the *single* most likely diagnosis? ★ ★ ★

A Bladder carcinoma

B IgA nephropathy

C Nephrotic syndrome

D Renal calculi

E Urinary tract infection

25. A 77-year-old man has been confused for the past 48h. The staff at his nursing home report that he has not been communicating or behaving as normal.

```
T 37.2°C, HR 110bpm, BP 90/66mmHg.
Urea 25mmol/L, creatinine 395µmol/L.
```

Which *single* further finding would indicate the need for aggressive resuscitation with IV fluids? ★ ★ ★

A Absent JVP

B Capillary refill time 2s

C Clear chest

D Gallop heart rhythm

E Reduced Glasgow Coma Scale score

26. A 58-year-old man attends his annual diabetes review. He has previously shown no signs of nephropathy but the registrar is keen to screen him for early signs of renal damage. His current medication is metformin 850mg PO twice daily. Which would be the *single* most appropriate test to perform at this stage? ★ ★ ★

A Creatinine clearance

B Early morning urine for albumin:creatinine ratio

C Renin

D Ultrasound scan of the kidneys

E Urine dipstick

27. A 66-year-old man attends a routine 6-monthly diabetes outpatient clinic. He remains asymptomatic and continues to control his blood sugars with metformin 850mg PO twice daily.

```
T 36.6°C, HR 75bpm, BP 135/95mmHg.

Urine dipstick: nothing abnormal detected.

24h urine collection: 150mg albumin.
```

His chest is clear, heart sounds are normal, and there is no peripheral oedema. Which is the *single* most appropriate next step in management? ★ ★ ★

A Bendroflumethiazide 2.5mg PO once daily

B Gliclazide 80mg PO once daily

C Lisinopril 2.5mg PO once daily

D Long-acting insulin SC once at night

E No alteration to management required

28. A 72-year-old woman has urinary sepsis and acute renal failure. She is a nursing home resident with severe frontal dementia and is clutching her lower abdomen and writhing around in pain. During her admission, she has repeatedly pulled out her urinary catheter and IV line and now tells the junior doctor that she does not want them replaced. During discussions, she is unable to retain information and cannot weigh up the relevant risks and benefits in order to formulate a decision. Which would be the *single* most appropriate next step? ★ ★ ★

A Contact her next of kin before making a decision

B Insert both, as passive euthanasia is illegal

C Insert both in her best interests, as she has no capacity to refuse

D Withhold treatment, as it is in her best interests to die

E Withhold treatment, as passive euthanasia is legal

EXTENDED MATCHING QUESTIONS

Causes of glomerular damage

For each patient with glomerular damage, choose the single most likely resulting pattern from the list of options below. Each option may be used once, more than once, or not at all. ★ ★ ★ ★

A Focal segmental glomerulosclerosis

B Henoch–Schonlein purpura

C IgA nephropathy

D Membranous nephropathy

E Minimal change glomerulonephritis

F Mesangial proliferation

G Mesangiocapillary glomerulonephritis

H Proliferative glomerulonephritis

I Rapidly progressive glomerulonephritis

J Thin basement membrane nephropathy

1. A 65-year-old woman has noticed her face becoming puffy, particularly around the eyes, over the past 6 months. She has regular monitoring of her rheumatoid arthritis for which she has been on intermittent immunosuppression, currently using azathioprine 150mg once daily.
Urea 9.2mmol/L, creatinine 112μmol/L, albumin 28g/L.
Urine dipstick: protein 3+.

2. A 22-year-old man has noticed his urine to be of small volumes and darker than usual. He has not felt his normal self since suffering a painful sore throat about a month ago. Prior to that, he had been completely well.
BP 145/90mmHg.
Urea 8.8mmol/L, creatinine 116μmol/L, albumin 45g/L.
Urine dipstick: protein 2+, blood 2+.

3. A 40-year-old man has had testicular pain for the past 2 weeks. It began gradually but is now extremely uncomfortable. He feels that both sides are swollen and become more so through the course of a day. He has previously tested positive for human immunodeficiency virus (HIV) but has taken no medications for this in the past 18 months.
BP 135/95mmHg.
Urea 7.9mmol/L, creatinine 98μmol/L, albumin 28g/L.
Urine dipstick: protein 3+.

4. A 27-year-old man has had regular nosebleeds for the past 3 months with crusting of the nose in the mornings. He has also felt intermittent eye pain with concurrent headaches and nasal congestion.
BP 140/90mmHg.
Urea 11mmol/L, creatinine 166μmol/L, albumin 37g/L.
Urine dipstick: protein 2+.

5. A 27-year-old man has noticed that his urine is discoloured for the third morning in succession. He has no other current complaints, but has recently recovered from a sore throat and fever that kept him off work for several days.
BP 120/80mmHg.
Urea 4.4mmol/L, creatinine 80μmol/L, albumin 48g/L.
Urine dipstick: blood 3+.

Single Best Answers

1. C ★

NICE guidance is that, if the fall in eGFR is <25% and the rise in serum creatinine is <30%, then the results can be rechecked within 2 weeks without altering the dose of the angiotensin-converting enzyme (ACE) inhibitor. If the fall is more precipitous, then other causes of acute renal failure (hypovolaemia, other drug side effects) need to be excluded. If no other cause can be found, then the ACE inhibitor should be stopped with an alternative antihypertensive added if required.

→ http://www.nice.org.uk/Guidance/CG73/NiceGuidance/doc/English

2. A ★

Hopefully, this is an obvious measure to take, but if in a rush on call, a reflex response to oliguria may be a quick fluid challenge (C) before rushing to another ward. However, before it can be assumed that the patient is not producing urine because of dehydration, a blocked catheter must be excluded. If examination of the abdomen reveals dullness to percussion up to the umbilicus, then the catheter itself and its patency need to be checked.

B This would be the route to go down if abdominal examination reveals a full bladder and the catheter seems patent but does not fill on flushing.

D Mixed venous saturations more than 75% and a CVP >8–10cmH$_2$O would suggest that the patient was well filled and are useful ways of assessing fluid status.

E Epidural analgesia typically lowers blood pressure, but switching it off is not the answer in suspected dehydration.

3. E ★

Although all options fit with the history, only E is present on the film. It is an IV urogram taken 20min after the injection of contrast dye. Immediately following this infusion, the contrast should be promptly taken up by a normal kidney and would create a distinct outline (or 'nephrogram') on the initial 1min film. A well-demarcated kidney on a 20min film, as in this case – a 'delayed nephrogram' – is a sensitive indicator of ureteral obstruction and renal function derangement. If the obstruction is acute, the delay is usually only for a few minutes, whilst in long-standing obstruction, the uptake of contrast by the kidney can be 1h or longer leading to a persistently dense nephrogram.

Schwartz DT and Residorff EF (eds) (2000). *Emergency Radiology*. McGraw-Hill, New York.

4. E ★   OHCM 8th edn → pp640–641

The symptoms described are those of colic: intermittent spasms caused by peristalsis down an obstructed viscus – in this case, the blockage is due to a ureteric calculus.

A This describes a cyst or – if infected – an abscess, or indeed any intra-abdominal fluid collection. Presentation depends on the site and size of the collection, but would usually be accompanied by systemic symptoms such as fever and vomiting.

B This is what happens in the early stages of appendicitis. As it has visceral rather than somatic nerves, inflammation of its walls causes pain that is felt in the epigastrium (midgut). Pain in the right iliac fossa, therefore, cannot be caused by inflammation of visceral peritoneum.

C This is the cause of the right iliac fossa pain (specifically over McBurney's point) in acute appendicitis. The pain is more constant than in renal colic and vomiting is less of a feature.

D Various parts of the bowel can become ischaemic, both acutely and chronically. Acute mesenteric ischaemia classically causes acute abdominal pain (usually around the right iliac fossa) but with an absence of clinical signs that masks how seriously unwell the patient can be. Chronic small bowel ischaemia causes colicky pain after meals, whilst chronic colonic ischaemia causes left-sided abdominal pain with bloody diarrhoea.

5. B ★   OHCM 8th edn → pp640–641

The results of a systematic review of 20 randomized controlled trials comparing non-steroidal anti-inflammatory drugs (NSAIDs) and opioids in the treatment of renal colic showed the following conclusions:

- Single doses of NSAIDs and opioids provide pain relief for patients with acute renal colic.

- Patients receiving NSAIDs achieve greater reduction in pain scores and are less likely to require further analgesia in the short term.

- Opioids, particularly pethidine, are associated with a higher rate of vomiting than NSAIDs.
- NSAIDs are therefore recommended ahead of opioids.
- If opioids are to be used, either because of contraindications to NSAIDs or ease of titratability, pethidine should be avoided.

Holdgate A and Pollock T (2004). Systematic review of the relative efficacy of non-steroidal anti-inflammatory drugs and opioids in the treatment of acute renal colic. *BMJ* **328**:1401.

→ http://www.bmj.com/cgi/content/full/328/7453/1401

6. A ★

This is a classical story of loin-to-groin renal colic (which in this case may have been precipitated by the loop diuretic, which can cause hypercalciuria). Once colic is suspected, further investigations hinge on the presence of blood in the urine. If there is blood detected on urinalysis, then, with a convincing story, it is reasonable to request an IV urogram (control, 5min post-injection of contrast, 20min post-injection, 60min post-injection and ideally, post-micturition). If there is no blood and yet the story and examination remain convincing, then either senior or specialist opinion should be sought for guidance (Figure 5.3).

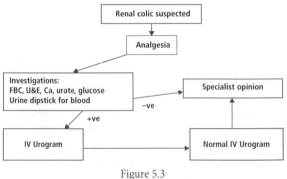

Figure 5.3

B Ketones can be present in the urine in both starvation and ketoacidosis.

C AND D   A urine sample positive for leucocytes and/or nitrites suggests a urinary tract infection.

E Proteinuria can occur in infection but may also suggest more chronic pathology as in diabetes or hypertension.

Kastner C and Tagg A (2003). Improving the effectiveness of the emergency management of renal colic in a district general hospital. *Emerg Med J* 20: 449–450.

→ http://emj.bmj.com/cgi/content/abstract/20/5/449

7. D ★

Low serum calcium and high phosphate cause parathyroid hormone (PTH) levels to rise, which leads to renal osteodystrophy. Activated vitamin D and phosphate binders limit this bone loss. Anaemia, normal potassium (hyperkalaemia is mostly due to acute renal failure) and a raised ALP would be expected.

8. D ★

In the acute phase after the relief of an obstruction, the kidneys kick back into action by producing a lot of urine: up to 1L within the first hour. It is therefore essential to provide concurrent rehydration therapy to avoid immediate dehydration. During this phase of diuresis, sodium and bicarbonate will also be lost in large quantities, so it is also important to keep a close eye on electrolyte levels and replace where necessary.

If the catheter does not relieve his distended abdomen, then imaging would be required (A and E). Given his chronic prostate problem, it would also be important to perform a rectal examination (B) and, once the catheter has been *in situ* for some time, to check serum prostate surface antigen. One-off doses of antibiotics (C) can be given at the time of catheterization as prophylaxis but should not be continued without good reason.

9. C ★

NICE guidance is that both potassium and estimated glomerular filtration rate (eGFR) should be checked prior to starting an angiotensin-converting enzyme (ACE) inhibitor (in this case for chronic renal failure in the setting of hypertension) and rechecked within 1–2 weeks. The drug should not be started if potassium >5mmol/L and should be stopped immediately if it rises >6mmol/L. See question 26 and the link below for more on the significance of the albumin:creatinine ratio.

→ http://www.nice.org.uk/nicemedia/pdf/CG073QuickRefGuide.pdf

10. D ★

The image shows a KUB film taken 20min after the injection of contrast dye. The bladder has filled and there is no obvious collection in the drainage system on the right. On the left, however, the calyces are clearly demarcated – in fact, they are dilated. The ureter itself appears to be ballooning from proximal to distal. It tapers as it reaches the bladder where there is a small calculus just visible. Even if it were not visible, the fact that there is a 'standing column' of dye in the drainage system suggests that there is a blockage distal to it: '*A normal ureter does not form a continuous contrast column because it tapers and disappears where it is contracted by peristalsis.*' (Schwartz and Residorff, 2000).

The indications for treatment of ureteric calculi are:

- Uncontrollable pain
- Renal impairment with single functioning renal units or bilateral calculi
- Stones >5mm diameter (as 90% of <5mm will pass spontaneously)
- Stones that have been *in situ* for up to 4 weeks (as previously normal kidneys can resist clinically significant damage from obstruction for up to 4 weeks)
- Recurrent urinary tract infection

Treatment is usually extracorporeal shock wave lithotripsy (ESWL) or ureteroscopy.

A This indicates a blameless part of the right pelvicalyceal junction.

B This shows a lateral part of a lower sacral vertebral body.

C This has picked out a phlebolith in the bladder.

E This indicates the most proximal part of the standing column. By definition, the obstruction must be located at its distal rather than its proximal end.

→ http://www.lua.co.uk/care-advice/kidney-stones/treatments

Schwartz DT and Residorff EF (eds) (2000). *Emergency Radiology*. McGraw-Hill, New York.

11.C ★ OHCM 8th edn → pp292, 294

IgA nephropathy is the commonest explanation for macroscopic haematuria in the western world. Most commonly affecting young men, it happens due to overproduction of IgA (classically in response to a throat infection), which then forms immune complexes that lodge in mesangial cells.

A This is the process behind Goodpasture's disease, which is very rare and also presents with haemoptysis (as antibodies also bind alveolar membranes).

B This occurs in polycystic kidney disease, which is more likely to present with abdominal pain from renal enlargement.

D Cystitis is more common in women and would be more likely to present with frequency and dysuria, as well as haematuria.

E These would be the biopsy findings in a rapidly progressive glomerulonephritis. It would present with acute renal failure following either vasculitic or infective processes.

Renal medicine

12. C ★

In the absence of risk factors for chronic kidney disease (hypertension, diabetes, cardiovascular disease, structural renal tract disease, or multi-system disease with renal involvement), age (A), gender (D) and ethnicity (B) should not be used as independent risk markers.

An often-forgotten risk factor for kidney disease, however, is metabolic syndrome, which is defined as:

Central obesity *or* BMI>30kg/m^2 *plus* two of the following:

- Triglycerides >1.7mmol/L
- High-density lipoprotein <1.03
- BP >130/85mmHg
- Fasting glucose >5.6mmol/L

→ http://www.nice.org.uk/Guidance/CG73/NiceGuidance/doc/English

13. C ★   OHCM 8th edn → pp296, 306, 308

Nephritic syndrome is proteinuria, haematuria, oliguria, and hypertension with rising urea and creatinine. In this case, it is most probably due to a post-streptococcal glomerulonephritis.

A Acute tubular necrosis is due to either ischaemia, drugs, or toxins, and presents as acute renal failure.

B Interstitial nephritis can occur secondary to drugs or infections and presents with either progressive renal impairment, acute renal failure, or hypertension.

D Nephrotic syndrome is the triad of proteinuria, hypoalbuminaemia, and oedema occurring most commonly in the wake of glomerular damage.

E If renovascular disease occurs in a 30-year-old, it is most likely to be due to fibromuscular dysplasia, which presents gradually with resistant hypertension. In those >50 years, it is most likely to be due to atherosclerosis.

14. E ★

This is a typical history of colic in the distribution of the right ureteric system. Supportive evidence should be sought via haematuria on urinalysis and a plain X-ray to screen for any obvious calculi before proceeding to an intravenous urogram (IVU).

A This is used to diagnose acute pancreatitis.

B This should be performed in most cases of the acute abdomen, particularly suspected bowel obstruction.

C After basic blood tests and a convincing history, the only way to diagnose an acute appendicitis is to proceed to theatre.

D This is useful for biliary colic or cholecystitis.

15. B ★

This man has features of urinary retention. Extremely painful and potentially very generally destabilizing, this is the first thing to treat as it may explain all of the symptoms (abdominal distension, confusion, and constipation).

Once the catheter has been passed, it would be sensible to dip and send the urine (D) and to treat with antibiotics (E) depending on the results. If the constipation does not improve, even after the bladder has emptied, then measures should be employed to investigate and treat it (A and C).

16. A ★

When confronted with proteinuria – particularly in a young person – it is always worth considering a vasculitis, and so it is important to find out: are there nosebleeds (as in this case, suggestive of Wegener's glomerulonephritis)? Joint pains? Eye pains? Rashes? It is just as important to screen for vasculitides in the setting of acute renal failure by sending off blood for erythrocyte sedimentation rate (ESR) and auto-antibodies.

B Tuberculosis can cause severe glomerular damage that presents with acute renal failure, but not via autoimmune destruction of blood vessels.

C Fever with an active urinalysis is more likely to signal a pyelonephritis.

D AND E Both of these can go on to cause a proliferative glomerulonephritis (usually presenting as the nephritic syndrome) due to general autoimmune processes rather than those specifically affecting the vasculature.

17. A ★ ★   OHCM 8th edn → p346

This woman has a septic arthritis and has become oliguric: she therefore has hypovolaemia-induced acute renal failure ('septic shock') and has clinically gone into disseminated intravascular coagulation (DIC) because of this. It is the wash-out of the joint that will get to the source of the sepsis (and as a result allow renal perfusion to gradually recover), but to enable this to proceed safely, any clotting defects should be speedily corrected beforehand. Oozing cannula sites should prompt screening for platelets, prothrombin time (PT), activated partial thromboplasin time (APTT), and D-dimers and an urgent conversation with a haematologist with the results to decide on the best way to correct any abnormality.

B   Extra antibiotics will not correct the clotting abnormalities.

C   There is not enough information in the scenario to know whether dialysis is indicated at this stage (potassium, pH, pulmonary oedema, and pericarditis). It is likely that she will need dialysis after the operation as her kidneys recover.

D   This would no doubt be useful and should happen at some stage to guide fluid balance, but it does not address the issue of coagulation. Incidentally, FFP can be given through a peripheral line.

E   There is no suggestion of acute blood loss.

18. A   ★ ★

The consultant is concerned that his patient has been receiving metformin while her kidneys are potentially poorly perfused: it is in this setting that the drug is very occasionally known to cause lactic acidosis (displayed by the laboured Kussmaul breathing, which tries to blow off the excess acid). An arterial blood gas should be performed immediately with the anion gap calculated (lactic acidosis causes a metabolic acidosis with a raised anion gap).

Of the others, E would have the most merit given the concern over poor renal perfusion in a diabetic, whilst D would also be useful.

Silvestre J, Carvalho S, Mendes V, et al. (2007). Metformin-induced lactic acidosis: a case series. *J Med Case Reports* 1:126.

→ http://www.jmedicalcasereports.com/jmedicalcasereports/article/view/5599/1199

19. C   ★ ★

The skeleton history along with the urine dip result is suggestive of systemic lupus erythematosus (SLE) with concurrent lupus-induced nephritis. In cases such as this where there is proteinuria, it is the glomerular filtrating apparatus that has been damaged, leading to a chronic leak of protein and/or blood. The treatment is threefold: reduce proteinuria with angiotensin-converting enzyme (ACE) inhibitors (and/or angiotensin II receptor blockers), manage hypertension (proteinuria is an independent risk factor for hypertension), and slow the renal disease process via immunosuppression (steroids ± cyclophosphamide).

20. C ★ ★

Why has this man gone into renal failure? The usual causes – hypovolaemia and distal obstruction – are not to blame. However, the absence of a palpable bladder does not rule out a more proximal obstruction as the cause, which could be shown by an ultrasound scan. When confronted with acute renal failure, it is the junior doctor's job to rule out the most likely causes, which will often involve arranging imaging of the renal tract.

A This is sensible if a catheter appears patent in the setting of a palpable bladder but is still not draining.

B CVP lines are useful for monitoring fluid balance (which is not a concern here) in acutely ill patients.

D There is no suggestion that there is an infective precipitant of the renal failure.

E Diuretics are not part of the management of acute renal failure, especially in someone who is well hydrated.

21. E ★ ★

This is an enzyme inhibitor and potentiates the effects of warfarin. It is widely used as first line treatment in urinary tract infections but is often forgotten as a source of important drug interactions. Although studies have failed to demonstrate an interaction with coumarin anticoagulants (such as warfarin) and penicillins, experience from anticoagulant clinics suggest that the INR can be altered by broad spectrum antibiotics such as amoxicillin.

22. C ★ ★ ★

Although low-molecular-weight heparin (B) can be given in severe renal impairment, monitoring of anti-factor Xa would be required because the patient would be at increased risk of bleeding. Therefore, unfractionated heparin would be a more appropriate choice.

A Aspirin has been shown to be less effective than anticoagulants in certain types of surgery (particularly major joint operations) and so heparins have been set as the gold standard.

D Compression stockings are often used in conjunction with a heparin injection as thromboprophylaxis but not on their own.

Thomas DP (2001). Thromboprophylaxis after replacement arthroplasty: anticoagulants are more effective than aspirin. *BMJ* 322:686–687.

→ http://findarticles.com/p/articles/mi_m0999/is_7288_322/
ai_73061939

Wille-Jørgensen P, Rasmussen MS, Andersen BR, and Borly L (2004).
Heparins and mechanical methods for thromboprophylaxis in
colorectal surgery. *Cochrane Database of Syst Rev* Issue 1: CD001217.

→ http://www.cochrane.org/reviews/en/ab001217.html

23. C ★ ★ ★

Although all of this man's parameters have deteriorated slightly,
it is only the anaemia that needs investigation at this stage. NICE
guidance states that management of anaemia should be considered
in chronic kidney disease (CKD) in those with Hb <11g/dL. If their
eGFR is <60ml/min, anaemia can be assumed to be due to the CKD.
If it is higher, then other causes need to be explored. Serum ferritin
levels are used to detect iron-deficiency anaemia in those with CKD:
levels <100μg/L are diagnostic in those with stage 5 CKD and are
highly suggestive in stages 3 and 4.

Note that NICE recommends the routine screening for osteoporosis
in those with stage 4 and 5 CKD (eGFR <30) but not before.

→ http://www.nice.org.uk/Guidance/CG73#documents

24. B ★ ★ ★   OHCM 8th edn → p294

This man is describing visible or macroscopic haematuria. Any one
single episode of macroscopic haematuria should be considered
significant. It is important to rule out transient causes (urinary
tract infection or drug side effects) and to then test for urea and
electrolytes and urinary protein:creatine ratio before referring to
either a urologist or a nephrologist.

He has developed haematuria soon after what sounds like an upper
respiratory tract infection – this is classical for IgA nephropathy
in which overproduction of IgA leads to immune complexes that
deposit in mesangial cells.

A If this man were older, then bladder carcinoma would be the
most likely diagnosis. It presents with painless macroscopic
haematuria and becomes more likely with age, especially if certain
environmental risk factors are in place (smoking; amines in some
dyes, paints, solvents, and textiles). It would need to be excluded
in this case (via an ultrasound scan and cystoscopy), but is not the
most likely diagnosis.

C Nephrotic syndrome is by definition proteinuria (>3g/24h),
hypoalbuminaemia (<30g/L), and oedema – this man has none
of these. Berger's disease can, however, cause the nephritic
syndrome – haematuria with proteinuria and hypertension.

D Stones do cause haematuria but this man has no pain to suggest that they are present.

E This man has no urinary symptoms, is afebrile, and not tachycardic, and his urine is nitrite negative. As part of the initial investigations, however, it would be important to send off a urine sample for microscopy, culture, and sensitivity.

→ http://www.renal.org/pages/media/Guidelines/RA-BAUS%20 Haematuria%20consensus%20guidelines%20July%202008.pdf

(*Renal Association and British Association of Urological Surgeons Guidelines on the Initial Assessment of Haematuria*, 2008.)

25. A ★ ★ ★

Before resuscitating, it is important to assess a patient's fluid status: are they over- or underfilled? Wet or dry? Soft signs such as tissue turgor and mucous membranes together with harder signs like the JVP, heart sounds, lung bases, capillary refill time, and peripheries should provide the answer. This man is in acute pre-renal failure, most likely due to hypoperfusion or sepsis. He is probably confused secondary to dehydration and will improve with IV fluids.

B This is a normal finding and is suggestive of adequate tissue perfusion.

C This is reassuring prior to starting aggressive fluid therapy but needs to be monitored, especially in those known to have ischaemic heart disease.

D This is indicative of heart failure and therefore the need for careful fluid therapy.

E This may also be a reason to start IV fluids, but does not inform about fluid balance.

26. B ★ ★ ★

The registrar is keen to catch the first signs of microalbuminuria, as this is the earliest sign of diabetic nephropathy (and predictive of increased total mortality, cardiovascular mortality and morbidity, and end-stage renal failure). The easiest way to do this is via a spot urine test before proceeding to 24h urine collection for protein and then treatment with either an angiotensin-converting enzyme (ACE) inhibitor or an angiotensin II receptor blocker as required. '*All patients with diabetes should have their urinary albumin concentration and serum creatinine measured at diagnosis and at regular intervals, usually annually*' (Management of Diabetes, Scottish Intercollegiate Guidelines Network).

A Creatinine clearance can be estimated via the Cockroft–Gault equation, or measured by collecting urine for 24h and taking a sample for plasma creatinine once during that time. It is

useful in those in whom a serum creatinine that is relatively
normal may be masking poor kidney function (e.g. in those with
low muscle mass).

C This is not indicated in the monitoring of diabetes. It is used
alongside aldosterone in the investigation of suspected
hyperaldosteronism.

D Imaging is not necessary as part of routine diabetes surveillance.
Once serum creatinine is >150μmol/L, it is advised that patients
are referred to a renal physician, at which point an ultrasound
scan of the kidneys would be useful to help guide treatment.

E This is not sensitive enough to be able to detect protein loss of
<300mg/day.

→ http://www.sign.ac.uk/guidelines/fulltext/55/section5.html

(*Management of Diabetes, Section 5. Management of Diabetic
Nephropathy.* Scottish Intercollegiate Guidelines Network.)

27. C ★ ★ ★

Microalbuminuria (albumin 30–300mg/24hf) should be tested
for every 6 months in type 2 diabetes for two reasons: it gives
early warning of impending renal disease and is an independent
risk factor for cardiovascular disease. Therefore, regardless of the
blood pressure, those who have it should start immediately on an
angiotensin-converting enzyme (ACE) inhibitor.

Strippoli GFM, Craig M, and Craig J (2006). Cochrane
review: antihypertensive agents for preventing diabetic kidney
disease. *Cochrane Database of Syst Rev* Issue 4: CD004136.

→ http://www.cochrane.org/reviews/en/ab004136.html

28. C ★ ★ ★

This is a difficult but common scenario. As the woman has no
capacity, she cannot refuse treatment (unless there is formal
documentation in the form of an advance directive). The doctors
need to weigh up what is in her best interests. In the short term,
that should normally include relieving pain by the minimal restraint
possible: in this case, this may entail giving low-dose sedation in
order to insert the catheter. In the medium term, answer A comes
in to play: to guide the doctors as to what may more generally be
in the woman's best interests, it would be useful to know how she
had been over the preceding months, whether she had expressed
thoughts about medical interventions, whether she was depressed or
indeed suicidal. Armed with this information, they would have some
basis for withholding treatment further down the line should she
continue to oppose it.

Extended Matching Questions

1. D ★★★★

This type of glomerular damage is associated with autoimmune conditions such as rheumatoid arthritis, as well as some of the drugs used to treat them. It tends to present in adults with nephrotic syndrome.

2. H ★★★★

This is damage to the glomerulus (actually an inflammatory reaction) occurring classically 1–12 weeks after a streptococcal infection of the skin or throat. It presents as nephritic syndrome but in most cases requires only supportive therapy.

3. A ★★★★

This man with currently untreated HIV infection is presenting with nephrotic syndrome. This is most likely to herald scarring of certain areas of glomeruli. In the setting of HIV, focal segmental glomerulosclerosis is known as HIV-associated nephropathy (HIVAN), a serious complication of advanced HIV that will need some or all of: highly active antiretroviral treatment (HAART), angiotensin-converting enzyme (ACE) inhibitors, steroids, and immunosuppression, but may still result in end-stage renal failure.

4. I ★★★★

This young man has varied symptoms – epistaxis with nasal crusting, sinusitis, and scleritis – which are suggestive of a vasculitic process. Concurrent with acute renal failure, this raises the possibility of rapidly progressive glomerulonephritis, the most aggressive of all glomerular diseases, with the potential to progress towards end-stage renal failure in a matter of days. If these kind of symptoms are present in a young person with acute renal failure, it is vital to perform a full autoimmune screen prior to involving the renal physicians who may opt for an urgent biopsy.

5. F ★★★★

IgA nephropathy (commonly occurring after virus infection) features immune complex deposition in mesangial cells, which respond by proliferating.

CHAPTER 6

HAEMATOLOGY

Tackling haematology is never easy. Revision can be a struggle as it may not always be obvious which topic areas will be directly relevant to clinical practice. As a result, for many, it founders on the nuances of the leukaemias and the myeloproliferative disorders.

In reality, diagnosis in these areas is performed by doctors at senior levels via means such as bone marrow aspiration and cytogenetics, and after consultation with other experienced colleagues.

We still, however, benefit from an understanding of these areas. Indeed, the first step in this direction is a useful one to take for a deeper general view of the specialty at large, as it allows a good visual to cling on to when dealing with a haematological puzzle. It is a trip right back to the beginning, right back to the stem cell (Figure 6.1).

A junior doctor's most frequent contact with haematology is interpreting a full blood count. In this task, the core skills of the chapter come to the fore: in response to an anaemia, we should be able to explore the possibilities of iron deficiency, vitamin deficiency, and haemolysis. On seeing a thrombocytopenia or abnormal clotting profile, we should be able to make a clinical assessment and perform further appropriate tests with a view to suggesting differential diagnoses. The questions in this chapter aim to build confidence in these tasks.

There is a lot more to haematology, however, than a blood count. As a junior doctor, there will be regular practical challenges such as prescribing and altering anticoagulation therapy, overseeing the safe delivery of a blood transfusion and managing acute situations such as sickle cell crises.

The way forward is to be able to master these basics and start to see the bigger picture. This means developing a feel for the more subtle symptoms and signs of haematological disease and becoming proactive in the face of abnormal blood results.

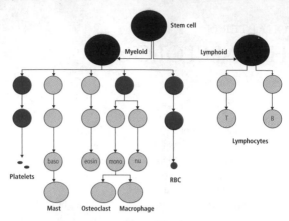

Figure 6.1

As with all of the chapters in this book, it is a way of thinking that is at stake: one that allows confident management of common situations and recognition of potentially catastrophic conditions, but also one that encourages creativity and initiative. When faced with a clinical conundrum, we should have the knowledge and confidence to ask appropriately, is the answer in the blood? ∎

SINGLE BEST ANSWERS

1. A 55-year-old man is receiving a transfusion of packed red cells during his recovery from colorectal surgery. He has suddenly developed a fever 30min into the transfusion.

```
T 38.3°C, HR 90bpm, BP 125/70mmHg, SaO₂ 98%
on air.
```

The transfusion has been stopped. Which *single* development should make the junior doctor most wary about restarting the transfusion? ★

A Pruritus

B Shivering

C Systolic BP <105mmHg

D Temperature >38.5°C

E Urticaria

2. A 23-year-old woman has been feeling tired and lethargic for the past 18 months. She occasionally feels dizzy on standing and is generally weak. She is otherwise well.

```
Hb 9.5g/dL, MCV 69fL.
```

Which is the *single* most appropriate further investigation to confirm the diagnosis? ★

A Hb electrophoresis

B HbA₂ level

C Serum iron + ferritin

D Thyroid function tests

E Vitamin B₁₂ + folate levels

3. A 72-year-old woman has been breathless and unwell for the past week. She is admitted to hospital and started on IV antibiotics for a chest infection. She has ischaemic heart disease and atrial fibrillation, and is on warfarin 2mg once daily. The on-call junior doctor is asked to check her blood results after she is moved to the medical ward. Her INR is 6.6. Which is the *single* most appropriate management? ★

A Fresh frozen plasma (FFP) 2U IV

B Reduce warfarin dose to 0.5mg

C Stop antibiotics

D Stop warfarin and monitor INR

E Vitamin K 5mg IV

4. A 68-year-old woman has had a swelling in her neck, weight loss, and night sweats for 6 months. Her family doctor refers her for investigations as an inpatient. After 72h on the ward she asks one of the doctors if she can read through her medical notes. Which is the *single* most appropriate response to her request? ★

A Allow the patient to take the notes whenever she likes

B Copy the parts of the notes that would be relevant to the patient

C Discuss the request with the hospital's information guardian

D Refuse as all medical notes are confidential

E Write a summary of the notes for the patient but withhold the original

5. A 52-year-old man has been feeling lethargic over the past year. He has had intermittent abdominal pain and has lost 5kg. His initial blood results are:

Hb 10.6g/dL, vitamin B$_{12}$ 305ng/L, folate 1.4μg/L, ferritin 110μg/L.

Which is the *single* most appropriate further investigation to establish the diagnosis? ★

A Anti-endomysial antibodies

B Anti-gastric parietal cell antibodies

C Liver function tests

D Peripheral blood film

E Thyroid function tests

6. A 75-year-old man has had lower back pain for over a year. It has got progressively worse and he has now noticed new pains in his right thigh and left arm. He is normally fit and well but has of late suffered repeated chest infections. Which *single* set of investigations would be the most likely to confirm the underlying diagnosis? ★

A Bone marrow aspirate + immunoglobulin profile

B Digital rectal examination + prostate specific antigen (PSA)

C Erythrocyte sedimentation rate + rheumatoid factor

D Full blood count + vitamin B$_{12}$, folate + ferritin

E Liver function tests + calcium

7. A 42-year-old woman has been increasingly tired over the past 6 months. She has felt faint on exertion with occasional palpitations. She admits to feeling irritable and rather low. Her skin and conjunctivae are pale.

```
Hb 9.2g/dL, MCV 102fL.
```

```
Film: hypersegmented polymorphs.
```

Which is the *single* most likely cause of the woman's symptoms? ★

A Alcoholism

B Liver disease

C Myxoedema

D Pernicious anaemia

E Pregnancy

8. A 66-year-old man has felt increasingly tired over the past 18 months. He has also been intermittently dizzy and complains of a sore tongue. He is pale and has a swollen red tongue.

```
Hb 9.9g/dL, MCV 105fL, WCC 6.2 × 10⁹/L,
platelets 265×10⁹/L.
```

Which *single* pair of investigations is most likely to confirm the diagnosis? ★

A Ferritin + total iron-binding capacity

B Folate + thyroid function tests

C Lactate dehydrogenase + reticulocytes

D Peripheral blood film + bone marrow aspirate

E Vitamin B$_{12}$ + anti-gastric parietal cell antibodies

9. A 72-year-old man has a sudden onset of pain in the right side of his chest. He recalls no trauma to the area and is surprised when he is told he has fractured ribs. He also has pain in his lower back and has had two admissions to hospital in the past 6 months with chest infections. Which *single* cell type is most likely to be proliferating? ★

A Germinal centre B cell

B IgM-secreting cell

C Mature B lymphocyte

D Myeloid cell

E Plasma cell

10. A 54-year-old woman has had bleeding from her gums daily for the past 2 weeks. She has also suffered four nosebleeds during this time. Over the past month or so, she has had a burning pain in her hands and feet with a throbbing in the tips of her fingers and toes, as well as an intermittent headache. Which *single* cell type is most likely to be proliferating? ★ ★

A Blast cell from marrow myeloid

B IgM-secreting cell

C Lymphoid progenitor cell

D Megakaryocyte

E Plasma cell

11. A 19-year-old woman has been in severe pain for the past 12h. It started in her left hip and has moved down her thigh. She is doubled over in agony and confined to bed. She has experienced similar episodes intermittently over the years. Paracetamol and codeine do little to relieve the pain and it is only after morphine 20mg SC that there is any improvement.

```
Hb 7.7g/dL, MCV 86fL.
```

Which is the *single* most appropriate explanation for her pain? ★

A Infarction of the bone marrow

B Localized tissue hypoxia due to anaemia

C Pathological bone fracture

D Pooling of red blood cells in the liver and spleen

E Sudden reduction in bone marrow production of red blood cells

12. A 59-year-old man is receiving a unit of packed red cells for bleeding oesophageal varices. Within an hour of the transfusion starting, he becomes agitated and appears very flushed. The site of his IV cannula is oozing blood.

```
T 38.4°C, HR 110bpm, BP 95/65mmHg.
```

Which is the *single* most likely explanation for his symptoms? ★ ★

A Acute haemolytic reaction

B Allergic reaction

C Anaphylaxis

D Bacterial contamination

E Non-haemolytic febrile transfusion reaction

13. A 72-year-old woman receives a unit of packed red cells as treatment for symptomatic anaemia. She has chronic renal and cardiac failure. Within an hour of the transfusion, she is even more breathless.

```
T 36.6°C, HR 95bpm, BP 145/80mmHg, SaO₂ 90%
on air.
```

Her JVP is raised and there are bibasal crepitations. The on-call registrar suggests that the woman should have received furosemide 40mg IV with the transfusion. Which *single* additional measure should have been taken to avoid the complication? ★ ★

A Inserting a urinary catheter

B Performing a chest X-ray

C Performing an ECG

D Putting her on high-flow oxygen

E Running the transfusion over 3h

14. A 62-year-old man has felt generally unwell for the past 3 months. His main problem is a widespread, intractable itch, but he has also lost his appetite and thus more than 5kg. He is lethargic and low in mood, and suffers from intermittent fevers with sweats at night. There is an enlarged, rubbery left cervical lymph node that is non-tender to palpation. Which is the *single* most likely cause of this man's symptoms? ★ ★

A B-cell malignancy

B Bone marrow malignancy

C Myeloid cell malignancy

D Plasma cell malignancy

E T-cell malignancy

15. A 33-year-old man has a routine pre-employment medical examination. He is asymptomatic but has sickle cell disease.

```
T 36.7°C, HR 65bpm, BP 122/78mmHg.

Hb 8.1g/dL, MCV 88fL.
```

His chest is clear and hearts sounds are normal. Which is the *single* most appropriate explanation for why he is not short of breath? ★ ★

A Due to chronic haemolysis, the Hb is diluted and actually much higher

B His cardiac output has been able to increase over time to compensate

C His MCV is within normal limits

D His oxygen dissociation curve is shifted to the right

E His vital capacity has been able to increase over time to compensate

16. A 39-year-old woman has received her second course of chemotherapy for a recently diagnosed acute myeloid leukaemia. She is a Jehovah's Witness and has a witnessed signed document stating that she would not accept supportive blood products at any stage. She has become breathless, weak and confused.

```
Hb 3.6g/dL.
```

The medical team caring for her feel that if she is not transfused with blood now, she will not survive.

Which is the *single* most appropriate next step? ★ ★ ★

A Apply for a court order to allow treatment to go ahead

B As she is now confused, they can treat her in her best interests

C Gain consent for the proposed treatment from her next of kin

D Reassess her capacity to decline the proposed treatment

E Respect her earlier wishes and withhold treatment

17. A 27-year-old woman is being treated in hospital for a chest infection. She has been switched to oral antibiotics with a view to completing the course at home. All her blood indices are improving, but her Hb levels have dropped by >4g/dL in the 5 days she has been in hospital. The registrar asks for a single blood test to assess the cause. Which is the *single* most appropriate explanation of the 'test' to which the registrar refers? ★ ★ ★

A Assessment of ability to absorb vitamin B₁₂

B Assessment of red cell fragility by placing in acid ~~Raised.~~

C Detection of levels of methaemalbumin ~~Loose — y~~

D Examination of a smeared drop of blood on a slide

E Identification of red cells coated with antibody or complement

18. A 41-year-old woman has had pain in her lower chest for 3 hours. It began while at rest and has been constant since. It is focused over the sternum and lower left ribs with radiation to under the left scapula. There is no associated breathlessness. In the preceding 2 weeks, she has experienced episodes of severe localized pain, most notably in her neck and shoulders but also in her thighs. She has also had several nose bleeds.

```
Hb 9.5g/dL, MCV 82fL, WCC 2.9 × 10⁹/L,
platelets 85 × 10⁹/L.
```

Which *single* investigation would be most likely to confirm the diagnosis? ★ ★ ★

A Auto-antibodies

B Haemoglobin electrophoresis

C Peripheral blood film

D Rheumatoid factor

E Vitamin B₁₂, folate, and ferritin

19. A 22-year-old woman attends an antenatal booking appointment. She has previously had three miscarriages at <24/40 weeks. She has recently had mouth ulcers and intermittent joint pains for which she is being investigated by the rheumatologists. Which *single* pair of results is most likely to confirm the underlying cause of her symptoms? ★ ★ ★

A ↑ activated partial thromboplastin time (aPTT) + ↓ platelets

B ↑ erythrocyte sedimentation rate (ESR) + ↑ rheumatoid factor

C ↓ Hb + ↓ MCV

D ↓ Hb + ↑ reticulocytes

E ↑ lactate dehydrogenase (LDH) + ↑ bilirubin

20. A 72-year-old man has had an acute non-ST-elevation myocardial infarction. He is being treated in hospital with a range of new medications. His renal function is moderately impaired and so he is given unfractionated heparin and monitored for signs of an adverse reaction. Which *single* subsequent episode is most likely to signal a reaction? ★ ★ ★

A Epistaxis

B Syncope

C Venous thrombosis

D Visual disturbance

E Widespread blanching rash

21. A 71-year-old man has noticed a change in sputum colour from clear to green and an increase in sputum volume over a 5-day period. He is started on 28% oxygen, antibiotics, steroids, and regular nebulizers. He has chronic obstructive pulmonary disease (COPD) and takes warfarin for atrial fibrillation. His INR is normally well controlled within the target range of 2–3. However, on the fourth day of his hospital stay, his INR is reported as 5.4. Which *single* drug is most likely to have caused his increased INR? ★ ★ ★

A Amoxicillin

B Clarithromycin

C Prednisolone

D Ipratropium

E Salbutamol

22. A 48-year-old man has a right inguinal hernia repair. A few days later, his right leg becomes tender and swollen and he is started on a treatment dose of subcutaneous low-molecular-weight heparin (LMWH). A Doppler ultrasound confirms a deep vein thrombosis (DVT) and he is started on warfarin. He asks why he needs to have both an injection and a tablet if the warfarin is replacing the LMWH on discharge. Which is the *single* most appropriate way to explain this strategy to the patient? ★ ★ ★

A Warfarin and the injection initially work together to give a greater clot-busting effect

B Warfarin can make the blood too thin too quickly, but the injection reduces the chances of this happening

C Warfarin initially increases the ability of the blood to clot so the injection is needed to keep the blood thin

D Warfarin takes a long time to reach a steady concentration in the blood, which is reduced by the injection

E Warfarin was started after the injection so has to be built up as the injection is weaned down

23. A 62-year-old man has had a headache coupled with dizziness intermittently for the past 6 months. He has also noticed an unpleasant burning sensation in his hands and feet. Both the big and first toes of his right foot are dusky in colour and tender to touch. Which *single* pathological process is most likely to be the cause of his symptoms? ★ ★ ★

A Bone marrow failure

B Chronic haemolysis

C Myeloproliferation

D Plasma cell proliferation

E Thrombophilia

24. A 21-year-old man has had severe chest pain for the last 4 hours. It is persistent and throbbing and has not been relieved by co-dydramol. It is typical of his sickle cell disease of which he has frequent crises.

```
T 37.1°C, HR 110bpm, BP 105/70mmHg, SaO₂ 95%
on air.
```

As per his analgesia protocol, he is prescribed morphine 10mg. Which is the *single* most appropriate route of administration? ★ ★ ★

A IM

B IV

C PO

D PR

E SC

25. A 52-year-old man has noticed increasing abdominal fullness over the past 18 months. He has no other symptoms. His abdomen is distended. There is a notched edge palpable in the right iliac fossa that moves further towards the anterior superior iliac spine on inspiration. There is dullness to percussion over the umbilicus. Which is the *single* most likely cause of the abdominal mass? ★ ★ ★

A Chronic myeloid leukaemia

B Idiopathic thrombocytopaenic purpura

C Myelodysplasia

D Polycythaemia rubra vera

E Portal hypertension

26. A 64-year-old man has had an increasingly full abdomen for the past year. He has felt lethargic but otherwise has been well. Initially, his blood results were normal. At his latest haematology appointment, he has the following blood results:

```
Hb 7.7g/dL, WCC 1.8 × 10⁹/L,
platelets 76 × 10⁹/L.
```

A bone marrow aspirate was reported as normal. Which is the *single* most likely explanation for the blood results? ★ ★ ★

A Bone marrow has stopped making cells

B Cells are trapped in the spleen's reticuloendothelial system

C DNA damage to a pluripotent haematopoietic stem cell

D Failure of normal differentiation of haematopoietic stem cells

E Immunoparesis due to monoclonal proliferation of plasma cells

27. A 77-year-old man is being treated for a chest infection. He has had multiple pulmonary emboli in the past and takes warfarin 4mg once daily. His last INR was 3.1 (target 3–3.5) 3 days ago. He is self-medicating on the ward, but, following his evening medications, is unsure whether or not he has taken his warfarin tonight. The nursing staff ask the junior doctor on call for advice. Which is the *single* most appropriate advice to give in this situation? ★ ★ ★

A Give the appropriate warfarin dose tonight + repeat the INR tonight

B No more warfarin tonight + request an INR for tomorrow

C No more warfarin tonight + send an urgent INR tonight

D Take 2mg warfarin tonight + request an INR for tomorrow

E Take 4mg warfarin tonight + request an INR for tomorrow

28. A 36-year-old woman has had intermittently heavy periods over the past 18 months. When they are heavy, they are no more painful than normal, but she does feel very weak and dizzy during them. She has also had nosebleeds at least two or three times a week for the past 6 months. There are numerous purple nodules on her buttocks, which do not disappear with pressure. Which is the *single* most likely explanation for this woman's symptoms? ★ ★ ★ ★

A Antibodies directed against the platelet membrane

B Bone marrow has been infiltrated

C Bone marrow has been suppressed

D Chronic haemolysis due to vitamin B_{12} deficiency

E Delayed hypersensitivity reaction to an unknown precipitant

EXTENDED MATCHING QUESTIONS

Causes of anaemia

For each patient with anaemia, choose the *single* best answer from the list of options below that is most likely to support the diagnosis. Each option may be used once, more than once, or not at all. ★ ★ ★

A Bilirubin

B Bone marrow aspirate + biopsy

C Direct antiglobulin test

D Ferritin + total iron-binding capacity (TIBC)

E Haemoglobin electrophoresis

F Haptoglobin

G Lactate dehydrogenase

H Parietal cell antibodies

I Peripheral blood film

J Reticulocytes

K Thyroid function tests

L Vitamin B_{12} + folate

1. A 41-year-old man is sweating and shaking 12 hours after a week-long alcoholic binge. He has had recurrent recent admissions to hospital in the same state. He is clammy, dishevelled, and slightly confused. His dentition is in a poor condition and he is covered in numerous partially healed cuts and skin blemishes. An abdominal ultrasound scan shows a small cirrhotic liver.
Hb 10.2g/dL, MCV 106fL, WCC 5.2 × 10⁹/L, platelets 85 × 10⁹/L.

2. A 50-year-old woman has had several nose bleeds over the last 3 weeks. She has also been easily tired and has noticed intermittent pains in her thighs and across her shoulders. Prior to these events, she has been fit and well.
Hb 9.4g/dL, MCV 84fL, WCC 2.8 × 10⁹/L, platelets 85 × 10⁹/L.

3. A 36-year-old woman has felt tired and lethargic for the past 18 months. She often has headaches and has even noticed an occasional buzzing sensation in her ears. She is otherwise fit and well, although her periods have been irregular and heavy since the birth of her second child last year.
Hb 8.8g/dL, MCV 69fL, WCC 8.2 × 10⁹/L, platelets 380 × 10⁹/L.

4. A 22-year-old woman is concerned that her skin is tinged yellow. She first noticed it in her eyes 3 or 4 days ago. She has no other symptoms, although she is still recovering from having 2 weeks off work for what her family doctor called 'glandular fever'. Both the liver edge and the splenic notch are palpable.
Hb 9.4g/dL, MCV 99fL, WCC 10.8 × 10⁹/L, platelets 550 × 10⁹/L.

5. A 52-year-old woman has felt increasingly lethargic for the past 3 years. She is occasionally dizzy and generally rather weak. She has gained 5kg, despite no increase in her appetite, and thinks her skin and hair are drier than they used to be. She is a non-smoker and does not drink alcohol.
Hb 9.8g/dL, MCV 104fL, WCC 8.4 × 10⁹/L, platelets 445 × 10⁹/L.

ANSWERS

Single Best Answers

1. C ★   OHCM 8th edn → p343

Increasing hypotension (with fever) is the most worrying sign as it heralds sepsis (i.e. bacterial contamination) or an acute haemolytic reaction and warrants stopping the transfusion and urgent discussion with a haematologist and a microbiologist. As this man's temperature is already raised, it would be the fall in blood pressure that would be the most concerning development.

A AND E   These most likely represent allergic reactions: in these cases, the transfusion could be slowed with the addition of chlorphenamine 10mg IM/IV and close monitoring.

B   Shivering is seen with fever in non-haemolytic reactions and can be treated by slowing the transfusion and giving paracetamol.

2. C ★   OHCM 8th edn → p318

It is not enough to know that a patient is anaemic. Before presenting such a finding on a ward round, it is vital to know what 'type' of anaemia it is. The first step to doing this is to look at the MCV. Different MCVs suggest different reasons behind the anaemia and so prompt the next stage in investigations:

- A raised MCV (>100fL) should be followed up with thyroid function tests (E), liver function tests, reticulocytes and vitamin B_{12} and folate levels (A).

- A normal MCV should prompt examination of the rest of the blood count including platelets along with renal function.

- A low MCV (<75fL) is most commonly indicative of iron deficiency, especially – as in this case – where it may be associated with menorrhagia. Low serum iron and ferritin with a raised total iron-binding capacity (TIBC) and transferrin would seal the diagnosis. If there is no convincing source of iron loss, then it is important to investigate the gastrointestinal tract: an incidental microcytic anaemia can be the way in which a tumour of the caecum or ascending colon presents.

A Hb electrophoresis would also be useful in the exploration of a possible thalassaemia, as it would in the diagnosis of sickle cell disease. Whilst thalassaemia minor can present with minor symptoms, it would be very unlikely for sickle cell disorders to do so (admittedly sickle cell trait might, but usually acutely in specific precipitating situations – such as hypoxic environments – rather than the more gradual presentation in this case).

B HbA_2 is one of the three main types of haemoglobin in adult blood. If iron studies were inconclusive in this case, then this may be a reasonable test to run as high levels of HbA_2 against a backdrop of a microcytic anaemia can occur in the relatively benign β-thalassaemia minor.

3. D ★

This is a common dilemma for the junior doctor. With such a high INR, it may be tempting to reverse it, but in the absence of bleeding, the British Society of Haematology guidelines state that readings <8 just need to be watched while warfarin is withheld. If the INR >8 and/or there is minor bleeding, then the agent of choice for reversal is vitamin K (0.5mg IV or 5mg PO). If there is major bleeding, then vitamin K 5–10mg may be needed.

A FFP has only a partial effect, is not the optimal treatment, and should never be used for the reversal of warfarin over anticoagulation in the absence of severe bleeding.

B Warfarin should be stopped and restarted once the INR <5.

C Some antibiotics do indeed interfere with the INR (ciprofloxacin and erythromycin (enzyme inhibitors) and rifampicin (enzyme inducer)), but this patient is in hospital for treatment of sepsis and it is the warfarin that should be stopped.

→ http://www.bcshguidelines.com/pdf/freshfrozen_280604.pdf

4. C ★

A patient has a right of access to their medical notes under the Data Protection Act 1998. There is no reason for this patient not to be allowed access to her notes and this should be made clear to her. It is also, however, important to weigh her right with the Caldicott principles. These were put in place to ensure maximum safety of confidential information. In order to implement these principles, every hospital should have a designated Caldicott guardian (often the medical director):

A Caldicott Guardian is a senior person responsible for protecting the confidentiality of patient and service-user information and

enabling appropriate information-sharing. The Guardian plays
a key role in ensuring that the NHS, Councils with Social Services
responsibilities and partner organizations satisfy the highest
practicable standards for handling patient identifiable
information.

In this case, therefore – as with all such cases – it is sensible to
contact the guardian for a brief discussion of the situation whilst
reassuring the patient that their rights will be respected.

→ http://www.dh.gov.uk/en/Managingyourorganisation/
Informationpolicy/Patientconfidentialityandcaldicottguardians/
DH_4100563

(*NHS Caldicott Guardians.* Department of Health.)

→ http://www.wales.nhs.uk/sites3/page.cfm?orgId=783&pid=31181

(*Caldicott: Principles into Practice.* NHS Wales.)

5. A ★　　　OHCM 8th edn → pp272, 318

This man is anaemic due to folate deficiency. In this age group, it is
important to exclude malabsorption, specifically coeliac disease, as
the cause.

B The presence of these antibodies is seen in pernicious anaemia,
in which there is a lack of intrinsic factor and thus an inability to
absorb vitamin B$_{12}$ in the terminal ileum.

C These are useful but would not be diagnostic.

D This is more useful in the investigation of a pancytopenia than
a folate deficiency.

E Hypothyroidism can cause symptoms of lethargy and a macrocytic
anaemia, but is not related to vitamin deficiencies.

6. A ★　　　OHCM 8th edn → p352

This man has worsening back pain with other bony pains
along with the suggestion of immunosuppression. C–E would
all provide useful but not diagnostic information for this
presentation. Option A would be desirable in the diagnosis
of myeloma, whilst B would detect the majority of prostate
malignancies. It is difficult to find reasons that totally exclude
prostate cancer as the cause here, but the lack of urinary
symptoms would certainly be one. The other would be that the
history is textbook for a myeloma (unexplained backache +
pathological fractures + recurrent bacterial infections). The work-up
of this patient should, however, certainly include a digital rectal
examination and a blood test for PSA, but diagnosis would be
confirmed by finding increased plasma cells on bone marrow
aspiration.

7. D ★   OHCM 8th edn → pp326–328

When anaemia with a high MCV is detected, the important tests to run include thyroid function tests, vitamin B$_{12}$ and folate levels, and reticulocytes. Added to these, a peripheral blood film can provide important information about the individual cells. Although all of the options given can cause a macrocytic anaemia, only D would show hypersegmented polymorphs on the blood film (all other options cause non-megaloblastic macrocytic anaemias, i.e. liver disease showing 'target cells' on the blood film).

The characteristic appearance of these polymorphs – large with multiple segments – is because the rate at which the nucleus develops is slower than the rate at which the cytoplasm develops. The delay in the nucleus developing is due to a lack of folate and/or vitamin B$_{12}$, which are necessary for DNA synthesis. When these cells are detected in the bone marrow, they are referred to as megaloblasts.

Pernicious anaemia is the most common cause of a macrocytosis with megaloblastic bone marrow. Symptoms stem from the inability of the gut to absorb vitamin B$_{12}$ due to a lack of secretion of intrinsic factor (following an autoimmune atrophic gastritis). Treatment is therefore to replenish stores of the vitamin by IM injections.

8. E ★   OHCM 8th edn → p328

A, B, C and E would all be reasonable and useful investigations into anaemia, although only B and E are targeted specifically at macrocytic anaemia (A would be useful in the microcytic anaemia of iron deficiency, whilst reticulocytes do cause a macrocytosis, but in response to other events such as haemolysis and haemorrhage). Given the specificity of the clinical signs (a 'beefy red sore tongue'), diagnosis would be confirmed by low vitamin B$_{12}$ levels and the antibodies to gastric parietal cells that characterize pernicious anaemia. Only D would be inappropriate in this instance: it would be indicated in a case of pancytopenia to explore the possibility of a haematological malignancy.

9. E ★   OHCM 8th edn → p362

Osteolytic bone lesions can cause unexplained backache with pathological fractures. Immunoparesis from monoclonal proliferation of plasma cells and marrow infiltration can lead to intermittent infections. Both of these features are suggestive of myeloma.

A This is Hodgkin's/non-Hodgkin's lymphoma.

B This is Waldenström's macroglobulinaemia.

C This is B-cell lymphoma.

D This is acute/chronic myeloid leukaemia.

10.D ★ ★   OHCM 8th edn → pp360–364

This woman is suffering with bleeding and the symptoms of microvascular occlusion. This is due to essential thrombocythaemia (high levels of platelets) that are derived from a clonal proliferation of megakaryocytes and so do not function normally.

A This is acute/chronic myeloid leukaemia.

B This is Waldenström's macroglobulinaemia.

C This is acute/chronic lymphoblastic leukaemia.

E This is myeloma.

11.A ★   OHCM 8th edn → p334

This woman is having a painful crisis, common to sickle cell disease (SCD). For some reason (often idiopathic, but can be hypoxaemia, dehydration, or infection), the microvasculature becomes occluded by a backlog of abnormally shaped red blood cells. This results in ischaemia and then infarction of the red bone marrow, and the characteristic deep-seated bone pain that can only be relieved by high-dose opioids. E refers to an aplastic crisis, whilst D refers to a sequestration crisis – both complications of SCD in which much more severe anaemia than in this case would be expected.

12.A ★ ★   OHCM 8th edn → p343

This man has a fever and hypotension and is showing evidence of haemolysis. In the setting of a blood transfusion, this is suggestive of a blood group incompatibility and is an emergency. The transfusion would clearly need to be stopped immediately, resuscitation commenced, and a haematologist contacted. If hypotension is prolonged, the patient may well need admission to the Intensive Therapy Unit for inotropic support.

If a red cell transfusion is accidentally given to the wrong patient, there is a 1 in 3 chance of an acute haemolytic reaction. Even a very low volume of ABO-incompatible blood is enough to cause symptoms. This should serve as a reminder in two ways:

1) As most ABO-incompatible infusions are given because of procedural errors (taking the sample, labelling it, collecting it, and cross-checking it before giving it), due care and attention must be given to every step of a transfusion. From the junior doctor's point of view, no matter how many tasks he may be juggling at once, this is the one to really put aside time for and to be rigorous over.

2) The process does not stop the moment the blood is connected to the patient. As the scenario illustrates, patients need to

be monitored closely as the transfusion is underway. This is particularly true of unconscious patients (or those not able to communicate), with whom the first signs of a reaction would be bleeding or worrying vitals. For this reason, many wards are not keen to run transfusions overnight as there is not the staffing power to meet the necessary level of vigilance.

B   In the context of a blood transfusion, an allergic reaction constitutes an itchy urticarial rash. It may be reasonable to give chlorpheniramine 10mg IM/IV and to slow the rate of transfusion and observe closely.

C   Anaphylaxis is an emergency due to the potential for rapid constriction of the airway. Symptoms follow a type I hypersensitivity reaction in which IgE leads to the release of histamine from mast cells. The patient becomes short of breath due to bronchospasm and hypotensive due to vasodilatation. In this setting, such symptoms demand immediate cessation of the transfusion and urgent attention to the patient's airway, probably with the assistance of an anaesthetist.

D AND E   Both of these cause the sudden onset of a fever, as in this case, but neither causes haemolysis. D is potentially more serious and would need treatment with antibiotics, whilst E should settle with antipyretics once the transfusion has been stopped.

McClelland DBF (2007). *Handbook of Transfusion Medicine*, 4th edn. The Stationery Office, London.

→ http://www.transfusionguidelines.org.uk/?Publication=HTM&Section=9&pageid=1145

13. E ★ ★   OHCM 8th edn → p342

In patients without heart failure, a unit of packed red cells can be run in quickly over 1–2h, or even STAT. In those with known disease, this should be slowed to around 3h; they should be given a diuretic with alternate units and monitored closely for signs of fluid overload. In some cases, a CVP line may even be necessary.

14. A ★ ★

The symptoms described are classical B-cell symptoms. These are found in malignancies of lymphocytes such as lymphoma and chronic lymphocytic leukaemia (CLL) and generally involves B cells more than T cells.

15. D ★ ★

The oxygen dissociation curve illustrates the relationship between PaO₂ and SaO₂ (Figure 6.2). The standard curve is calculated for

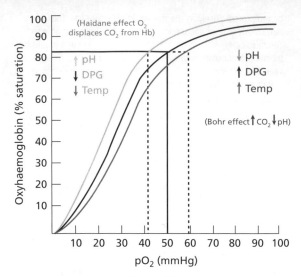

Figure 6.2

normal adult HbA. The curves for foetal HbF and HbSS in sickle cell disease (SCD) occupy different positions.

In SCD, the dissociation curve is shifted to the right, indicating that the Hb has a lower affinity for oxygen and can therefore more easily release it to the tissues. As a result, lower levels of Hb can be well tolerated.

A There is chronic haemolysis in SCD but this does not cause haemodilution; rather, it causes a rise in bilirubin and reticulocytes.

B An increase in cardiac output is seen in some conditions (e.g. hyperthyroidism, Paget's disease, and multiple myeloma) as a response to increased demands but not in SCD.

C Having a 'normal' MCV does not preclude breathlessness.

E If anything, a man this age with SCD is likely to have a restrictive lung defect due to recurrent episodes of pulmonary vaso-occlusion.

Sylvester K, Patey RA, Milligan P, *et al.* (2004). Pulmonary function abnormalities in children with sickle cell disease. *Thorax* **59**:67–70.

→ http://thorax.bmj.com/cgi/content/abstract/59/1/67

16. E ★★★

This woman has made an advance decision to refuse a particular treatment based on some strongly held personal beliefs. When the proposed treatment is life-sustaining, the advance decision – as in this woman's case – needs to be 'formally' recorded; under the new Mental Capacity Act 2005, this means that she needs to have signed it and to have been witnessed doing so by a responsible healthcare professional. This then overrides any change in the patient's capacity or any desire for the medical team to treat her in her best interests.

→ http://www.gmc-uk.org/guidance/ethical_guidance/consent_guidance/advanced_care_planning.asp

(*Consent: Patients and Doctors Making Decisions Together.* Advance Care Planning, paragraphs 57–61. General Medical Council, 2008.)

17. E ★★★ OHCM 8th edn → pp330–333

The registrar is referring to the possibility of an autoimmune haemolytic anaemia (AIHA) as a complication of a *Mycoplasma pneumoniae* infection. The test he has in mind is Coombs' test, which would confirm the presence or absence of a direct anti-globulin reaction characteristic of AIHAs. AIHAs are mediated by auto-antibodies and are most commonly idiopathic but can occur following infections (e.g. *Mycoplasma*, or Epstein–Barr virus) and cause extravascular haemolysis and spherocytosis.

A This is the basis of the Schilling test. It is used in megaloblastic macrocytic anaemias to determine whether a low serum vitamin B_{12} level is due to reduced absorption at the terminal ileum or to decreased secretion of intrinsic factor.

B This describes Ham's test for paroxysmal nocturnal haemoglobinuria (PNH) in which acidified serum activates an alternative complement pathway, which induces lysis of erythrocytes (the diagnosis of choice is now flow cytometry). PNH causes a chronic intravascular haemolysis with pancytopenia and an increased risk of thrombosis.

C Methaemalbumin is formed when Hb is broken down to haematin, which then combines with albumin. It is raised in severe intravascular haemolysis.

D This is a basic description of how a peripheral blood film is performed. Although it often provides useful information in cases where any of the cell lines are depleted, it is not the specific test referred to here.

With a presenting complaint of chest pain, it would be right at first to exclude a cardiac cause. This would involve taking some routine bloods. When these reveal a pancytopenia, the recent history of aches, pains, and epistaxis become important. This woman's problems stem from decreased cell counts across the lineages: the first diagnostic test would be a peripheral blood film before the haematologists proceed to bone marrow aspiration and immunophenotyping.

A This would be reasonable based on the history of pain, which is suggestive of some kind of chronic inflammatory process. Conditions such as systemic lupus erythematosus (SLE) can also suppress some of the cell lines. A rheumatological disease probably comes in second place as the likely cause of this scenario.

B This is useful in diagnosing haemoglobinopathies but would not explain the lymphopenia and thrombocytopenia.

D This would be an unusual presentation of the disease, which, although it may cause an anaemia of chronic disease over time, would be more likely to raise the platelets in response to chronic inflammation.

E These are useful in most anaemias but are unlikely to explain the complex set of symptoms.

The history is suggestive of anti-phospholipid syndrome, which most commonly occurs on its own, but can occur – as here – with systemic lupus erythematosus (SLE). As well as the presence of the antibodies anti-cardiolipin and lupus anticoagulant, results also show thrombocytopenia and a paradoxically prolonged aPTT (as a result of a reaction between the lupus anticoagulant and phospholipids involved in the coagulation cascade).

B These are most commonly raised together in rheumatoid arthritis.

C This woman may have a microcytic anaemia, but this would not be the confirmatory finding in the search for a diagnosis.

D AND E These are suggestive of a haemolytic anaemia (↓ Hb, ↑ LDH, ↑ bilirubin = increased red cell break down, ↑ reticulocytes = increased red cell production).

The reaction to heparin referred to is heparin-induced thrombocytopenia (HIT). In HIT (occurring in 1–5% of patients on heparin), the platelet count falls, although not usually enough for bleeding to occur. The most common symptom is enlargement of a pre-existing blood clot or the development of a new one. This reaction takes a minimum of 4 days to develop: this is how long it takes for antibodies against heparin to be produced, which then bind to the molecule and cause platelet activation and subsequent thrombosis. As well as monitoring symptoms, it is important to take serial full blood counts over the first week to 10 days of the initiation of heparin therapy.

When HIT is suspected clinically, heparin treatment needs to be stopped immediately. However, this alone does not halt the fall in platelets or reduce the risk of thrombosis. To achieve this, treatment with non-heparin anti-coagulants that do not cross-react with the HIT antibodies is required to dampen the storm of thrombin, as well as a more protracted course (2–3 months) of warfarin to prevent the recurrence of thrombosis.

A This is unusual in HIT as platelet levels tend not to drop far enough.

B This would be more suggestive of orthostatic hypotension due to decreased blood volume following haemorrhage.

D Rather than a thrombocytopenia, this would be more suggestive of a hyperviscosity syndrome such as polycythaemia rubra vera or myeloma.

E A proportion of patients who suffer HIT will develop a rash, but this would be a non-blanching petechial rash caused by the low platelet count.

Franchini M (2005). Heparin-induced thrombocytopenia: an update. *Thombosis J* 3:14.

→ http://www.thrombosisjournal.com/content/3/1/14

21.B ★ ★ ★ OHCM 8th edn → p702

As warfarin is metabolized via the cytochrome P450 system, any concurrent drugs that inhibit this system will potentiate anticoagulation (increase INR), whilst those that induce the system will impair anticoagulation (decrease INR). Of the drugs listed, only clarithromycin has been shown to definitely act as an enzyme inhibitor. Prednisolone has been shown both to induce and inhibit, whilst the others have no effect.

→ http://www.nhssb.n-i.nhs.uk/prescribing/documents/Drugs%20 to%20Watch%20with%20Warfarin%20Nov06.pdf

22. C ★★★

Warfarin is a vitamin K antagonist. The level of protein S is dependent on vitamin K activity and, because it acts as a co-factor for protein C, there is a reduction in the breakdown of factors Va and VIIIa. This causes the clotting cascade to favour the formation of clots and produces a transient pro-thrombotic state. To cover this period, LMWH is employed as an anticoagulant and can be discontinued once the warfarin has been through its pro-thrombotic state and the INR is within target range.

It can be a challenge to summarize such concepts in easily digestible lay terms. Doctors will develop their own strategies for doing so, but a useful tip is to be consistent with the terms employed, for example always using 'the injection' when referring to LMWH and the 'thinness of the blood' to invoke the INR. Other ways to aid understanding (and with understanding comes concordance) include writing down key points for the patient to take home and asking the patient to repeat back a summary of the key points.

23. C ★★★ OHCM 8th edn → p360

The symptoms described – headaches and erythromelalgia – could be due to either hyperviscosity (as in polycythaemia rubra vera where there are excess red and white blood cells and platelets) or microvascular occlusion (as in essential thrombocytosis where there is a persistently high platelet count). The other myeloproliferative disorders – myelofibrosis and chronic myeloid leukaemia – tend to present with general symptoms of lethargy or the discomfort of an enlarged spleen.

A This describes what happens in aplastic anaemia, which would be more likely to present with anaemia, bleeding, or infection.

B This occurs in, for example, sickle cell disease.

D This is the process behind myeloma, which, due to marrow infiltration, can also present with anaemia, bleeding, or infection, but also with backache and pathological fractures.

E Although thromboses are features of myeloproliferative disorders, this is due to thrombocytosis (i.e. the sheer number of platelets) rather than thrombophilia (an innate tendency towards clotting due to defects in the coagulation pathway).

24. E ★★★

According to the British Committee for Standards in Haematology, SC is probably the route of choice in sickle cell crises. Although absorption is slightly unpredictable, it is the safest for the short- and long-term health of the patient. Sites should be varied between the abdomen and upper arms and legs.

A This route used to be widely used, particularly in the administration of pethidine. However, due to the risk of muscle fibrosis, this is now contraindicated.

B The IV route allows rapid absorption, but in a patient who has regular crises, access may be a problem; indeed, repeated attempts may continue to compromise this, which could become a very serious problem if a life-saving transfusion were ever needed.

C The oral route is used for moderate pain or once pain has been controlled by other means.

D The rectal route is used for non-steroidal anti-inflammatory drugs (NSAIDs) in ureteric and pelvic pain, but is not commonly used to administer opioids.

→ http://www.bcshguidelines.com/pdf/SICKLE.V4_0802.pdf

(*Guidelines for the Management of the Acute Painful Crisis in Sickle Cell Disease.* The British Committee for Standards in Haematology.)

25. A ★ ★ ★

When confronted with a vague history, it is important to perform a rigorous examination. The findings elicited here suggest that the mass palpated in the abdomen is a spleen. The fact that its notched edge is felt in the right iliac fossa confirms this as a case of massive splenomegaly.

As chronic myeloid leukaemia (CML) presents insidiously, the finding of the enlarged spleen often predates any symptoms. In 50% of cases, it extends >5cm below the left costal margin at the time of first discovery, and interestingly, its size actually correlates with the full blood count, i.e. patients with the largest spleens are those with the highest white cell counts.

It can be useful to think of splenomegaly as being due to three main causes:

1) Increased workload (e.g. red blood cell turnover, extramedullary haematopoiesis).

2) Infiltration (e.g. leukaemias, metabolic diseases).

3) Abnormal circulation (e.g. portal hypertension, cardiac failure).

Of the options, portal hypertension (E) is the only other that can cause moderate to large splenomegaly, but this would be in association with hepatomegaly.

ITP (B) does not increase the workload of the spleen and although myelodysplasia (C) and polycythaemia (D) both do, they cause a more subtle splenomegaly than seen in this case of CML.

→ http://emedicine.medscape.com/article/199425-overview

26. B ★ ★ ★

The scenario outlines splenomegaly with pancytopenia but a normal bone marrow. Pancytopenia is due either to reduced cell production or to increased cell destruction. Only B refers to the increased destruction that is the hallmark of hypersplenism, whilst all of the others refer to decreased production and implicate the bone marrow in some way: aplastic anaemia (A), myelodysplasia (C), acute myeloid leukaemia (D), and myeloma (E).

Hypersplenism is pancytopenia caused by splenomegaly. When a spleen is large enough, it causes sequestration of all blood groups passing through its system and thus reduced counts. It does not exist on its own but as a secondary process to almost any cause of splenomegaly.

27. B ★ ★ ★

This is a common dilemma for the on-call junior doctor. It can feel like a difficult decision, but really just one thing needs to be remembered: if there are any uncertainties about whether a dose of warfarin has been given, no further doses should be given on that occasion and an INR should be taken the next day. Taking an INR on the same night would not leave long enough for any doses that had been given earlier that evening to be evident and as a result an extra dose may then be given.

28. A ★ ★ ★ ★ OHCM 8th edn → p338

The scenario describes menorrhagia, epistaxis, and purpura – collectively evidence of platelet dysfunction. In this demographic, the most likely cause is idiopathic thrombocytopaenic purpura (ITP). ITP is a relatively common autoimmune disorder in which platelets that are coated in antibody are removed from the reticuloendothelial system, thus reducing their lifespan to a few hours. The purpuric rash is as a result of thrombocytopaenia causing the breakdown of capillaries and bleeding into the skin. This type of rash (as well as petechiae and ecchymoses, which are just smaller and larger versions, respectively) is due to disorders of platelets or the vasculature. Coagulation disorders (including deficiencies of any factors – Factor VIII here is haemophilia A) are more likely to cause bleeding into joints (haemarthrosis) or muscle.

B This occurs, for example, in acute leukaemias, lymphoma, myeloma, and myelodysplasia, all of which would be most likely to present with more symptoms than just those due to platelet dysfunction.

C The most extreme example of this is aplastic anaemia, a rare stem-cell disease in which the bone marrow becomes hypoplastic and stops making cells, therefore affecting all cell lineages.

D This refers to the lemon tinge that those with B_{12} deficiency can acquire; they are anaemic but do not suffer with platelet dysfunction and the symptoms that accompany it.

E This refers to a non-specific haemolytic anaemia that, although it could present with platelet dysfunction, would also present with symptoms of anaemia.

Extended Matching Questions

1. L ★★★

This man presents in withdrawal from alcohol. His cirrhotic liver is the cause of the thrombocytopenia and it is nutritional deficiency that causes the non-megaloblastic macrocytic anaemia.

2. I ★★★

Pancytopenia with symptoms suggestive of dysfunction of cell lineages – epistaxis and fatigue – warrants immediate investigation due to the possibility of an acute leukaemia.

3. D ★★★

This is iron-deficiency anaemia due to menorrhagia.

4. C ★★★

This woman has autoimmune haemolytic anaemia following infection with Epstein–Barr virus (EBV) – Coombs' test identifies red blood cells coated with antibody or complement.

5. K ★★★

This woman has signs and symptoms of hypothyroidism, which causes a non-megaloblastic macrocytic anaemia.

CHAPTER 7
INFECTIOUS DISEASES

The term 'infectious diseases' brings to mind tropical illnesses contracted following travel to remote parts of the globe. Although these are important, they are thankfully not that common. The approach, however, to a febrile patient should largely be the same, no matter where they have been, with a number of questions always meriting consideration:

The patient

- Is this an unusual infection?
- Are they immunocompromised? Pregnant? Taking steroids? Diabetic? HIV-positive? Undergoing chemotherapy?
- Is anyone else unwell?
- Are they taking antibiotics or have they been in hospital recently?
- Has there been IV drug use or unprotected intercourse?

The travel

- Have they been abroad in the last 6 months?
- Where, and what is endemic?
- Are they appropriately vaccinated?
- Have they taken antimalarials?
- Have they been bitten by animals or insects?
- Have they swum in the rivers or lakes?

Of course, it is important to know of the flukes, nematodes, trematodes, and cestodes, but most of the day-to-day infections we will come across will have less exotic backgrounds.

This chapter focuses on the recognition of malaria, typical and atypical pneumonias, tuberculosis, and human immunodeficiency virus (HIV)-related infections.

Over the last century, targeted immunization programmes and the discovery of antibiotics have enabled the eradication of a number of infectious diseases and the effective treatment of many more. With the development of treatments – particularly antibiotics – we now face new challenges in infectious disease in Western medicine. Our patients do not always respond to the treatment we have relied on in the past (e.g. growing MRSA resistance) and are now becoming unwell and dying following treatment (e.g. *C. difficile* colitis).

Although we have a duty to ensure that infectious patients are not knowingly putting their partner's life at risk with their infections, many others who are friends or work colleagues will visit and may not know the reason for the patient's admission. The stigma associated with many infectious diseases and the effects that these infections can potentially have on relationships with family and friends requires us as health professionals to be tactful at all times.

A few further rules for infectious disease and sepsis can make things easier in the long run. The temptation to start antimicrobials is high, but we must culture everything – urine, sputum, blood, and wound discharge – to give us insight if the empirical therapy does not work. We must also recognize the opportunity for health promotion and prevention of disease by encouraging the uptake of vaccinations, anti-malarial usage, and hygiene: something as simple as hand washing after each patient contact may do more for the greater good than any other act we undertake. ∎

SINGLE BEST ANSWERS

1. A 36-year-old man has been recently diagnosed with human HIV and commenced on antiretroviral treatment. He is seen in the sexual health centre a month later to discuss the diagnosis with his partner, who has been HIV-positive for about 10 years. They have no other casual partners but have not used condoms during sexual intercourse since his HIV diagnosis. The doctor informs the man that his recent blood tests show that his CD4 level is normal and his viral load is undetectable.
Which is the *single* most appropriate sexual health advice? ★

A CD4 levels should be above 350 if no barrier contraception is used

B There are different viral resistance patterns; therefore barrier contraception is advised

C They are both HIV-positive, so will not be infected by the virus again

D Viral load should be checked monthly if no barrier contraception is used

E With an undetectable viral load, they are safe not using barrier contraception

2. A 37-year-old HIV-positive man has had difficulty reading road signs while driving over the last 5 days. He says he can see shadows float across his field of vision in his right eye and he is not sure that he can see everything. Which *single* type of virus is responsible for this condition? ★

A Adenovirus

B Herpes virus

C Papovirus

D Paramyxovirus

E Pox virus

3. A 31-year-old man attends a sexual health clinic for an HIV test. He is concerned that he may have contracted the illness after an ex-partner was diagnosed with the virus. He last had sexual intercourse with him 8 weeks ago. The test is performed and is negative. Which is the *single* most appropriate advice? ★

A Advise him to retake the HIV test in a month or so

B Reassure him about the negative test result

C Repeat the test as soon as possible if his ex-partner has a high viral load

D Return to the clinic if he has any flu-like symptoms in the next 6 months

E Start a month of antiretroviral medication as post-exposure prophylaxis

4. A 43-year-old man is very unwell in hospital with a disseminated fungal infection. He has been recently diagnosed with HIV. His family have come to visit him from abroad and know nothing of his diagnosis or likely prognosis. The on-call junior doctor, who has not met the man before but who knows the basics of his history, is asked by a nurse to bring the family to up to date. Which is the *single* most appropriate next step? ★

A Ask the nurse caring for him to bring the family up to date

B Bring them up to date at the bedside

C Invite the family to read through the medical notes

D Refuse to talk to them because the doctor has never met the patient

E Suggest they arrange a meeting with his usual doctors in the morning

5. A 17-year-old man is complaining of abdominal pain. He has vomited several times and is shivering uncontrollably. He has just returned from a month-long trip home to see his parents in Nigeria.

```
T 38.0°C, HR 110bpm, BP 105/65mmHg.

Random capillary blood glucose 3.2mmol/L.
```

He is slightly confused and has yellow sclerae. Which is the *single* most likely diagnosis? ★

A HIV

B Malaria

C Sickle cell crisis

D Typhoid

E Yellow fever

6. A junior doctor is taking blood from an IV drug user and accidentally pricks herself with the used needle. She is worried about the risks of contracting hepatitis and HIV and asks the on-call registrar for some advice about what to do next. Which is the *single* most appropriate next step? ★

A Check the doctor's liver function now and repeat it in a month's time

B Discuss the situation with Occupational Health as soon as possible

C Request an HIV test with the blood already taken from the patient

D Speak to the infectious diseases consultant in the morning

E Wait for 3 months and then take an HIV test

7. A 36-year-old woman is behaving erratically on the ward. She has developed a headache, confusion, and violent and aggressive behaviour. She is known to have HIV. The on-call registrar has asked one of the junior doctors to perform a lumbar puncture urgently. Which is the *single* most appropriate next step? ★ ★

A Perform the procedure but only after the woman is sectioned

B Refuse to perform the procedure if the doctor feels he may be at risk

C Restrain the woman and perform the procedure immediately

D Take all steps to minimize risk before performing the procedure

E Wait for the woman to calm down before performing the procedure

8. A 19-year-old woman has had a productive cough and chest pain for the past 2 months. She has lost 10kg in this time. She is cachectic and has raised cervical and inguinal lymph nodes. After initial tests, she is diagnosed with an atypical pneumonia and a large pleural effusion. The admitting consultant has asked that the team make it a priority to establish her HIV status. Which would be the *single* most appropriate way to do this? ★ ★ ★

A As it is in her best interests, send her blood without informing her

B Contact a specialist and ask them to secure written consent

C Gain consent from one of her family members

D Have a pre-test discussion and secure informed verbal consent

E Organize pre-test HIV counselling before seeking consent

9. A 38-year-old man has felt feverish with diarrhoea for the last 6 days. He recently returned from a month long trip around West Africa. He took regular antimalarial medications and had received all of his travel vaccines. Blood tests confirm he has *Plasmodium falciparum* malaria. The doctor decides that there are no features to suggest that this is a severe case and selects oral drug treatment. Which is the *single* most appropriate next step? ★ ★ ★

A Atovaquone + proguanil

B Chloroquine + proguanil

C Clindamycin + artemether

D Mefloquine + doxycycline

E Quinine + ciprofloxacin

10. A 48-year-old man is diagnosed with pulmonary tuberculosis. He discusses the future treatment plan with the respiratory consultant. He is informed that ethambutol is not required because the risk of isoniazid resistance is low, and he is commenced on rifampicin, pyrazinamide, and isoniazid. Which is the *single* most appropriate test that should be done before treatment is commenced? ★ ★ ★

A Blood pressure

B Echocardiogram

C Pulmonary function tests

D Hepatic function

E Visual acuity

11. A 28-year-old man has been newly diagnosed with pulmonary tuberculosis. He is due to start a 6-month course of quadruple drug therapy with rifampicin, isoniazid, pyrazinamide, and ethambutol. Which *single* pair of tests should be carried out prior to starting treatment? ★ ★ ★

A Audiometry + otoscopy

B INR + ultrasound scan of the liver

C Ishihara plates + Snellen chart tests

D Oral glucose tolerance test (OGTT) + random venous blood glucose

E Peak flow + spirometry

12. A 32-year-old woman has had profuse green diarrhoea and a headache for 3 days. For the last week, she has had a non-productive cough and has felt increasingly lethargic. She has recently returned from a 3-week tour of rural Thailand. ★ ★ ★

T 39.8°C, HR 58bpm, BP 110/62mmHg, SaO₂ 97% on air.

She is tender in the right and left upper quadrants. Which is the *single* most likely cause of her symptoms?

A Dengue fever

B Leptospirosis

C Malaria

D Shigella dysentery

E Typhoid

13. A 31-year-old homeless man has had a productive cough for the last 2 months. He feels lethargic and has lost about half a stone in weight. He drinks 30–40 units of alcohol per week and smokes crack cocaine. Which is the *single* most appropriate initial treatment? ★ ★ ★ ★

A Rifampicin and isoniazid twice weekly

B Rifampicin and pyrazinamide once daily

C Rifampicin, isoniazid, and ethambutol once daily

D Rifampicin, isoniazid, pyrazinamide, and ethambutol three times weekly

E Rifampicin, streptomycin, and clarithromycin three times weekly

14. A 36-year-old woman has been HIV-positive for 4 years and takes a three-drug combination of antiretroviral therapy. She has recently found out she is 8 weeks pregnant. She has not had any children previously and seeks advice from her doctor about her forthcoming pregnancy. Her viral load is undetectable and her CD4 count normal. Which is the *single* most appropriate advice she should be given? ★ ★ ★ ★

A Change her antiretroviral therapy to zidovudine monotherapy before the end of the first trimester to prevent teratogenic side effects

B She should have a pre-labour caesarean section to protect the baby from the mother's blood and body fluids

C She should not breastfeed her baby, as the virus is present in the milk and she will transmit this to the baby

D She should stop all her antiretroviral drugs during pregnancy to avoid immunosuppressing the baby

E There is no risk of HIV transmission during a vaginal delivery because her viral load is undetectable and her CD4 count is normal

EXTENDED MATCHING QUESTIONS

Causes of bacterial infection

For each patient, choose the *single* most likely causative bacteria from the list of options below. Each option may be used once, more than once, or not at all. ★

A Bacillus cereus

B Bacteroides fragilis

C Campylobacter jejuni

D Clostridium difficile

E Escherichia coli

F Haemophilus influenzae

G Klebsiella pneumoniae

H Listeria monocytogenes

I Pseudomonas aeruginosa

J Salmonella enteritidis

K Shigella dysenteriae

L Staphylococcus aureus

M Streptococcus mutans

N Streptococcus pneumoniae

1. A 22-year-old woman has felt tired, feverish, and unwell over the last 2 days. She has passed urine every few hours, although she still feels like she could pass more urine immediately afterwards.
T 37.2°C, HR 75bpm, BP 125/70mmHg.
Urine dipstick: blood 2+, nitrites 1+, leukocytes 1+.

2. A 17-year-old man has felt increasingly unwell for the last 6 days. He has cystic fibrosis and usually has a productive cough. However, his sputum, which is normally clear, is now thick and green in colour.
T 37.9°C, HR 90bpm, BP 130/75mmHg.

3. A 18-year-old man has had a red sore area on his face for the last week. He has tried a benzoyl peroxide cream, which he normally uses for his acne, but this has not helped. He says it produced a lot of serous fluid initially but has now crusted over.
T 36.2°C, HR 66bpm, BP 120/65mmHg.

4. A 19-year-old man has had a headache, stiff neck and photophobia for the last 12h. He flexes his hip and knee when asked to flex his neck.
T 38.2°C, BP 110/77mmHg, HR 90bpm
Lumbar puncture results- opening pressure 280mmCSF (normal range: 0–250mmCSF), glucose 1.8mmol/L, protein 2.1g/ L.

5. A 23-year-old woman has developed colicky lower abdominal pain and profuse diarrhoea over the last 12h. She has only recently left hospital following an admission for cellulitis.
T 37.4°C, BP 130/76mmHg, HR 88bpm.
Stool: offensive odour, loose with streaks of mucus and blood.

Drug side effects

For each patient, choose the *single* most likely drug from the above list to have caused the side effects outlined. Each option may be used once, more than once, or not at all. ★ ★

A Amoxicillin

B Cefalexin

C Ceftazidime

D Ceftriaxone

E Ciprofloxacin

F Clarithromycin

G Ethambutol

H Flucloxacillin

I Gentamicin

J Isoniazid

K Metronidazole

L Pyrazinamide

M Rifampicin

N Teicoplanin

O Trimethoprim

P Vancomycin

6. A 28-year-old woman has a terrible headache, nausea, and vomiting. At lunchtime, she went to a restaurant but only consumed 2 units of alcohol. She is midway through a 10-day course of antibiotics.

7. A 38-year-old man is worried after noticing that his urine and contact lenses have been coloured red. Two weeks ago, he was started on combination therapy for tuberculosis.

8. A 68-year-old man has been feeling itchy for the past few days and his wife thinks that his eyes are slightly yellow. Four weeks ago, he was diagnosed with osteomyelitis of his right calcaneus and started on a high-dose antibiotic. He has type 1 diabetes mellitus.

9. A 73-year-old woman has a chest infection and is given a week of antibiotics. She has atrial fibrillation and takes warfarin. Her INR is normally well controlled but when next checked is 5.3.

10. A 52-year-old man has a Gram-positive infection. The antibiotic that he has been prescribed should be given by infusion over an hour and a half, but has been given as a bolus by mistake. He has developed a red, itchy rash over his face, neck, and chest.

Use of antibiotics

For each patient, choose the *single* most appropriate
antibiotic from the list of options below. Each option
may be used once, more than once, or not at all. ★ ★ ★

A Ceftazidime 1g IV

B Cefuroxime 1.5g IV

C Chloramphenicol 250mg PO

D Erythromycin 500mg PO

E Flucloxacillin 500mg PO

F Fusidic acid 500mg PO

G Gentamicin 4mg/kg IV

H Linezolid 600mg PO

I Phenoxymethylpenicillin 500mg PO

J Piperacillin/tazobactam 4.5g IV

K Rifampicin 600mg PO

L Trimethoprim 200mg PO

M Vancomycin 125mg PO

N Vancomycin 1g IV

11. A 62-year-old woman has had suprapubic pain over the last 4 days. She has been passing urine more often than before and describes the sensation as 'burning'.

12. A 61-year-old man has an emergency laparotomy and repair of a perforated duodenal ulcer with an omental patch. A week later, he begins to feel very unwell and discharge from the laparotomy wound detects meticillin-resistant *Staphylococcus aureus* (MRSA).

13. A 64-year-old woman has developed profuse diarrhoea a week after being successfully treated for a severe hospital-acquired pneumonia. The microbiology department analyse a stool sample and contact the ward 4h later asking them to isolate the patient and start treatment.

14. A 62-year-old man undergoes a three-vessel coronary bypass operation. He is anaesthetized, and, during induction, given an antibiotic as prophylaxis against infection during the procedure.

15. A 64-year-old woman has had joint and muscle aches for the last 4 days. Initially she had a dry cough but latterly this has become productive of green sputum. She has been taking amoxicillin for 3 days but feels she is getting worse.

Causes of opportunistic infection

For each patient, choose the *single* most likely cause of the opportunistic infection from the list of options below. All patients are HIV-positive. Each option may be used once, more than once, or not at all. ★ ★ ★ ★

A Candida albicans

B Coccidioides immitis

C Cryptococcus neoformans

D Cytomegalovirus

E Epstein–Barr virus

F Herpes simplex virus

G Histoplasma capsulatum

H Mycobacterium avium

I Mycobacterium tuberculosis

J Neisseria meningitidis

K Pneumocystis jirovecii

L Shigella dysenteriae

M Toxoplasma gondii

16. A 44-year-old man has been brought to the Emergency Department after a seizure. His family feel he has become confused and more aggressive over the last 3 weeks. He has no history of epilepsy and is not currently taking any medications.
Glasgow Coma Scale (GCS) score 12/15.
CD4 count: 80/mm³.

17. A 51-year-old man has had abdominal pain and profuse diarrhoea over the last 3 weeks. He has lost almost 5kg in weight and is getting regular night sweats.
Hb 9.5g/dL, WCC 2.1 ×10⁹/L, CD4 count 50/mm³.

18. A 55-year-old woman has been getting more confused over the last 3 months. Over the last 2 days, she has been vomiting and has had double vision. She has no neck stiffness but has a right lateral rectus palsy.
CD4 count: 100/mm³.

19. A 39-year-old woman has recently found some white patches on the side of her tongue, which she was unable to remove with her tooth brush. She does not complain of any discomfort in her oral cavity.
CD4 count: 180/mm³.

20. A 45-year-old man describes small dark specks moving into his visual field over the last 2 months. This started in his right eye but more recently has also begun to affect his left eye. Confrontation testing shows some loss of peripheral vision in both eyes. On the Snellen chart, both eyes score 4/6.
CD4 count: 45/mm³.

ANSWERS

Single Best Answers

1. B ⋆

The risk is that the man and his partner will be re-infected by each other's virus, which may have different resistance patterns. This could make their current antiretroviral therapy less effective.

2. B ⋆

This is caused by human herpes virus 5 (cytomegalovirus) infection. It usually causes a retinitis, which will lead to blindness without treatment with ganciclovir. It can affect multiple organ systems including the skin, gastrointestinal tract, peripheral nerves, and brain.

→ http://emedicine.medscape.com/article/1227228-overview

3. A ⋆

Taking an HIV test before he has seroconverted (has detectable HIV antibodies in the serum) will produce a false-negative result. To be sure of the result, he should be advised to retake the test 3 months after the last possible infectious encounter to be sure that he has definitely not been infected. In rare cases, seroconversion can take up to a year.

→ http://www.umm.edu/ency/article/000604.htm

4. E ⋆

It is a common occurrence during an on-call shift that a junior doctor will be asked to speak to the family of a patient who is unknown to them. There are occasions when it is appropriate to do so: for example, when a patient has just been admitted to hospital and is yet to come under the care of a team, or in an emergency when conditions have changed dramatically and time is of the essence. However, in cases such as those outlined in the scenario, more caution needs to be shown. A careful scroll through the notes is likely to show the junior doctor that the man's medical team have specific plans for handling such delicate information. Whilst it may be hard to resist the questioning of concerned relatives, in sensitive cases like this, it is important to do so: for the benefit of the patient, his family, and the medical team.

5. B ★   OHCM 8th edn → pp394–397

This is a classic history for malaria: a fever that peaks every third day with rigors, jaundice, and general malaise. It should be suspected in all those who have a fever of unknown origin after recent travel to an endemic area. There is a suggestion that this man actually has severe malaria – he has mild hypoglycaemia and confusion – and so requires urgent treatment.

Yellow fever (E) and typhus (D) should certainly be on the differential diagnosis list (severe typhus can cause confusion and jaundice after a sudden onset of fever, and yellow fever in its most severe form can cause fever and jaundice), but common things being common, it is malaria that should be tested for and treated in the first instance.

Sickle cell crises (C) can present in a similar way – abdominal pain and a tachycardia with jaundice – but are less likely to cause fevers and rigors, whilst there is no suggestion that this could be HIV seroconversion (A) or indeed any presentation of an AIDS-defining illness.

6. B ★

Every hospital is different. Some advise discussing these types of incident with a Consultant in Infectious Disease and others recommend contacting the Occupational Health Department. However, the most important thing is that you act immediately following the needle-stick injury, making this choice the most important.

A It might be useful to get baseline bloods but is not the most important.

C Consent is needed before this should happen.

D Action needs to be taken today.

E An HIV test in 3 months may well be needed but is not the first choice.

7. D ★ ★

All patients are entitled to care and treatment to meet their clinical needs. You must not refuse to treat a patient because their medical condition may put you at risk. If a patient poses a risk to your health or safety, you should take all available steps to minimize the risk before providing treatment or making suitable alternative arrangements for treatment.

→ http://www.gmc-uk.org/guidance/good_medical_practice/
GMC_GMP.pdf

(Good Medical Practice, p11, paragraph 10. General Medical Council.)

8. D ★ ★ ★

The aim here is to establish informed consent from the patient.
In a competent patient, A and C are therefore inappropriate. The
British Association for Sexual Health and HIV (BASHH) guidelines
(consistent with General Medical Council guidance) state that
consent does not have to be written. They also state that it is not
essential to offer lengthy counselling, rather an open discussion in
which two main areas are addressed:

1) The benefits of testing to the individual.

2) Details of how the result will be given.

It is the patient's right to refuse testing and the healthcare
professional's responsibility to record the offer of a test in the notes
along with any relevant discussions.

→ http://www.bashh.org/guidelines

(UK National Guidelines for HIV Testing 2008. BASHH.)

9. A ★ ★ ★

Oral quinine 600mg three times daily followed by or together with
doxycycline 200mg for 5–7 days is appropriate treatment but is not
an option available in the list. Alternatives include Malarone®, which
is atovaquone and proguanil combined and can be given as a 3-day
course of four tablets daily.

Lalloo DG, Shingadia D, Pasvol G, et al. (2007). UK malaria treatment
guideline. J Infect **54**:111–121.

→ http://www.elsevier.com/framework_products/promis_misc/
malaria_guidelines.pdf

10. D ★ ★ ★

The three drugs that are being started are all associated with liver
failure. If there is no evidence of pre-treatment liver disease and
liver function tests are normal, they only need to be checked again
if there are complaints of malaise, fever, or vomiting, or if jaundice
develops. Those with pre-existing liver disease should be monitored
frequently especially during the first 2 months.

Ethambutol is used when isoniazid resistance is considered high.
Where possible, visual acuity (E) should be checked beforehand as
ethambutol is known to cause a toxic optic neuropathy.
This is largely reversible, although on occasion it has been known to
produce irreversible loss of vision.

Melamud A, Kosmorsky GS, and Lee MS (2003). Case report: ocular
ethambutol toxicity. Mayo Clin Proc **78**:1409–1411.

11. C ★★★

All the antituberculosis drugs have side effects. However, not all of them need to be actively monitored. In order to detect whether ethambutol is causing a reduction in visual acuity or reduced colour vision, it is important to get baseline functioning in these areas before the drug is started. (See answer to question 10.)

12. E ★★★

This is caused by faecal–oral transmission of Salmonella typhi. In the early stages, it typically features a headache and a slow rising fever, but with a relative bradycardia. As the illness progresses, hepatosplenomegaly and green 'pea-soup' diarrhoea commonly occur. Intestinal haemorrhage/perforation and neurological complications can occur.

A In dengue fever, a headache, rash, myalgia, and arthralgia predominate.

B There is no suggestion of this. It is transmitted via rat urine.

C Gastrointestinal symptoms do not usually feature in malaria.

D This does not usually lead to green stools.

13. D ★★★★

In 2006, NICE recommended that:

Directly Observed Therapy (DOT) should be considered for patients who have adverse factors on their risk assessment, in particular:

- street- or shelter-dwelling homeless people and prisoners with active TB

- patients with likely poor adherence and those who have a history of non-adherence.

→ http://www.nice.org.uk/nicemedia/pdf/CG033FullGuideline.pdf

(Tuberculosis. Clinical diagnosis and management of tuberculosis and measures for its prevention and control. NICE, 2006.)

14. C ★★★★

Research suggests that a caesarean section is unnecessary (although not risk-free) in a woman who has an undetectable viral load and is taking antiretroviral therapy. However, she should still avoid breastfeeding the child.

→ http://findarticles.com/p/articles/mi_m0CYD/is_10_37/ ai_87014863/

Extended Matching Questions

1. E ★

Uropathogenic E. coli is responsible for between 75 and 90% of urinary tract infections. Other causes include Staphylococcus saprophyticus, Klebsiella, Enterococcus, and Proteus.

2. I ★

This is the major pathogen in cyctic fibrosis. Patients are initially infected by S. aureus and H. influenzae but the majority of sufferers are infected with P. aeruginosa or Burkholderia cepacia by their mid-teens.

3. L ★

This is impetigo, which is mainly caused by S. aureus. It can be treated with fusidic acid cream or, in more severe cases, oral flucloxacillin.

4. N ★

In an adult in the developed world more than 75% of meningitis is due to Neisseria meningitidis and Streptococcus pneumoniae. The sign elicited is Brudzinski's neck sign.

→ http://www.turner-white.com/pdf/hp_jul99_signs.pdf

5. D ★

Diarrhoea in association with recent antibiotic use and a hospital stay makes this the most likely diagnosis. The first-line treatment is metronidazole.

6. K ★★

This pro-drug is activated by an enzyme found in anaerobic bacteria and protozoal organisms. When alcohol is consumed at the same time, a disulphiram-like reaction can occur with nausea, vomiting, flushing, tachycardia, and shortness of breath. Disulphiram was originally designed to encourage abstinence from chronic alcohol use and works by inhibiting the metabolism of acetaldehyde, which is one of the major causes of a 'hangover'.

7. M ★★

This is a well-known hepatic cytochrome P450 enzyme inducer and has numerous side effects, the most serious of which is probably hepatitis and in some cases liver failure. Although the orange-red colouring of bodily fluids is harmless, patients should be warned about it to prevent unnecessary worry and damage of contact lenses, which may be permanently stained.

8. H ★ ★

This drug-induced cholestasis usually presents with a painless jaundice 2–6 weeks after use but can occur up to 3 weeks after the drug has been stopped. Studies estimate a frequency of about 7 per 100,000 first-time users and most patients recover within a few months.

Russmann S, Kaye JA, Jick SS, and Jick H (2005). Risk of cholestatic liver disease associated with flucloxacillin and flucloxacillin prescribing habits in the UK: cohort study using data from the UK General Practice Research Database. Br J Clin Pharmacol **60**:76–82.

9. F ★ ★

Although metronidazole, ciprofloxacin, and clarithromycin inhibit the metabolism of warfarin and thus increase the INR, the latter is the most appropriate choice to treat her chest infection.

10. P ★ ★

'Red man syndrome' is an anaphylactoid reaction due to vancomycin-induced mast cell degranulation and release of histamine. This is usually associated with a rapid infusion rate and results in pruritus and an erythematous rash over the face, neck, and upper torso. Symptoms usually disappear shortly after discontinuation of the infusion, with the most severe reactions inversely proportional to the age of the patient.

Sivagnanam S and Deleu D (2003). Red man syndrome. Crit Care **7**:119–120.

11. L ★ ★ ★

This is the first-line treatment for a urinary tract infection. A urine dip can be performed looking for nitrites (Gram-negative bacteria convert nitrates to nitrites) and leukocytes and blood. A midstream urine sample can be sent for microscopy, culture, and sensitivity analysis if this is positive.

12. N ★ ★ ★

This glycopeptide antibiotic is the first-line treatment for MRSA infection. It is renally cleared, has a narrow therapeutic range, and requires trough-level monitoring to prevent nephro- and ototoxicity. Teicoplanin is an alternative requiring no monitoring.

Infectious diseases

13. M ★ ★ ★

This is Clostridium difficile infection, and first-line treatment is oral metronidazole but this is not an option. Oral vancomycin 125mg four times daily is the second-line treatment.

14. B ★ ★ ★

This is deemed 'clean' surgery and only needs to protect against Staphylococcus aureus and other skin flora. IV vancomycin is used in cases of resistance.

15. D ★ ★ ★

'Atypical' pneumonia often starts with an initial 'flu-like illness with a dry cough, which can become productive. Amoxicillin will not treat this type of infection caused by bacteria such as Mycoplasma and Legionella. Macrolides and tetracyclines are used as treatment.

16. M ★ ★ ★ ★

Cats are the primary host of this parasitic infection, which spreads following ingestion of infected meat or cat faeces or via transplacental transmission. In immunocompetence, the infection causes a 'flu-like illness, but is usually self-limiting and enters a latent stage. In immunodeficient individuals, the infection can be reactivated or, more severely, can develop acutely and can lead to encephalitis and chorioretinitis. Treatment often involves the use of sulphadiazine and pyrimethamine.

17. H ★ ★ ★ ★

This man has disseminated Mycobacterium avium complex infection, which usually involves M. avium and M. intracellulare and often presents with symptoms suggestive of tuberculosis. Prophylactic use of the macrolide antibiotics clarithromycin and azithromycin, or rifabutin can be used when the CD4 levels drop below 50/mm^3. In acute infection, ethambutol is often combined with one of the macrolides.

18. C ★ ★ ★ ★

Cryptococcal meningitis is caused by an encapsulated yeast-like fungus, which does not always produce the classic finding of meningism. Acutely, it can be treated with amphotericin and flucytosine and is often followed by fluconazole prophylaxis.

19. E ★ ★ ★ ★

This is oral hairy leukoplakia (OHL) and can indicate progression of the HIV infection. It often appears as white plaques on the lateral side of the tongue. Although it is named 'hairy' (to describe the folded hair-like appearance), it can also appear as smooth flat lesions and is often confused with Candida infection. The difference between the two infections is that OHL cannot be removed, whereas when Candida is removed it leaves red sore patches. As in this case, OHL is usually asymptomatic, but if it requires treatment, acyclovir is often used and it usually improves with antiretroviral treatment.

20.D ★★★★

Cytomegalo virus (CMV) is a type of herpes virus (human herpes virus 5). Between 50 and 80% of immunocompetent adults are infected with CMV but most show no symptoms of the acute infection, with a small number having a glandular fever-like syndrome before the infection becomes latent. In immunodeficiency, this can be reactivated and can cause an associated colitis, hepatitis, or, as in this case, bilateral retinitis ('pizza-pie' retina). It is often treated with ganciclovir or the pro-drug valganciclovir.

CHAPTER 8
NEUROLOGY

While cardiac, hepatic, and renal disease can be suffered privately, hidden from the outside world, neurological impairment often leads to a profound visible disability: the professional with a lifetime of facial asymmetry following a Bell's palsy, the young mother reliant on a wheelchair because of multiple sclerosis, or the grandfather with a stiff, weak arm and facial droop after a stroke. These people cannot cover up their dialysis fistulae, ascites, or midline sternotomy scars. Theirs are eye-catching abnormalities betraying dysfunction deep within.

Diagnosis of neurological disorders is often considered by junior doctors to be highly complex and, as such, is responsible for a great deal of anxiety. One of the most difficult challenges can be determining the location of the lesion, which often results in cranial nerve dysfunction, as well as a motor and sensory deficit.

A helpful approach to this is by analysis of the patterns that each lesion produces. The table below describes the pattern of motor deficit, which should be followed by a sensory examination to isolate the location of the lesion.

Location of lesion	Signs
Cortex	Normal or increased tone Weakness of all movements of hand or foot
Internal capsule/ corticospinal tract	Contralateral hemiplegia with upper motor neurone weakness
Spinal cord	Para- or tetraplegia Lower motor neurone signs at level of the lesion Upper motor neurone signs below the lesion
Peripheral nerve	Distal weakness (although can also be proximal weakness)

It is the 'regular' patterns of dysfunction – upper and lower motor neurone lesions and those involving the dorsal columns and spinothalamic tract – that are tested throughout this chapter.

An 'unmissable' neurological deficit presenting as hemiplegia, dysphasia, or loss of consciousness is rapidly and intensively managed. However, things are often rather more subtle. Sentinel headaches warn of impending subarachnoid haemorrhage, whilst transient weakness can pre-date a disabling stroke. If these signs and symptoms can be detected, then appropriate interventions can be tried to avoid a major neurological event from developing.

As well as sharpening skills in symptom recognition and management planning, the goal of this chapter is to approach neurology via a thorough assessment of cognitive, cranial, motor, and sensory modalities. It is then possible to describe the loss of function and suggest a location for the lesion and the type of pathology that may be causative, even if – as is often the case – the specific diagnosis remains immediately elusive. ■

NEUROLOGY
SINGLE BEST ANSWERS

1. A 72-year-old woman is recovering from an episode of temporal arteritis. She is due to be discharged on a gradually reducing dose of prednisolone tablets. She is being counselled on the risks of stopping the tablets suddenly. Which *single* symptom should this patient be warned to expect if she stops her tablets suddenly? ★

A Abdominal pain

B Depression

C Dizziness on standing

D Fits

E Weakness in upper arms and thighs

2. An 18-year-old man has recently been diagnosed with idiopathic generalized epilepsy. He lives with his parents who have not witnessed any of his three previous fits and are concerned about what to do if he has another one and ask their doctor for advice. Which *single* course of action should be stressed to the parents? ★

A Call the emergency services immediately

B Clear local danger and wait for the seizure to pass

C Give diazepam 20mg PR

D Give lorazepam 10mg PR

E Hold him down to prevent injury until the seizure passes

3. A 60-year-old woman has lost the ability to pick up small objects with her right hand. She also finds it difficult to fasten buttons. There is no other weakness. She is unable to copy one particular movement made by the doctor examining her (Figure 8.1). Which *single* nerve is most likely to have been compromised? ⋆

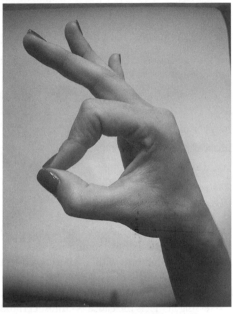

Figure 8.1

A Anterior interosseous

B Median

C Musculocutaneous

D Radial

E Ulnar

4. A 76-year-old man has collapsed. This has happened increasingly over the past year and tends to happen when he stands from sitting. This is not associated with any residual ill effects, but he also reports mild lower abdominal pain. He has hypertension and type 2 diabetes.

Abdomen: soft with mild supra-pubic tenderness that is dull to percussion.

Digital rectal examination: hard impacted stool.

Which is the *single* most likely underlying cause of this man's symptoms? ★

A Accumulation of cerebrospinal fluid with normal intracranial pressure

B Degeneration of basal ganglia

C Disturbance of autonomic nerve function

D Permanent loss of cerebral neurones

E Temporary loss of local cerebral blood flow

5. A 66-year-old woman has awoken to find that the right side of her mouth is sagging and she has difficulty eating on that side, with food getting trapped. She has a very watery right eye, her speech is impaired, and she is hypersensitive to sounds in her right ear. The doctor assessing her feels the cause is almost certainly 'idiopathic'. Which is the *single* most likely factor in her history that influenced her judgement? ★

A Hypersensitivity to sounds

B Speech impairment

C Trapping of food

D Unilateral sagging of mouth

E Watery eye

6. A 32-year-old man has been dribbling saliva from the right side of his mouth and having difficulty closing his right eye over the last 48h. His wife has noticed that his face is drooping on the same side. He has normal facial sensation but cannot raise his eyebrow on the right side. Which is the *single* most appropriate next step? ★

A No treatment

B Start oral aciclovir

C Start oral aciclovir + oral prednisolone

D Start oral prednisolone

E Urgent MRI head scan

7. A 68-year-old man has had a worsening tremor of his hands for 9 months. He says his father and brother were troubled with the same problem and that they both noticed improvement after treatment with a β-blocker. Which *single* additional feature in the history would be consistent with the most likely diagnosis? ★

A He uses two types of inhaler for his asthma

B His writing seems smaller than it used to be

C It disappears when he moves his hands

D It is only noticeable when his hands are still

E It seems to improve with alcohol

8. A 24-year-old woman has had a headache and double vision for 2 weeks. She is nauseous and has vomited on two occasions, but finds that her symptoms get better as the day progresses. An MRI scan of her head is normal. A lumbar puncture is performed and has an opening pressure of 36mmCSF (normal range: 0–250mmCSF). Which *single* additional feature from her history is most relevant to the likely diagnosis? ★

A Her father had chemotherapy 2 years ago for a glioma

B She drinks five or six cups of strong coffee each day

C She has a family history of migraine

D She smokes 20 cigarettes per day

E She takes orlistat 120mg PO three times daily

9. A 22-year-old man has had a headache increasing in intensity over the past 48h. He has started to feel nauseous and rather drowsy.

`T 37.8°C, HR 100bpm, BP 125/70mmHg.`

When the junior doctor asks him to lift his head from the pillow, the man is seen to involuntarily lift both legs in the air. Which is the *single* most accurate explanation for this finding? ★

A Limb girdle weakness

B Meningeal irritation

C Muscle spasm

D Raised intracranial pressure

E Sciatic nerve inflammation

10. A 49-year-old woman has weakness in her right arm and her right leg. She has been finding it increasingly difficult to find words. These symptoms have developed gradually over a 2-week period.

```
T 37.1°C, HR 85bpm, BP 105/70mmHg.
```

She has reduced power on the right with brisk reflexes and upgoing plantars. Which is the *single* most likely underlying diagnosis? ★

A Cerebral infarct

B Cerebral metastases

C Hemiplegic migraine

D Subarachnoid haemorrhage

E Transient ischaemic attack

11. A 77-year-old man has felt 'muddled' for the last 5 days. He cannot put his finger on what is wrong but neighbours say he has been talking and acting inappropriately.

```
T 37.5°C, HR 110bpm, BP 95/70mmHg, RR 26/
min, SaO₂ 92% on air.
```

He is pale, clammy, and agitated and in an abbreviated mental test he scores 5/10. Which *single* set of investigations would be the most likely to support the diagnosis? ★

A CT head + carotid Doppler ultrasound scan

B CT of the head, thyroid function tests + mini mental state examination

C ECG, 12h troponin level + echocardiogram

D Full blood count, blood cultures + chest X-ray

E Random venous blood glucose + glycosylated haemoglobin (HbA1C)

12. A 50-year-old woman has had an aching pain and numbness in her right hand and arm for 5 months. She finds that shaking her arm vigorously relieves the symptoms. She takes levothyroxine although she admits that she often forgets to take it. Which is the *single* most appropriate instruction to confirm the diagnosis? ★

A Cross your middle finger over the dorsal surface of the index finger

B Move your wrist towards the thumb laterally

C Place the thumb in a closed fist and tilt hand towards the little finger

D Raise your thumb vertically out of an open palmar surface

E Spread your extended fingers open horizontally

13. A 48-year-old man has undergone a 10h intra-abdominal operation. After the operation, he has some numbness in his ring and little finger of his right hand. The doctor thinks he may have damaged a nerve and examines him to confirm the diagnosis. Which is the *single* most appropriate instruction to confirm the diagnosis? ★

A Cross your middle finger over the dorsal surface of the index finger

B Move your thumb across the palm and touch the base of the little finger

C With the palm facing downwards, bend the wrist up towards your forearm

D With the palm facing sideways, keep your hand in this position against resistance

E With the palm facing upwards, bend the wrist up towards your forearm

14. The junior doctor on-call receives a bleep from a nurse during a busy night shift. A 78-year-old man has been found on the floor. He did not lose consciousness but was unable to get back on his feet, despite normally being fully independent. He is hoisted back into bed. He has no pain in his hips or wrists. He was admitted 3 days ago with a urinary tract infection and in atrial fibrillation. Which is the *single* most important detail from the nurse, in isolation, that should prompt an immediate review of the patient, i.e. in the next 5min? ★

A Alcohol dependence

B Headache

C Large swelling over his occiput

D Slurred speech

E Temperature 37.7°C

15. A 58-year-old man has double vision, especially while reading. He has hypertension and type 2 diabetes. As he is talking, he tilts his head to the right, but when asked to straighten up, his left eye appears to be slightly higher vertically than the right. Which is the *single* most likely diagnosis? ★

A Left inferior oblique palsy

B Left inferior rectus palsy

C Left lateral rectus palsy

D Left superior oblique palsy

E Left superior rectus palsy

16. A 39-year-old man has suffered a seizure while out shopping. He is admitted to hospital where he is drowsy and confused. This is his third such episode in the past 6 months. He has idiopathic generalized epilepsy and has been through a variety of treatment regimens. He currently takes phenytoin 300mg PO once daily. Which is the *single* most appropriate investigation to determine the trigger? ★

A Blood levels of phenytoin

B Calcium and phosphate

C Full blood count

D Random capillary blood glucose

E Urea and electrolytes

17. A 26-year-old man lost consciousness 30min ago at work. He was found on the floor shaking; this lasted for 10min. He had a similar attack 1 month ago. He drinks only occasional alcohol and takes no medications.

```
T 36.1°C, HR 88bpm, BP 142/78mmHg, SaO₂ 99%
on air.

Glasgow Coma Scale (GCS) score 12/15
```

A CT head scan is reported as 'normal'. Which is the *single* most likely diagnosis? ★

A Cataplexy

B Drop attacks

C Non-epileptiform attack disorder

D Primary generalized epilepsy

E Vasovagal syncope

$18.$ A 77-year-old woman has fallen 15ft from a balcony. Her cervical spine is immobilized and she has a non-rebreather mask on, with 15L/min of oxygen running. She is agitated and groaning and grabs the doctor's hand and opens her eyes as he rubs her sternum. She is awaiting a CT scan of her head and neck, but within a few minutes she starts to make snoring sounds and her oxygen saturation drops. Which is the *single* most appropriate next step? ★

A Head tilt and chin lift manoeuvre

B Jaw thrust

C Laryngeal mask airway

D Oropharyngeal airway

E Tracheostomy

19. A 77-year-old man has had a headache for the past 24h. He has vomited and is increasingly drowsy and confused. An urgent CT scan of his head is performed (Figure 8.2). Which *single* further detail from the history would be most supportive of the likely diagnosis? ★

A He has had a high fever for several days

B He sustained a head injury 3 days previously

C His level of consciousness has fluctuated for many weeks

D Onset of headache was sudden and devastating

E Reported personality change over the past few months

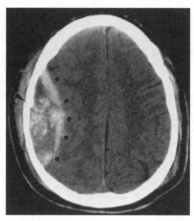

Figure 8.2

20. A 55-year-old man has had a headache for the last 3 days. The pain is over the occipital region and associated with nausea and vomiting.

```
T 36.5°C, HR 80bpm, BP 150/80mmHg.
```

He is unable to abduct his right eye on lateral gaze, but otherwise examination of his cranial nerves is unremarkable. He has grade 5/5 power in his limbs and down-going plantar reflexes. Which *single* pathological process is most likely to explain these symptoms? ★

A Demyelination

B Hydrocephalus

C Ischaemia of cerebral arteries

D Ruptured cerebral aneurysm

E Subdural haematoma

21. A 38-year-old woman has fractured her right fibula. She says that she has some numbness on the top of her right foot. The junior doctor thinks she may have damaged a nerve and examines her to confirm the diagnosis. Which is the *single* most appropriate instruction to confirm the diagnosis? ★

A Bend your foot up towards your knees

B Make the sole of your foot into a cup

C Point your toes and place the soles of your feet together

D Stand up on your tiptoes

E While I hold your foot, bend the furthermost joints in your toes

22. A 34-year-old man has been dribbling out of the right side of his mouth for 12h. He thought the television was particularly loud this morning, whilst his wife has commented that his face is lopsided and that he looks like he is grimacing rather than smiling. Which *single* feature in the examination confirms the most likely diagnosis? ★

A Asymmetry of the oropharynx

B Difficulty balancing

C Discharge from his ear

D Ipsilateral limb weakness

E Unilateral eyebrow raise

23. A 44-year-old man attends pre-assessment clinic prior to the laparoscopic repair of his umbilical hernia. He has epilepsy and has been taking sodium valproate 600mg PO twice daily for the past 5 years. Which *single* investigation should be performed prior to surgery? ★

A Blood levels of sodium valproate

B Clotting profile

C Fasting venous blood glucose

D Full blood count

E Urea and electrolytes

24. A 30-year-old man has weakness of his right hand, shown in Figure 8.3. He has been involved in a road traffic collision and is being assessed for other injuries. Which is the *single* most likely point of injury? ★

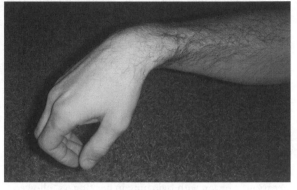

Figure 8.3

A Between the two heads of the pronator teres

B Epicondylar groove

C Flexor retinaculum

D Lateral to medial epicondyle

E Middle third of humeral shaft

25. A 72-year-old woman loses function in her right arm for a 12h period. She is assessed overnight in hospital and by the morning she is back to her normal self. Which is the *single* most appropriate treatment? ★

A Aspirin 75mg PO once daily + dipyridamole modified release (MR) 200mg PO twice daily

B Aspirin 300mg once daily

C Clopidogrel 75mg PO daily + dipyridamole MR 200mg PO twice daily

D No ongoing treatment required

E Warfarin (variable doses, target INR of 2–3)

26. An 80-year-old woman's speech has suddenly become slurred. She can find words without trouble but has difficulty enunciating them. A similar thing happened 2 weeks previously. She takes bendroflumethiazide 2.5mg PO once daily. Which *single* further detail in the history would be most supportive of the likely diagnosis? ★

A Concurrent tingling spreading from fingers to face

B Difficulty swallowing

C Photophobia

D Symptoms followed a severe occipital headache

E Symptoms resolved after 1h

27. A 72-year-old woman has had three episodes of left arm weakness in the last week. On each occasion, it began with twitching in her fingers followed by a sudden inability to move her whole arm lasting for around 30min. Her daughter says that during these periods, her speech was noticeably slurred. Which *single* examination finding would be most likely to support the diagnosis? ★

A Atrial fibrillation

B Fingers that turn pale, then blue, then red when cold

C Horizontal nystagmus

D Tenderness over the left temple

E Weak left radial pulse

28. A 66-year-old man has suffered sudden-onset weakness of his left arm and left leg. An urgent CT scan of his head is performed and is suggestive of an acute ischaemic event. He is admitted to a medical ward where his care is handed over to the on-call junior doctor.

```
T 38.4°C, HR 100bpm, BP 195/110mmHg, SaO₂ 96%
on air.

Random capillary blood glucose: 3.4mmol/L.
```

Which *single* reading listed above warrants the most urgent attention? ★

A Blood glucose

B Blood pressure

C Heart rate

D Oxygen saturation

E Temperature

29. An 81-year-old woman is found groaning and coughing in bed. She was admitted the previous week following a large left middle cerebral artery infarct.

```
T 39.4°C, BP 110/50mmHg, SaO₂ 92% on 15L O₂.
```

Her chest has coarse crepitations bilaterally, her JVP is not seen, and she has no peripheral oedema. Which is the *single* most likely cause of her sudden deterioration? ★

A Aspiration pneumonia

B Myocardial infarction

C Pleural effusion

D Pulmonary embolism

E Pulmonary oedema

30. A 30-year-old woman has had a seizure at home. Within 15min, she has arrived at the Emergency Department but is still fitting. The ambulance crew have given diazepam 10mg PR. She is given oxygen 15L via a Hudson™ mask and IV access is secured via a peripheral vein. Which is the *single* most appropriate next step? ★

A Arrange electroencephalogram monitoring

B Contact Intensive Care for intubation

C Lorazepam 4mg IV slow bolus

D Phenytoin 15mg/kg at 50mg/h IV

E Thiamine 250mg IV over 10min

31. A 55-year-old man has had muscle pains for about 2 weeks, mainly affecting his thighs and which is particularly bad when he climbs stairs. He has type 2 diabetes and high blood pressure. He started simvastatin 40mg PO once at night a month ago. He has 5/5 power in both legs. Which is the *single* most appropriate investigation? ★

A Creatine kinase

B Troponin

C Urea and electrolytes

D Erythrocyte sedimentation rate

E Lactate dehydrogenase

32. A 23-year-old man has pain in his right shoulder after a heavy tackle while playing rugby. He has no neurovascular deficit of the upper limb, but he has some soft-tissue swelling and tenderness over the head of the humerus. His range of movement is slightly reduced globally and he is unable to abduct his right arm without first leaning to the right. Which is the *single* muscle most likely to have been affected? ★

A Infraspinatus

B Subscapularis

C Supraspinatus

D Teres major

E Teres minor

33. A 48-year-old man has a mid-shaft fracture of the right humerus. He has some numbness on his right hand and forearm. The junior doctor thinks he may have damaged a nerve and examines him to confirm the diagnosis. Which is the *single* most appropriate instruction to confirm the diagnosis? ★

A Move your thumb across your palm to the base of the little finger

B Resist displacement of a piece of paper between middle and ring finger

C Spread your fingers open increasing the space between them

D With the palm facing downwards, bend the wrist up towards your forearm

E With the palm facing upwards, bend the wrist up towards your forearm

34. A 22-year-old man has sustained a sports injury. He scuffs the top of his right shoe along the floor as he walks and cannot turn his foot outwards against resistance. Which is the *single* most likely distribution of sensory compromise? ★

A Dorsum of foot

B Lateral calf

C Lateral calf + dorsum of foot

D Medial calf

E Medial calf + dorsum of foot

35. A 66-year-old man has been feeling 'slowed down' over a 6-month period. He is struggling to cope around the house and is becoming increasingly reliant on his wife. She has noticed him to be lower in mood and less expressive and effusive generally. He has a resting tremor and a slow gait of small steps. Which *single* further feature would be suggestive of Parkinson's disease rather than Parkinsonism? ★

A Asymmetrical symptoms

B Inability to look up

C Postural dizziness

D Short-term memory problems

E Urinary retention

36. A 74-year-old man visits his family doctor due to increasing difficulty walking over the past 6 months. He has a fixed facial expression and a unilateral tremor of his right hand. Which is the *single* most appropriate next step? ★

A Check serum dopamine levels

B Refer to a neurologist

C Request a CT head scan

D Start a dopamine agonist

E Start levodopa

37. A 30-year-old woman has been reported to have had a seizure. It happened in the standing area at the end of a 2h concert. She remembers feeling nauseous and sweaty beforehand. Her partner describes her falling to the ground where she jerked her limbs for several seconds. She did not bite her tongue and was not incontinent of urine. Two hours later in the Emergency Department, she is lucid although distressed. The junior doctor examines her, refers her for an electroencephalogram (EEG), and sends her home. The registrar feels it is unlikely to be a seizure. Which *single* detail from the history is most likely to have made the registrar reach this conclusion? ★

A Lack of tongue biting

B Lack of urinary incontinence

C Nausea beforehand

D Prolonged standing

E Sweating beforehand

38. A 31-year-old woman lost consciousness 30min ago. A collateral history describes her falling to the floor and jerking for 10min. She had another attack in the ambulance and was given diazepam 10mg PR, but she has three more attacks in the Emergency Department. She has no past medical history of note, drinks minimal alcohol, and takes no medications. The attacks last 2–3min and she feels her finger twitch before they start.

```
T 36.1°C, HR 88bpm, BP 125/68mmHg, SaO₂ 99%
on air.

Glasgow Coma Scale (GCS) score 15/15.
```

A CT head scan is reported as 'normal'. Which is the *single* most likely diagnosis? ★

A Cerebral glioma

B Complex partial epilepsy

C Drop attacks

D Secondary generalized epilepsy

E Non-epileptiform attack disorder

39. A 42-year-old woman has been feeling more and more tired at the end of her days at work. When she gets home, she struggles to lift anything and is too weak to eat or even use the telephone. She has bilateral ptosis and on counting down from 50 her voice becomes increasingly quiet. Which *single* pathological process most accurately explains all of this woman's symptoms? ★

A Demyelination

B Mononeuritis multiplex

C Myopathy

D Neuronal degeneration

E Space-occupying lesion

40. A 30-year-old woman has had difficulty walking for the past 12h. She first noticed it when she left work the previous night: her walk to the station, which usually takes only a few minutes, on this occasion took over an hour. She has grade 3 power in her lower limbs and an extensor plantar response bilaterally. Her range of eye movements is normal but painful. Which is the *single* most likely cause of her symptoms? ★

A Amyotrophic lateral sclerosis

B Guillain–Barré syndrome

C Multiple sclerosis (MS)

D Syphilis

E Vitamin B_{12} deficiency

41. A 27-year-old woman has been having regular headaches over the last few months. She describes the presence of stripes across her field of vision before the onset of the headache. She is otherwise well and takes only the oral contraceptive pill. Which *single* additional patient narrative from the history would be consistent with the most likely diagnosis? ★

A 'I have intense shooting pain around my eye and across my cheek'

B 'It's one side of my head. I feel nauseous and the light hurts my eyes'

C 'My eye looks blood shot, the eye-lid swells, and I produce more tears'

D 'The pain has started to wake me up and is worse when I lie down'

E 'Work has been very busy recently and I rarely have a chance to relax'

42. A 25-year-old woman has had uncontrolled headaches over a period of 6 months. These are unilateral and associated with nausea and photosensitivity. She has tried a number of simple analgesics with no effect. After seeing a neurologist, she unsuccessfully tried an oral triptan. She is having to take large amounts of time off work now and asks if she can take anything to prevent the headaches. Which is the *single* most appropriate prophylaxis? ★

A Amitriptyline

B Codeine phosphate

C Propranolol

D Sodium valproate

E Topiramate

43. A 53-year-old man has had recurrent headaches for 3 weeks. These are accompanied by feelings of nausea and aggravated by lifting heavy boxes at work. His mother suffered with migraines for many years. A neurological examination is normal. Fundoscopy reveals no evidence of papilloedoema. Which is the *single* most appropriate initial management? ★

A Referral to a neurologist within 2 weeks

B Send off urine for 5-hydroxyindoleacetic acid (5-HIAA) levels

C Start oral codeine

D Start high-dose prednisolone

E Trial of oral sumatriptan

44. A 24-year-old man has fallen off a 2m high wall onto grass. He thinks he landed on his head. He has not lost consciousness at any time. His story, however, is unclear as he has drunk over 20 units of alcohol. Aside from the effects of the drinking, he seems well and reports no drowsiness or nausea. The junior doctor is keen to discharge the man home. Which *single* examination finding should prompt the junior doctor to arrange a CT scan first? ★

A Bleeding from scalp

B Bruising behind the ears

C Coarse tremor in hands

D Past pointing

E Romberg's test positive

45. A 30-year-old man has suffered a head injury. He was hit by a blunt object about 2h prior to coming to the Emergency Department. He remembers the incident well and has not been nauseous or vomited and has no real headache. He was keen to stay at home and sleep it off, but his wife was concerned as she felt he was falling in and out of sleep and was rather confused. Which is the *single* most appropriate management? ★

A CT head scan

B Discharge home

C MRI head scan

D Observe for 12h

E Skull X-ray

46. A 50-year-old man is having increasing difficulty walking. For the past week, his legs and arms have weakened such that he cannot stand from sitting and is unable to dress himself. His sensation is unaffected. Prior to this episode, he has been well, although he does recall a bout of diarrhoea and vomiting around 6 weeks ago. Which is the *single* most likely pathological process to have caused his symptoms? ★

A Infection

B Inflammation

C Malignancy

D Metabolic dysfunction

E Vasculitis

47. A 26-year-old man has had successive seizures without regaining consciousness between them. After arriving at the Emergency Department, he had lorazepam 4mg IV and was started on an infusion of phenytoin 15mg/kg. It is now 40min since the first seizure began. Which is the *single* most appropriate next step? ★

A Arrange for electroencephalogram (EEG) monitoring

B Diazepam 10mg IV

C Fast bleep the anaesthetist

D Second dose of lorazepam 4mg IV

E Thiamine 250mg IV

48. A 28-year-old woman lost consciousness at home an hour ago and is brought in to the Emergency Department. She has no previous medical history and this has never happened previously. Her mother is worried that she has had a 'fit'. Which *single* feature from the history is most likely to confirm her mother's concerns? ★

A Biting the end of her tongue

B Feeling tired and wanting to sleep

C Incontinence of urine

D Still being confused when the ambulance arrived

E Twitching after she fell to the ground

49. A 20-year-old woman has had one seizure at home. She and her partner, with whom she lives, attend an appointment with an epilepsy specialist 3 weeks later. The decision is made to postpone starting any treatment. The couple remain concerned about the prospect of having another seizure and in particular about when they should contact the emergency services. Which *single* feature should prompt her partner to call the emergency services? ★

A A second fit starts before she has regained consciousness

B She experiences an 'aura' prior to the seizure

C She is incontinent of urine

D The clonic phase lasts for more than 10min

E There is evidence of tongue biting

50.

A 75-year-old woman has had a headache for a number of days. She cannot remember when it started but feels that it is getting worse. Her husband reports that she has had intermittent episodes of being vacant and rather drowsy. He says that she has fallen several times in the past few months and he feels she is unsafe in their current accommodation. The on-call registrar asks the junior doctor to arrange a CT scan of her head (Figure 8.4). Which is the *single* most appropriate next step? ★

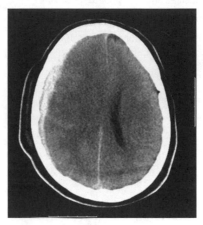

Figure 8.4

A Ceftriaxone 2gm IV STAT

B Contact the neurosurgeons

C Dexamethasone 8mg PO STAT

D Lumbar puncture

E MRI of the brain

$51.$ An 81-year-old woman has suffered a stroke. The most striking examination finding is a speech deficit. A CT head scan is carried out (Figure 8.5). Which would be the *single* most accurate description of her speech? ★

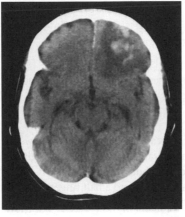

Figure 8.5

A Effortful with limited vocabulary

B Fluent but empty

C Low volume and monotonous

D Slow, indistinct, and effortful

E Slurred and staccato

52. A 38-year-old man has been shot in the back of his right thigh. He says that the sole of his right foot feels numb. The junior doctor thinks he has damaged a nerve and examines him to confirm the diagnosis. Which is the *single* most appropriate instruction to confirm the diagnosis? ★

A Lift your foot up towards your knee

B Point your toes and place the soles of your feet together

C Turn the sole of your foot out to the side

D With a straight leg, bury your heel into the couch

E With your leg bent at the knee, straighten your leg against resistance

53. A 36-year-old woman who is 34 weeks pregnant has a strange sensation in her right hand. She has weakness of her abductor pollicis brevis and sensory loss over her radial three and a half fingers and palm. Which *single* anatomical site is most likely to be the source of her symptoms? ★

A Between the brachialis and brachioradialis

B Between the two heads of the flexor carpi ulnaris

C Deep to the flexor retinaculum

D Medial to the brachial artery in the forearm

E Posterior to the medial humeral epicondyle

54. A 43-year-old woman has had an increasingly severe headache for the last 6 weeks. She has latterly become nauseated and confined to a darkened room. Three months previously, she completed chemo- and radiotherapy for a recurrent breast carcinoma.

T 37.6°C, HR 100 bpm, BP 95/70mmHg.

Which *single* pathological process is most likely to have caused these symptoms? ★ ★

A Haemorrhage

B Infection

C Inflammation

D Metastasis

E Thrombosis

55. A 65-year-old woman has fallen at home. She has had increasingly regular headaches for several weeks. She has hypertension, type 2 diabetes, and Crohn's disease and takes bendroflumethiazide, amlodipine, metformin, gliclazide, prednisolone, and azathioprine. A CT head scan is carried out (Figure 8.6). Which is the *single* most likely pathological process at the root of this woman's condition? ★ ★

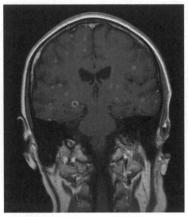

Figure 8.6

A Atherosclerosis

B Immunosuppression

C Inflammation

D Malignancy

E Seroconversion

56. A 66-year-old man has noticed that one of his eyelids will not open properly. He also complains of pain and tingling in the shoulder and arm on the same side. He has hypertension, gout, and a chronic cough having quit smoking 5 years previously. The right pupil is constricted and the right side of the face is dry from sweat. Which *single* pathological process most accurately explains all of this man's symptoms? ★ ★

A Autonomic neuropathy

B Infection

C Mononeuritis multiplex

D Paraneoplastic syndrome

E Venous sinus thrombosis

57. A 70-year-old woman has begun dragging her right foot along as she walks. Two weeks previously, her left wrist felt weak such that she could not straighten it. She has had rheumatoid arthritis for 35 years and is currently using methotrexate 12.5mg once weekly. Which is the *single* most likely neuropathological process to explain her symptoms? ★ ★

A Autonomic neuropathy

B Demyelination

C Entrapment

D Inflammatory peripheral neuropathy

E Mononeuritis multiplex

58. A 59-year-old woman has been unable to speak for the last 24h. Her daughter has noticed her to be irritable and slightly confused for most of the past week. She has also fallen several times in this period and complained of a headache that is worse in the mornings. Which *single* management option would be most likely to improve this woman's symptoms? ★ ★

A Alteplase 0.9mg/kg IV

B Aspirin 300mg PO once a day

C Dexamethasone 8mg PO twice a day

D Nimodipine 60mg PO six times a day

E Therapeutic lumbar puncture

59. A 78-year-old woman has a sudden onset of weakness in her right arm and right leg. She also has difficulty speaking, managing only a few isolated words. There is no discernible visual or sensory loss. The on-call registrar asks the junior doctor to organize an urgent CT head scan, telling her to classify the presumed stroke for the benefit of the radiologist. Which would be the *single* most accurate way to classify this woman's neurological deficits? ★ ★

A Dominant circulation infarct

B Lacunar infarct

C Partial anterior circulation infarct

D Posterior circulation infarct

E Total anterior circulation infarct

60. A 58-year-old man is confused. He has no recollection of the events that brought him into hospital but says he has never been unwell before. Records show that this is his fifth admission within a 6-month period.

```
T 35.6°C, HR 110bpm, BP 90/55mmHg.
```

His eyes flicker from side to side and when asked to walk he can only stagger. He scores 0/10 in an abbreviated mental test. Which is the *single* most appropriate course of action? ★ ★

A Aspirin 300mg PO once daily

B Dexamethasone 8mg PO twice daily

C Glucagon 1mg IM STAT

D Donepezil 5mg PO at night

E Thiamine IV three times a day

61. A 78-year-old woman has had increasingly regular diarrhoea for the last 2 weeks. She has also noticed some blood mixed in with the stool. As she is awaiting a colonoscopy, she develops sudden-onset weakness of her left foot. She finds that she cannot pick her foot up properly but drags it behind her, her toes scraping along the floor. She is otherwise only treated for asthma, which she developed in her 50s. Which is the *single* most likely pathological process that would explain this woman's symptoms? ★ ★

A Immunosuppression

B Infection

C Inflammation

D Malignancy

E Vasculitis

62. A 24-year-old woman has had 4 months of right-sided parietal headaches with intermittent blurred vision. The headaches are most severe in the morning and get better through the course of the day. Which is the *single* most likely diagnosis? ★ ★ ★

A Benign intracranial hypertension

B Cluster headache

C Giant cell arteritis

D Migraine

E Tension headache

63. An 81-year-old man has collapsed. When he comes round, he says he felt dizzy immediately prior to falling but does not remember exactly what happened. He recovers quickly and feels back to his normal self. He has hypertension, asthma, type 2 diabetes, and osteoporosis, and had been started on a new medication the previous day. Which *single* medication is the most likely cause of the collapse? ★ ★ ★

A Alendronate

B Doxazosin

C Metformin

D Rosiglitazone

E Salbutamol

64. A 67-year-old woman had an extended right hemi-colectomy with a primary anastomosis 2 days ago. She started eating a light diet today and was recovering well. At 1am, the nursing staff call the junior doctor on call because she is confused and tremulous and has been trying to climb out of bed for 2h. The patient says that she wants to get out of bed '*to find her dog, which ran past the end of the bed earlier*'.

```
T 37.4°C, HR 90bpm, BP 105/88mmHg, SaO₂ 95%
on air, capillary blood glucose 5.5mmol/L.

Sodium 131mmol/L, potassium 4.1mmol/L,
creatinine 88µmol/L, Hb 9.5g/dL, MCV 104fL.
```

Which is the *single* most appropriate next step in management? ★ ★ ★

A Administer 2L of oxygen via nasal cannulae

B Cross-match for a 2U blood transfusion

C Start haloperidol 2.5mg PO

D Start a reducing regime of chlordiazepoxide

E Start trimethoprim for a presumed urinary tract infection

65. A 60-year-old woman has a sudden episode of weakness in her left arm. It lasts for no more than 3 or 4h but is associated with slurring of her speech. She has hypertension and takes bendroflumethiazide 2.5mg PO once daily and simvastatin 20mg PO once daily. A neurological examination reveals no residual deficit. An ECG is carried out (Figure 8.7). Which is the *single* most appropriate course of action? ★ ★ ★

A CT head scan, then start warfarin if appropriate

B Review in clinic in 3 months and start warfarin if appropriate

C Start warfarin immediately

D Start warfarin only if there are further episodes of weakness

E Start warfarin only if the pulse rate not adequately controlled

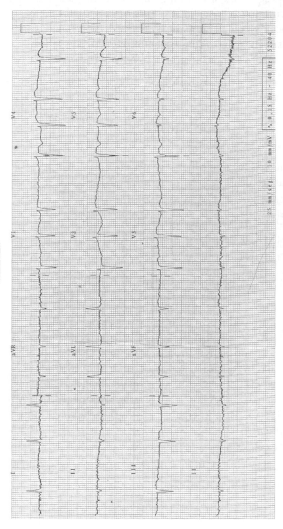

Figure 8.7

66. A 17-year-old woman has had a seizure at home, having felt sick for the preceding 2h. It was witnessed by her father who describes 1min of her stretching her arms and legs out followed by 10min of all four limbs shaking. She was incontinent of urine and bleeding from the side of her tongue. This is her first such episode. No specific trigger can be detected. Twelve hours later, she has recovered well apart from being unable to lift her left arm. The consultant suggests starting sodium valproate 200mg PO twice daily. Which *single* factor is most likely to have influenced the consultant's decision? ★ ★ ★

A Lack of a specific trigger

B Left arm weakness

C Pre-seizure sickness

D Tongue biting

E Urinary incontinence

67. A 67-year-old man has been brought into the Emergency Department in the early hours of the morning with a head injury following a fall at home 30min ago. All he remembers is finding himself on the floor; he is not sure whether he lost consciousness. Which *single* feature should prompt a request for an urgent CT head scan? ★ ★ ★

A He fell down two flights of stairs

B He has vomited twice since the fall

C He is more than 65 years old

D He suffers from epilepsy

E His Glasgow Coma Scale score (GCS) is currently 14

$68.$ A 45-year-old woman has had a headache and has felt increasingly anxious over the last week. Her family report that she has been acting aggressively and saying bizarre things. The on-call junior doctor is called to the medical ward where she has been admitted. The woman is behaving erratically: she has made threatening remarks to staff, disturbed fellow patients, and now wants to self-discharge. She is due to be reviewed by a psychiatrist in the morning. Which is the *single* most appropriate next step? ★ ★ ★

A Allow her to self-discharge

B Arrange for her to be detained under Section 5(2) of the Mental Health Act 2007

C Ask the police to detain her under Section 136 of the Mental Health Act 2007

D Await review by a psychiatrist in the morning

E Sedate her

$69.$ A 33-year-old woman has had recurrent spells of tingling in her arms for the past 6 months. The tingling is noticeably worse when she is trying to use her arms and often seems to come on after she has had a hot bath. She has otherwise been well and does not smoke or drink alcohol. Which *single* investigation or pair of investigations would be the most likely to support the diagnosis? ★ ★ ★

A Anti-acetylcholine receptor antibodies

B CT thoracic outlet

C MRI brain + spinal cord

D Nerve conduction studies

E Vitamin B_{12} + folate

70. A 78-year-old man has become acutely confused over the last few hours. He is recovering from a lower respiratory tract infection and is awaiting a rehabilitation placement. He has hypertension, chronic obstructive pulmonary disease (COPD), Parkinson's disease, and type 2 diabetes. He is unsteady on his feet and has increased tone in all four limbs, more so than is usual for him. Which *single* medication is most likely to have caused his deterioration? ★ ★ ★

A Amoxicillin

B Cyclizine

C Diazepam

D Prednisolone

E Rosiglitazone

71. A 28-year-old woman has had a severe headache for the past 2 weeks. Her family doctor examines her eyes. The left eye constricts directly to light with a consensual response in the right. However, as he swings the torch from the left to the right eye, he notes that both pupils appear to dilate. Which would be the *single* most accurate explanation of this finding? ★ ★ ★

A Argyll Robertson's pupil on the right

B Myotonic right pupil

C Normal variation

D Raised intracranial pressure

E Relative afferent pupillary defect on the right

72. A 32-year-old man claims he has taken 30 temazepam 20mg tablets 5h ago. He has a long history of depression and recurrent suicide attempts. He smells of alcohol, his speech is slurred, and he has an unsteady gait.

```
RR 12/min, SaO₂ 96% on air.
```

```
Chest: scattered crepitations.
```

Which is the *single* most appropriate next step? ★ ★ ★ ★

A Activated charcoal

B Flumazenil IV

C Neurological observations until consciousness level improves

D Urgent referral to the Intensive Therapy Unit for intubation and ventilation

E Urinary alkalinization

73. An 82-year-old woman has rapidly become unable to speak. Her family report that she has been increasingly tired over the last 3 weeks and latterly has been restricted to sitting in a chair. Prior to this, she walked with a stick and was independent with regard to all activities of daily living. She is awake but not able to follow commands and is therefore difficult to examine.

```
T 38.4°C, HR 105bpm, BP 100/65mmHg.
```

Tone and reflexes are globally increased with equivocal plantars but no focal neurology. Which *single* investigation is the most likely to produce a definitive diagnosis? ★ ★ ★ ★

A Blood culture

B CT scan of the brain

C Electroencephalogram (EEG)

D Lumbar puncture

E MRI of the brain

EXTENDED MATCHING QUESTIONS

Collapse ?cause

For each patient, choose the *single* most likely diagnosis from the list of options below. Each option may be used once, more than once, or not at all. ★

A Aortic stenosis

B Arrhythmia

C Carotid sinus syncope

D Drop attack

E Epileptic seizure

F Hypertrophic obstructive cardiomyopathy

G Hypoglycaemic attack

H Micturition syncope

I Narcolepsy

J Non-epileptiform attack disorder

K Orthostatic hypotension

L Transient ischaemic attack

M Vasovagal syncope

1. A 35-year-old man collapsed but remembers nothing of the event, which happened 20min ago. This is the third time it has happened this week. His wife says he fell to the ground and his body jerked for several minutes during which time he was unresponsive. He did not bite his tongue or wet himself and he has no external injuries. He takes no prescribed or recreational drugs.
T 36.2°C, HR 80bpm BP 125/70mmHg.
Glasgow Coma Scale score (GCS): 15/15.
CT head: normal.
Blood tests: normal.

2. A 71-year-old man collapsed getting off the bus and was unable to regain his feet. He did not lose consciousness and remembers the whole event. He takes metformin for type 2 diabetes and has hypertension.
T 36.0°C, HR 70bpm, BP 105/70mmHg.

3. A 63-year-old man collapsed while running across the road and lost consciousness for a short period. He thinks he has been more breathless recently and has started to use sublingual glyceryl trinitrate while out walking.
T 36.3°C, HR 75bpm, BP 140/100mmHg.

4. A 42-year-old woman lost consciousness while standing on a busy train. She became hot and nauseated and her vision 'closed in' before she collapsed. She was witnessed to have jerked a few times on the ground before she regained consciousness. She has never had anything like this before and feels fine now.
T 36.2°C, HR 72bpm, BP 130/70mmHg.

5. A 66-year-old man has collapsed at home. He is still unable to communicate with the staff in the Emergency Department 1h later. His wife reports that he has been more argumentative and aggressive in recent months.
T 36.4°C, HR 77bpm, BP 140/80mmHg.
GCS: 11/15.

Causes of speech deficits

For each patient with a speech deficit, choose the *single* most likely anatomical site for the lesion responsible from the list of options below. Each option may be used once, more than once, or not at all. ★ ★ ★

A Basal ganglia

B Cerebellum

C Corpus callosum

D Frontal lobe

E Inferior parietal lobe (dominant)

F Inferior temporal lobe (dominant)

G Inferolateral frontal lobe (dominant)

H Internal capsule

I Lower motor neurone

J Neuromuscular junction

K Occipital lobe

L Posterior temporoparietal lobe (dominant)

M Superior parietal lobe (dominant)

N Superior temporal lobe (dominant)

6. A 72-year-old man can produce only a limited range of words with a great deal of effort. He uses the same few words for many different situations. He struggles to get the exact pronunciations right and appears very frustrated by his shortcomings.

7. A 42-year-old woman talks in short, clipped sentences. She tries hard to enunciate every syllable but does run some together – particularly the last sounds of longer words. Her speech is irregular in volume but of a regular, almost automated rhythm and tone.

8. A 48-year-old man talks very slowly and quietly. He is unable to enunciate his words correctly. His speech is nasal with air coming out of his nose as he talks.

9. An 81-year-old woman appears to have no problems with the production of speech. She talks fluently and at a good rate. However, on closer listening, there are lots of grammatical errors and inappropriate – often made-up – words used. She does not correct herself and responds to questions inappropriately.

10. A 47-year-old woman has difficulty controlling the pitch of her voice. The longer she speaks the quieter her voice becomes. As it quietens, it also becomes more slurred and of one tone.

Investigating a collapse

For each patient, choose the *single* option that is most likely to determine the underlying diagnosis, from the list of options below. Each option may be used once, more than once, or not at all. ★

A 0.5ml of 1:1000 epinephrine IM

B 12-lead ECG

C 24h ECG

D Abdominal ultrasound scan

E Blood alcohol level

F Blood glucose level

G Chest X-ray

H CT scan of the head

I Echocardiogram

J Electroencephalogram (EEG)

K Full blood count

L Full neurological assessment

M Intercostal chest drain

N Lumbar puncture

O Pulse oximetry

P Thoracic needle decompression

Q Treatment dose low molecular weight heparin

R Video telemetry

11. A 24-year-old man has been found slumped on the floor of his office. His colleagues say that in the past month he has lost quite a lot of weight, looked very tired, and at times been quite confused and aggressive. He feels sweaty and is slurring his words.

12. A 63-year-old man collapses on the way to his renal outpatients appointment. He has a packet of alfacalcidol in his pocket.
BP 110/65mmHg (sitting), 88/60mmHg (standing).

13. A 72-year-old man has lost consciousness and has fallen a number of times in the last month. He has no chest pain and gets no warning that these are going to occur. His wife says he goes white and his arms twitch and about 30s later he goes pink again.

14. A 68-year-old man is undergoing a CT scan of his chest with contrast to investigate a suspicious-looking lesion on his chest X-ray. Soon after the scan begins, he feels very short of breath and faint.

15. A 28-year-old woman has collapsed while playing tennis. She felt very short of breath before the event but recovered quickly. This is the fourth time this has happened in recent weeks. Her father died in his sleep 18 years ago at the age of 32.

Causes of headache

For each patient with a headache, choose the *single* most likely diagnosis from the list of options below. Each option may be used once, more than once, or not at all. ★ ★ ★

A Benign intracranial hypertension

B Cervical spondylosis

C Cluster headache

D Giant cell arteritis

E Meningitis

F Migraine

G Sinusitis

H Space-occupying lesion

I Subarachnoid haemorrhage

J Tension headache

K Trigeminal neuralgia

16. A 40-year-old man has pain around his right eye. It develops rapidly, lasts 30–40min and has happened once or twice daily for the last 2 weeks. His eye becomes watery and bloodshot. He had similar headaches 6 months ago, but they resolved without treatment after a month.

17. A 30-year-old woman has a headache over her right eye. She feels nauseated and has vomited several times. Loud sounds and brushing her hair produce pain. These headaches have been happening for the last 2 years, often at times of increased stress at work.

18. A 52-year-old man develops a headache after shaving. It starts as a sharp, stabbing pain but only lasts for a few seconds. The same problem occurs later that evening as he is eating his dinner.

19. A 29-year-old woman has had a frontal headache for the last 12h. She is also feeling increasingly drowsy. She has not felt well for the last 24h, initially complaining of pains in her legs and cold hands and feet.

20. A 33-year-old woman has woken in the morning with a headache for the last 3 weeks. It generally improves as the day goes on, but is aggravated by coughing. She has started vomiting once or twice daily.

ANSWERS

Single Best Answers

1. C ★   OHCM 8th edn → p370

Feeling faint or dizzy on standing up is suggestive of postural hypotension. It is a feature of hypovolaemia, autonomic dysfunction, and – as here – adrenal gland dysfunction. After long-term steroid use, normal hormone production by the adrenals is suppressed. As it will take some time for endogenous production to restart, patients need to be gradually weaned off steroids to avoid a period of 'hypo-adrenalism' and the dangerous symptoms that go with it.

The other options are all features of prolonged steroid use.

2. C ★

Rectal diazepam remains the first-line therapy for seizures occurring outside the hospital setting. They are usually kept at home by the family in case they are needed. It has very short-acting anticonvulsant properties (20min as opposed to 12h for lorazepam) and can therefore be given again after 15min if status is threatening. An alternative – but currently unlicensed – treatment is buccal midazolam, which may be easier to administer.

A It may be necessary to contact help if the seizure continues for longer than 30min or another seizure starts straight after the first.

B It is certainly sensible to move anything out of the path of someone having a seizure.

D This is not given PR.

E Holding the person down is liable to cause more harm than good and may result in injury and greater post-ictal muscle fatigue.

→ http://www.nice.org.uk/Guidance/CG20 (Epilepsy. NICE Clinical Guideline 20, 2004.)

3. A ★

The anterior interosseous nerve arises from the median nerve about 5cm above the medial epicondyle supplying the flexor digitorum profundus and the flexor pollicis longus muscles. It can be compromised by direct trauma or by compression by surrounding muscles (pronator teres), ligaments, or scar tissue. The result is the inability to pinch the thumb and forefinger together (in the way shown in Figure 8.1) and thus difficulty with fine motor pincer movements.

4. C ★

There are three symptoms described: postural falls, urinary retention, and constipation. Whilst they may occur in someone who is cognitively impaired, dementia itself does not cause them. They are all processes modulated by the autonomic system and likely to be affected by diabetes. Whilst they can co-exist with Parkinson's disease in the 'Parkinson's plus' syndrome multisystem atrophy, there is no hint of Parkinsonism in this patient.

5. A ★   OHCM 8th edn → p504

All the other options can occur in any case of facial nerve palsy. Only A is seen in Bell's (idiopathic) palsy due to hyperacusis from stapedius palsy.

6. C ★

In the treatment of Bell's palsy, there is moderate quality evidence that, for presentation within 72h of the onset of symptoms, there is improved function at 4 months if prednisolone is given with aciclovir as opposed to prednisolone alone.

BMJ Clinical Evidence Handbook. United Health Foundation, 2008.

7. E ★

This is benign essential tremor, a rhythmic tremor (4–12Hz) that is only present when the affected muscle groups are moved. It can be worsened by stress, demands to perform a task under pressure, the cold, caffeine, and some drugs. It usually improves following small amounts of alcohol and β-blockers.

A This can be a side effect of salbutamol, but is more likely to occur intermittently after overuse of the drug rather than progressively and constantly.

B AND D Micrographia and resting tremor are features of Parkinson's disease, which would be more likely to begin in just one hand.

C This is also true of Parkinson's disease, whilst the opposite is true in essential tremor.

8. E ★   OHCM 8th edn → p502

The gradual presentation together with a 'normal' MRI scan of the brain and raised intracranial pressure suggest a diagnosis of benign intracranial hypertension. This is associated with obesity in young women and would be consistent with use of the pancreatic lipase inhibitor orlistat, which is used as a drug treatment for obesity.

Caffeine (B), smoking (D), and a strong family history (C) would all add weight to a convincing history of migraine, whilst a family history of a cerebral tumour at a much older age (A) is unlikely to be relevant at this stage.

9. B ★

The junior doctor has elicited Brudzinski's neck sign. As with Kernig's sign, this a notoriously insensitive marker of meningeal irritation. Even though it is very specific, the fact that it has been absent in 95% of proven cases of meningitis in some studies has led people to question its value in the pre-treatment work-up of meningitis. It is however, quick to perform, non-invasive, and may be of use in borderline cases.

Thomas KE, Hasbun R, Jekel J, and Quagliarello VJ (2002). The diagnostic accuracy of Kernig's sign, Bruzinski's sign, and nuchal rigidity in adults with suspected meningitis. Clin Infect Dis **35**:46–52.

10. B ★   OHCM 8th edn → p502

It can be difficult to consider metastatic disease as a diagnosis if there is no knowledge of a primary. However, the gradual onset of neurological symptoms over a 2-week period essentially rules out a vascular process and thus all other options. They would all cause symptoms much more suddenly than in this case: in minutes for A, minutes to hours for C, seconds for D and minutes to hours (resolving <24h) for E.

The fact that symptoms continue to develop suggests that there is an ongoing process. In this case, it is due to the worsening oedema surrounding the mass. Given the discovery of an intracerebral mass, it would be essential to try to identify a primary (e.g. breast, bowel, skin), although the intracerebral mass may itself be the primary.

11. D ★   OHCM 8th edn → p488

This man presents with confusion. He has a temperature and is tachycardic, tachypnoeic, and hypoxic. Even before examining his chest, he should be suspected of having a chest infection causing systemic upset and an acute confusional state.

A These are used in the work-up after a transient ischaemic attack, which is unlikely to present with confusion as, by definition, sufferers return to normal very quickly.

B These are part of a dementia screen; dementia is unlikely to present so suddenly and should not be suspected until sepsis has been excluded.

C An acute coronary syndrome can present with delirium but there is no suggestion of cardiac dysfunction in this case.

E These are used to investigate diabetic ketoacidosis; hypoglycaemia is more likely to cause delirium.

12. D ★

This is often weakened in carpal tunnel syndrome and tests abductor pollicis brevis innervated by the median nerve.

A This tests the dorsal interossei (ulnar nerve).

B This tests the extensor carpi radialis longus (radial nerve).

C This is Finkelstein's test for De Quervain's tenosynovitis.

E This tests the dorsal interossei/abductor digiti minimi (ulnar nerve).

13. A ★   OHCM 8th edn → p506

This is 'cubital tunnel syndrome', which has been caused by intra-operative compromise and compression of the ulnar nerve at the elbow. The second commonest entrapment neuropathy to carpal tunnel syndrome, the ulnar nerve is particularly vulnerable around the elbow.

B This tests the opponens pollicis (median nerve).

C This tests wrist extension (radial nerve).

D This tests the pronator teres (median nerve).

E This tests wrist flexion (median nerve).

14. D ★

The sudden-onset weakness in combination with slurred speech in an elderly patient who has been admitted with atrial fibrillation should serve as an alert to a possible stroke.

A This might explain some of the nocturnal delirium.

B AND C   These are consistent with a fall.

E This is due to the urinary tract infection.

15. D ★

This man's head tilt is characteristic of a trochlear nerve lesion: patients usually tilt away from the side of the lesion in order to reduce their diplopia. The trochlear nerve has three roles: intorsion, depression, and abduction of the globe. It is most commonly disturbed by head trauma, but can be affected – as here – in microvasculopathies such as diabetes. The diplopia is worse on downward gaze and gaze away from the affected muscle.

A, B AND E These occur together in palsies of the oculomotor nerve and result in an eye resting in the 'down and out' position.

C Patients with left lateral rectus palsy cannot fully abduct the affected eye and so develop an esotropia (convergent squint) and resulting diplopia.

16.A ★

In someone with poorly controlled seizures, there should always be rigorous discussion as to the levels of concordance. If there remain doubts as to the patient's adherence to the prescribed medication, then NICE guidance is that this is an indication for monitoring the blood levels of the medication. Ideally, this should happen in the outpatient setting with the aim of preventing admission to hospital.

→ http://www.nice.org.uk/Guidance/CG20 (Epilepsy. NICE Clinical Guideline 20, 2004.)

17.D ★   OHCM 8th edn → pp494–497

This man has had his second tonic–clonic seizure and has presented with a reduced GCS, in the post-ictal phase.

A This usually occurs against a background of daytime somnolence (narcolepsy).

B This generally occurs in older people, usually women.

C This was known previously as 'pseudoseizures'. It is often difficult to tell apart from primary generalized epilepsy, but would not be the case in a man with a low GCS score following the seizure.

E He would not be as drowsy following a simple faint.

18.B ★   OHCM 8th edn → p802

This woman's Glasgow Coma Scale score is 9 (E2, V2, M5). Her airway has become partially obstructed and this simple manoeuvre will help open it. A head tilt should not be attempted, to protect the cervical spine, which has not been cleared following a significant fall from height.

19.B ★   OHCM 8th edn → p486

The man is showing the symptoms of a rising intracranial pressure (ICP). The CT scan shows blood in the extradural space. Typical of this type of bleed is the 'lucid interval' in which consciousness holds steady for several days after the initial insult before the rising ICP takes its toll. Unlike a subdural bleed, extradural bleeds cannot take weeks or months to declare themselves.

A This could be due to any infective cause.

C This could occur in a subdural bleed.

D This indicates a subarachnoid hemorrhage.

E This indicates a space-occupying lesion.

20. D ★   OHCM 8th edn → p482

It can be difficult to assess the severity of headaches, especially if there are no associated symptoms. In this case, however, the continued nausea and vomiting and the focal neurology suggest a serious cause. The lateral rectus palsy may suggest the site of the aneurysm (but could also suggest an intracerebral haematoma).

A This process affects the central nervous system in multiple sclerosis; although this can present with 'eye signs', it is unlikely to do so with a headache and a mononeuropathy in a man in his 60s.

B Normal pressure hydrocephalus is the clinical triad of nystagmus + ataxia + urinary incontinence, none of which are features of this case.

C This is the pathological process behind >80% of strokes; it is unlikely to be accompanied by headache and nausea as in a bleed. An ischaemic stroke leads to infarction of upper motor neurones and would be more likely to cause some combination of motor or sensory loss.

E This can present with a headache but is usually associated with drowsiness and fluctuating consciousness. Intracerebral haematoma can cause localizing neurological signs (e.g. sixth nerve palsy), but this tends to happen long after the injury and onset of the headache.

21. A ★   OHCM 8th edn → p506

This is a common peroneal nerve injury, which runs a course around the neck of the fibula and has been damaged by the fracture. The other movements are all the function of the tibial nerve.

B This tests the small muscles of the foot.

C This tests the tibialis posterior (inverts the foot at the ankle).

D This tests the gastrocnemius.

E This tests the flexor digitorum longus.

22. E ★   OHCM 8th edn → p504

The scenario describes a Bell's palsy due to malfunction of all branches of the facial nerve (CN VII). Lack of frontal sparing would suggest a lower motor neurone lesion.

A Together with asymmetry of the ipsilateral tonsil, this might suggest a parotid tumour.

B AND C   Together with bleeding, headaches, and tinnitus, these might suggest a cholesteatoma.

D This suggests an upper motor neurone lesion.

23. B ★

Due to its effects on the liver, NICE guidance is that clotting studies should be performed prior to any surgery in those on sodium valproate.

→ http://www.nice.org.uk/Guidance/CG20 (Epilepsy. NICE Clinical Guideline 20, 2004.)

24. E ★

The image shows both wrist and finger drop, depicting a radial nerve injury. Up to 18% of humeral fractures are associated with radial nerve palsy, most commonly middle shaft fractures.

→ http://www.wheelessonline.com/ortho/radial_nerve_palsy_following_frx_of_the_humerus

25. A ★

After both transient ischaemic attacks (TIAs) and ischaemic strokes, two antiplatelet agents should be prescribed for the prevention of further vascular events. An alternative is clopidogrel monotherapy (but not clopidogrel + dipyridamole as in C).

B High-dose aspirin should be started after an ischaemic stroke and continued for at least 14 days.

E Patients who are in atrial fibrillation and suffer either a TIA or an ischaemic stroke should be offered anticoagulation therapy.

→ http://www.sign.ac.uk/pdf/qrg108.pdf

26. E ★

Recurrent episodes of neurological disturbance in someone with hypertension are highly suggestive of transient ischaemic attacks (TIAs). The diagnosis would be clinched by the rapid resolution of symptoms (<24h). Given the high rates of stroke in those who suffer TIAs, this woman needs to have an ultrasound scan of her carotids with a view to an urgent endarterectomy.

27. A ★   OHCM 8th edn → p480

A neurological disturbance that lasts <24h is the definition of a transient ischaemic attack (TIA). The temporary occlusion of the cerebrovasculature is either due to an embolus from the carotids or from a heart that has valve disease, a post-myocardial infarction thrombus, or – as in this case – is fibrillating.

B This describes Raynaud's phenomenon.

C If >2 beats and not just at the extremities of gaze, this is suggestive of a cerebellar or vestibular lesion.

D This is found in giant cell arteritis, which can mimic a TIA but only rarely.

E This is a non-specific finding, although unilateral pulse weakness has been described in patients with systemic sclerosis, thoracic outlet syndrome, and Takayasu's arteritis.

28. E ★

Do not attempt to drop blood pressure acutely (due to the risk of inadequate cerebral perfusion). Instead, concentrate on diagnosing and treating fevers and discrepancies in blood sugar.

29. A ★

Aspiration signifies the inhalation of gastric contents into the lower airways, which then causes an infective process. Most at risk are those who cannot protect their own airway, as in the early stages after a stroke. Whilst this patient is at risk of all options after a stroke, her chest signs and hypoxia are most suggestive of A: the doctor who sees her in this condition should certainly investigate her with blood cultures and a chest X-ray and treat her with IV antibiotics to include cover for anaerobes.

30. C ★

At 15min, this woman is still in 'early' status. According to NICE guidelines, she therefore needs a bolus of lorazepam along with her usual anti-epileptic drugs (if she is on any). Only when her status becomes 'established' (30–60min) should a phenytoin infusion be started. Fifteen minutes is too early to contact an anaesthetist, but may be appropriate if the team are particularly concerned or lacking in experience.

→ http://www.nice.org.uk/nicemedia/pdf/CG020fullguideline_appendixC_corrected.pdf

31. A ★

When starting a statin, patients should be made aware of the risks of developing a myopathy and advised to report any muscle weakness or pain as soon as it develops. In this event, it is important to measure the creatine kinase (CK) promptly. If it is more than five times the upper limit or if myopathy is suspected on clinical grounds (as in this case), then treatment should be discontinued. If symptoms resolve and levels of CK return to normal, then the statin could be tentatively reintroduced, or an alternative could be considered.

Wierzbicki AS (2002). Statins: myalgia and myositis. Brit J Cardiol 9:193–194.

→ http://www.bjcardio.co.uk/pdf/709/Vol9_Num4_April_2002_p193-194.pdf

32. C ★

Rupture of supraspinatus is the most common rotator cuff injury. The supraspinatus muscle arises from the supraspinous fossa on the scapula and inserts into the greater tubercle of the humerus. The infraspinatus and teres minor insert here as well, with the subscapularis inserting into the lesser tubercle.

33. D ★   OHCM 8th edn → p506

This is a radial nerve injury which runs a course in a groove around the mid-shaft of the humerus and has been damaged by the fracture.

A This tests the opponens pollicis (median nerve).

B AND C These test the palmar interossei (ADductors) and dorsal interossei (ABductors) (both ulnar nerve).

E This tests the forearm flexors (median nerve).

34. C ★

This man has a foot drop and weak eversion: symptoms of a common peroneal nerve lesion. The common peroneal nerve is commonly damaged by trauma to the lateral side of the knee. It is here that it winds around the head of the fibula covered only by skin and subcutaneous tissue. After entering the peroneus longus muscle, it divides into deep and superficial branches. It is the superficial branch that provides sensory innervation to the skin of the lower lateral calf and dorsum of the foot. The deep branch is primarily a motor nerve.

→ http://emedicine.medscape.com/article/1141734-overview

35. A ★

C and E suggest the autonomic complications associated with multisystem atrophy, whilst B and D reflect two symptoms (defective vertical gaze and dementia) common in progressive supranuclear palsy. Parkinsonism is a syndrome of tremor, rigidity, bradykinesis and loss of postural reflexes. Parkinson's disease is one cause of Parkinsonism.

36. B ★

NICE recommend that, if there is any suspicion of a patient having Parkinson's disease, they should be referred to a neurologist or a physician with an interest in Parkinson's disease, before drug treatment is initiated. This is to reduce misdiagnosis, unnecessary treatment, and the use of increasingly complex drug regimes.

37. D ★

Both C and E could represent the aura prior to a partial seizure, whilst neither tongue biting nor urinary incontinence occur in every case of an epileptic seizure. The history certainly suggests a case of vasovagal syncope and, although the brief jerks may have made the junior doctor think of epilepsy, the story as a whole is not concerning for this. In cases of probable syncope, NICE guidelines state that an EEG should not be performed (due to possible false positives). An EEG should only be used to support a diagnosis of epilepsy in those in whom the history is suggestive.

→ http://www.nice.org.uk/Guidance/CG20 (Epilepsy. NICE Clinical Guideline 20, 2004.)

38. E ★

These used to be called 'pseudoseizures' and although the diagnosis of NEAD is one of exclusion, this presentation with rapid recovery (GCS 15/15) very soon after the attack is suggestive. It is commoner in females and young adults and occurs more often in those who have family members who have seizures or if they suffer from depression or anxiety. Childhood sexual abuse has also been shown to be associated.

B AND D These would be associated with a much slower recovery and in this age group would be most likely to have happened before (although of course, first fits are possible at any age).

A A space-occupying lesion would be likely to have caused some symptoms before this episode.

C These are more common in the older population and feature sudden leg weakness and instant recovery.

39. C ★   OHCM 8th edn → p516

The scenario describes fatiguable weakness affecting several muscle groups: extraocular (ptosis), bulbar ('too tired to eat'), and limb girdle ('struggles to lift anything'). This pattern is strongly suggestive of myasthenia gravis, which is above all a disease of muscles.

This woman has acute lower limb weakness and what sounds like an optic neuritis. Although MS can present in a variety of ways, these are two of the most common initial symptoms. More commonly, patients present with one symptom that improves only for another different problem to develop some time later. Anyone in this demographic who gives a history of flitting, seemingly unlinked (by time and space) neurological problems should raise suspicions and prompt an in-depth history and careful examination.

A Amyotrophic lateral sclerosis is a pattern of motor neurone disease. It typically begins with insidious muscle weakness that develops into twitching, cramping, and then stiffness. The sequence of symptoms varies from person to person, but it would be unlikely that a sufferer would deteriorate as rapidly as the woman in this case.

B Guillain–Barré syndrome could cause such rapid weakness but not with upgoing plantars and it would not affect eye movements. It often occurs following a viral illness.

D Quaternary syphilis can cause an ataxic gait and numbness but not such rapidly weak legs.

E This can give rise to paraesthesia and a peripheral neuropathy, but these are likely to develop gradually and not cause weakness.

Classical migraine (which can be triggered by the oral contraceptive pill) is associated with an aura, which is often teichopsia (a transient visual sensation of flashing lights/colours), usually followed by the headache within the hour.

A This indicates trigeminal neuralgia; it can be associated with multiple sclerosis and tumours, usually in older women.

C This indicates a cluster headache, occurring once or twice in a 24h period for 4–12 weeks but then followed by sometimes 1–2 years without symptoms.

D This indicates raised intracranial pressure; it is also associated with vomiting, personality changes, seizures, and progressive focal neurology.

E This indicates a tension headache, 'like a tight band around the head' and often provoked by home/work stress and associated with low mood.

This is appropriate first-line treatment for migraine prophylaxis at a dose of 80–240mg daily. Opioids (B) can cause a medication overuse headache and dependence and should not be used. The other options are useful second-line options: tricyclic antidepressants (A) and antiepileptics (D and E).

Duncan CW, Watson DPB, and Stein A (2008). Diagnosis and management of headache in adults: summary of SIGN guidelines. BMJ **337**:a2329.

43. A ★

This man has headaches of recent onset with features of raised intracranial pressure. A 'normal' fundoscopy examination will not be able to definitively rule out papilloedema and with this history an urgent referral for investigations is warranted.

B This is raised in carcinoid syndrome.

C AND E   These are reasonable treatments for migraines.

D This would be indicated if temporal arteritis was suspected.

44. B ★

It is difficult to assess for neurological deficits in those that have been drinking. Guidance is therefore that these people should be admitted. Furthermore, if there are any signs of a basal skull fracture, then a CT head scan should be performed. B refers to Battle's sign (ecchymosis of the mastoid process) and along with periorbital ecchymosis, cerebrospinal fluid rhino/otorrhoea, and haemotympanum should prompt urgent imaging.

A This is not a significant finding in assessment of a head injury.

C This might suggest alcohol withdrawal but is unlikely in this situation.

D This is a cerebellar sign.

E This is positive in conditions causing sensory ataxia

→ http://www.nice.org.uk/Guidance/CG56#documents

(Head Injury. NICE Clinical Guideline 56, 2007.)

45. A ★

It can be difficult to be clear about the management of head injuries, but, broadly summarized, CT scans should be performed on those with normal consciousness but a skull fracture and all those with abnormal consciousness. (Note that it is not just skull fractures that demand imaging in those with a Glasgow Coma Scale score of 15/15; others are persisting severe headache, nausea and vomiting, irritability or altered behaviour, and a seizure.)

By this rationale, the patient in this case deserves a CT head scan. This is because the chances of finding intracranial pathology in someone with disturbed consciousness is 20% whilst in someone who is fully conscious and has no other features, the chances are <1%.

C This is not used in the acute setting for head injuries

D In those who are drowsy or confused, it might be acceptable to observe them for at most 4h from the time of injury; if they have still failed to recover full consciousness, it would then be appropriate to request a CT head scan.

E If a CT is planned, there is no need to carry out a skull X-ray. These are used in those situations where a CT is not planned but there is evidence of skull fracture.

→ http://www.sign.ac.uk/guidelines/fulltext/46/section5.html

46. B ★   OHCM 8th edn → p716

The history given is suggestive of Guillain–Barré syndrome, a peripheral neuropathy triggered by infection but actually caused by the inflammatory response that follows (antibodies attacking nerve cells).

47. C ★

This man is now in established status epilepticus. He has received the necessary drug treatments (bolus + subsequent infusion of antiepileptic drugs) and is heading towards the general anaesthesia phase. Prior to this, an anaesthetist and thus the Intensive Therapy Unit (ITU) should be contacted. An anaesthetist will be needed to protect this man's airway and oversee the administration of a drug like propofol, whilst the ITU should be preparing itself to accept this man who will need close monitoring and possibly EEG monitoring.

→ http://www.nice.org.uk/Guidance/CG20

(Epilepsy. NICE Clinical Guidelines 20, 2004.)

48. D ★

Although tiredness and fatigue can occur with syncope, confusion lasting more than 2min after regaining consciousness should be regarded as a sign that this woman may well have had a seizure. Urinary incontinence can occur with syncope if the bladder was full at the time of the attack. A deep bite of the lateral border of the tongue is suggestive of a seizure but the tongue can also be bitten during a syncopal episode. Twitching and jerking can occur due to simple hypoxia but tonic and then clonic movements for more than 1min should be regarded as suspicious of a seizure.

McCory D and McCorry A (2007). Collapse with loss of awareness. BMJ **334**:153.

49. A ★

According to NICE guidelines, there are four circumstances in which the emergency services should be contacted:

1) If seizures develop into status epilepticus.

2) If there is a high risk of recurrence.

3) If it is a first fit.

4) If there is difficulty monitoring the individual's condition.

A second fit starting before the person has regained consciousness is one of the definitions of status, the other being seizures lasting >30min.

→ http://www.nice.org.uk/guidance/index.jsp?action=download&o=29530

(Epilepsy in Children and Young People: Quick Reference Guide. NICE Clinical Guideline 20, 2004.)

50. B ★   OHCM 8th edn → p486

The history suggests and the image confirms the diagnosis of a subdural haematoma. The only immediate course of action for the junior doctor is to ask for a neurosurgical opinion with a view to irrigating the clot. A lumbar puncture (D) would be dangerous in this setting (probable raised intracranial pressure), steroids (C) would not reduce the raised intracranial pressure (they just reduce oedema around tumours), there is no suggestion of meningo-encephalitis (A), and there is no need for further imaging (E).

51. A ★

The image shows a lesion at Broca's area causing an expressive dysphasia, characterized by slow and non-fluent speech.

B This would indicate receptive dysphasia.

C This would indicate Parkinson's disease.

D This would indicate pseudobulbar palsy.

E This is cerebellar speech.

52. B ★   OHCM 8th edn → p506

This man is unable to plantar flex or invert his foot due to an injury to the tibial nerve. The tibial nerve supplies a sensory branch to the sole of the foot and a motor branch to the hamstrings, tibialis posterior, gastrocnemius, flexor digitorum longus, and the small muscles of the foot.

A AND C   Both movements – dorsiflexion and eversion of the
foot – are powered by the common peroneal nerve.

E   This tests the quadriceps femoris (femoral nerve).

D   This tests the gluteus maximus (inferior gluteus nerve).

53. C ★

This is carpal tunnel syndrome and can occur in pregnancy as
a result of fluid retention causing compression of the median nerve
in the carpal tunnel below the flexor retinaculum.

A   This is the radial nerve.

B   This is the ulnar nerve.

D   This is the anterior interosseus branch of the median nerve,
but if the site of symptoms arose from here, there would be
weakness of wrist flexion due to the innervations of the
forearm flexors.

E   This is the ulnar nerve.

54. D ★★

This is carcinomatous meningitis whereby metastasis has occurred
from the primary to the meninges; imaging may show the suggestion
of meningeal uptake – an MRI is more likely to do so than a CT
scan – but the best way to detect malignant cells in the meninges is
via a lumbar puncture.

Chamberlain MC and Kormanik PR (1997). Carcinomatous
meningitis secondary to breast cancer: predictors of response to
combined modality therapy. J Neurooncol **35**:55–64.

55. B ★★

The brief history is suggestive of cerebral space-occupying masses.
The MRI scan (coronal view) shows multiple discrete ring enhancing
lesions. Differentials for these appearances include metastases
(most commonly from lung, kidney, breast, melanoma, and colon),
demyelination, multiple infarcts, and in patients who are HIV
positive, lymphoma. However, in those who have been on long-term
immunosuppression like this woman, the most likely cause
are abscesses. They are different from metastases in that they
cause surrounding oedema and have thinner walls. The most
common infections that can cause multiple small lesions are
toxoplasmosis, cryptococcosis, and cysticercosis.

Chapman S and Nakielny R (eds) (2003). Aids to Radiological
Differential Diagnosis, 4th edn. Saunders.

56. D ★★

The symptoms and signs (ptosis, miosis, and anhidrosis) described are those of Horner's syndrome and of nerve impingement (C8–T2). In an ex-smoker who continues to cough, this could be explained by an apical lung tumour (Pancoast's tumour) that is impacting on both brachial and cervical sympathetic plexuses.

57. E ★★   OHCM 8th edn → p506

When two peripheral nerves are compromised, the confusing term mononeuritis multiplex is used. It is rare but is associated with diabetes, some vasculitides, and rheumatoid arthritis.

A This does not affect peripheral nerves, rather a range of functions including postural blood pressure, sweating, and bladder and bowel function.

B The main example of this is multiple sclerosis.

C This would be the most likely cause of an isolated nerve lesion.

D The classical inflammatory neuropathy is Guillain–Barré syndrome: an acute, mainly motor demyelinating neuropathy.

58. C ★★   OHCM 8th edn → p502

Evolving neurological signs against a background of headache and personality changes are highly suspicious of an intracranial space-occupying lesion. Immediate management should consist of treating the associated cerebral oedema with steroids.

A This is used for thrombolysis of those presenting within 4.5h with the symptoms of an ischaemic stroke (see link below).

B This is used in the acute treatment of transient ischaemic attack and stroke.

D This is a calcium channel blocker used occasionally in the treatment of malignant hypertension. A headache and visual disturbance is possible with a BP >200/140mmHg, but it is unlikely to be associated with other gross neurological changes.

E This can be used to relieve the symptoms of benign intracranial hypertension; this is a key differential diagnosis in these cases and may turn out to be the cause if brain imaging is normal. Whilst investigations are pending, however, cases of raised intracranial pressure together with evolving neurology and personality changes need to be treated as if for a space-occupying lesion.

→ http://www.sign.ac.uk/pdf/qrg108.pdf

59. C ★★

The registrar wants his junior to use the Bamford classification system. This woman has motor weakness and higher cortical dysfunction (dysphasia), therefore scoring 2/3 (she doesn't score for hemianopia). Cerebellar or brain stem signs indicate a posterior circulation infarct, whilst A does not exist. The system is quick and easy to use, adds weight to out-of-hours radiology or neurology referrals ('Hi, I have a 78-year-old who's having what looks like an acute PACI on the ward…') and is informative with regard to prognosis. The definitions according to the Bamford classification system are:

- Total anterior circulation infarct (TACI). All of the following:
  - Higher dysfunction (decreased level of consciousness, dysphasia, visuospatial)
  - Homonymous hemianopia
  - Motor/sensory deficit (>2/3 face/arm/leg).
- Partial anterior circulation infarct (PACI).
  - Any two of the three features of TACI or
  - Higher dysfunction alone or
  - Limited motor sensory deficit.
- Posterior circulation infarct (POCI). Any of the following:
  - Cranial nerve palsy and CL motor/sensory deficit
  - Bilateral motor/sensory deficit
  - Conjugate eye movement problems
  - Cerebellar dysfunction
  - Isolated homonymous hemianopia.
- Lacunar infarct (LACI). Any of the following (all affecting >2/3 face/arm/leg):
  - Pure sensory deficit
  - Pure motor deficit
  - Sensorimotor deficit
  - Ataxic hemiparesis.

Must not have new dysphasia/visuospatial problem/proprioceptive loss/any vertebrobasilar features.

60. E ★★ OHCM 8th edn → p728

The acute onset of ophthalmoplegia (nystagmus as here or lateral rectus or conjugate gaze palsies), an ataxic gait, and global confusion is known as Wernicke's encephalopathy: it results from thiamine deficiency (which is common in heavy alcohol users) and can proceed to the more serious Korsakoff's syndrome (characterized by a retrograde amnesia resulting in confabulation). Untreated, mortality rates are 20% in Wernicke's and 85% in Korsakoff's. Apart from arresting the decline into Korsakoff's, thiamine has been shown variously to reverse all three clinical problems within hours.

Therefore, in any patient with one or more of the three symptoms and no other more likely cause, give two pairs of thiamine ampoules IV in 50–100mL 0.9% saline over 30min three times a day for 3–7 days before converting to oral thiamine.

A Aspirin is started after a transient ischaemic attack or stroke.

B This is used to treat cerebral oedema in space-occupying lesions.

C This may have a role to play in the treatment in Korsakoff's syndrome and also in Alzheimer's dementia.

D Glucagon can be used to treat hypoglycaemia, although it does not work as well in patients who have been drinking alcohol.

Day E, Bentham P, Callaghan R, Kuruvilla T, and George S (2009). Thiamine for Wernicke–Korsakoff Syndrome in people at risk from alcohol abuse. Cochrane Database Syst Rev Issue 2:CD004033.

→ http://mrw.interscience.wiley.com/cochrane/clsysrev/articles/CD004033/pdf_standard_fs.html

61. E ★★

The scenario describes a case of Churg–Strauss syndrome, which is not important: what is important is realizing that a vasculitic process should be considered as an explanation for any multisystem presentation. Churg–Strauss syndrome is a medium- and small-vessel autoimmune vasculitis that often affects the lungs, gastrointestinal system, and peripheral nerves.

62. A ★★★ OHCM 8th edn → pp460, 502

Benign intracranial hypertension presents as a mass might: headache and signs of raised intracranial pressure. Because of this, sufferers typically suffer most in the mornings.

B A cluster headache can last for this long and the pain is almost always unilateral. However, the pain comes at night more often than the morning and is accompanied by watering of the eye, which can become bloodshot and swollen.

C This is not really the right demographic: it should be suspected in those >50 years who have a persistent headache.

D Migraine is often unilateral and is probably the best differential here as it does present with strong neurological signs but it is unlikely to follow such a regular protracted course.

E Tension headache is unlikely to present as a unilateral pain: it is classically a 'tight band around the head'.

63. B ★ ★ ★

Doxazocin is an α_1 antagonist and is used in the treatment of benign prostatic hypertrophy and hypertension, although it is usually the third- or fourth-line treatment. The most likely cause of the collapse is a postural drop in blood pressure, which can occur after the first dose.

A Alendronate is associated largely with gastrointestinal side effects.

C Metformin cannot cause hypoglycaemic attacks.

D Rosiglitazone is associated with fluid retention and can precipitate heart failure, but not chest pain or shortness of breath in this scenario.

E Salbutamol in high doses can cause tremor, tachycardia, and agitation, but is unlikely to cause a collapse.

64. D ★ ★ ★

Confusion is common following surgery, especially in the elderly. This woman has a few features particular to the diagnosis: alcohol withdrawal. This classically presents between 10 and 72h after admission with hypotension, tachycardia, and visual/tactile hallucinations. She should be given generous amounts of chlordiazepoxide (a benzodiazepine) for the first 3 days, which is then gradually reduced.

65. A ★ ★ ★

This woman has had a transient ischaemic attack (TIA) and is in atrial fibrillation (AF). According to NICE guidelines, she needs to be anticoagulated, but before this can happen, a recent infarct and a haemorrhagic cerebral event need to be excluded, hence the CT. If she had had a stroke, then the guidance is that a CT scan is performed to exclude haemorrhage, and warfarin is started 2 weeks later.

The decision to anticoagulate is not based on neurological findings (D) or the rate of AF (E) and should not be postponed (B). All those in AF should be risk stratified for stroke. As this woman has just had a TIA, she immediately becomes high risk. Other high risk criteria are:

1) Previous ischaemic stroke or thromboembolic event.

2) Age >75 years with hypertension, diabetes, or vascular disease.

3) Clinical evidence of valve disease, or heart failure of left ventricular dysfunction on echocardiography.

Unless there are contraindications, all those in the high-risk group should be anticoagulated with warfarin to a target INR of 2.5.

→ http://www.nice.org.uk/nicemedia/pdf/word/CG036niceguideline word.doc

(Atrial Fibrillation. NICE Clinical Guideline 36, 2006.)

66. B ★ ★ ★

In most cases, anti-epileptic treatment does not start until after a second seizure. However, NICE guidance highlights four situations in which it should be started after the first seizure:

1) The individual has a neurological deficit.

2) The electroencephalogram (EEG) shows unequivocal epileptiform activity.

3) The individual considers risk of further seizures unacceptable.

4) Imaging shows a structural abnormality.

Although this woman's deficit is likely to be temporary (Todd's paresis following a seizure involving the motor cortex), it is a sign that the seizure was likely to be epileptic in origin and that the risk of recurrence is high.

→ http://www.nice.org.uk/guidance/index.jsp?action=download&o= 29530

67. B ★ ★ ★

Vomiting more than once should prompt a request for an urgent CT head scan, i.e. within 1h of arrival. Following a head injury but no immediate triggers for an urgent scan, anyone >65 years, with a dangerous mechanism of injury and amnesia of events >30min, can wait for up to 8h before the scan if out of hours.

→ http://www.nice.org.uk/CG56

(Head Injury: Triage, Assessment, Investigation and Early Management of Head Injury in Infants, Children and Adults. NICE Clinical Guideline 56, 2007.)

68. B ★ ★ ★

The relevant Sections of the section 136 of the Mental Health Act 2007 are:

Section 5(2): Doctors' Holding Power. This allows the doctor in charge of the patient's care (or an alternative nominated by this doctor) to legally detain a voluntary patient in hospital for 72h.

Section 2: Admission for Assessment. This allows assessment (and treatment) for a period of 28 days. It is often used to detain a patient during their first compulsory mental health admission to hospital.

Section 3: Admission for Treatment. This is used if continued detention and treatment is required for a patient on a Section 2 or a patient who has previously been admitted and has a firm treatment plan. Initially it is valid for 6 months, but it can be renewed for another 6 months and then a year at a time.

Section 4: Emergency Admission for Assessment. This requires only one doctor (unlike a Section 2, which requires two) and should only be used when there is not judged to be enough time to organize a Section 2. It allows admission for 72h during which time, if warranted, a second doctor can convert it into a Section 2.

Section 136: Removal of People from Public Places. Allows a police officer to take someone who they feel has a mental disorder and in need of immediate care or in the interests of the person or others, to a 'place of safety'. This allows a period of up to 72h to assess the need for an admission under Section 2.

A She might be a danger to herself or others and should not be allowed to self-discharge.

C This is not an appropriate Section in this case.

D She does not sound like she would be prepared to wait.

E Sedating her against her consent would be battery.

→ http://www.opsi.gov.uk/acts/acts2007/pdf/ukpga_20070012_en.pdf

69. C ★ ★ ★

Multiple sclerosis (MS) remains a clinical diagnosis due to an absence of pathognomonic findings. An MRI will detect plaques in the central nervous system but is non-specific. Symptoms are often seen to worsen or even present for the first time when body temperature rises, as it is thought that this slows conduction, especially through already demyelinated nerves.

A This test is used if myaesthenia gravis is suspected: this would be more likely to present with muscle weakness than paraesthesia.

B Thoracic outlet syndrome usually follows neck trauma and presents with paraesthesia and weakness in an arm due to compression of neurovascular structures at the thoracic outlet. It would be unlikely to cause such a flitting picture that attacks both arms, as in this case.

D Guillain–Barré syndrome, like MS, is a demyelinating disease. Nerve studies therefore show slowing of conduction. It is unlikely to run a course as long as this case – it runs a progressive rather than a fluctuant pattern and is more likely to affect the lower rather than the upper limbs.

E Subacute combined degeneration of the spinal cord is a reasonable differential diagnosis in cases of lower limb paraesthesia as it causes a peripheral neuropathy. It is, however, progressive rather than relapsing and remitting and unlikely in someone so young.

70. B ★ ★ ★

Cyclizine will exacerbate the extra-pyramidal symptoms of Parkinson's disease due to its central anticholinergic effects. This manifests as confusion, difficulty walking, and an increase in tone.

71. E ★ ★ ★

The 'swinging flashlight test' reveals an abnormal response in the right pupil. The fact that the right eye produces less pupillary constriction suggests an afferent defect on that side. Although it may appear that both pupils are dilating, this is just relative: they are, in fact, both trying to constrict, but failing to do so fully due to the partial afferent nerve damage that distinguishes this condition. In this case – a young woman with concurrent headache – the damage may have occurred following an optic neuritis and may be indicative of a history of multiple sclerosis. Full dilation and lack of a subsequent response would suggest a total CN II lesion.

72. C ★ ★ ★ ★

Treatment of benzodiazepine overdose is supportive with maintenance of the airway, regular assessment of consciousness level, and IV fluids.

A This and gastric lavage are no use in pure benzodiazepine overdose.

B Although flumazenil is a benzodiazepine antagonist, it is not used to reverse purposeful overdose because there is no way of being sure how much of the hypnotic has been taken. Flumazenil can trigger seizures via the benzodiazepine receptor as a result of the reduction in the seizure threshold. It is only used if the overdose has been caused during a procedure in the hospital environment.

D There is no indication for this at the moment.

E This uses sodium bicarbonate to produce urine with a pH between 7.5 and 8. This can enhance elimination of weak acids such as cocaine, tricyclic antidepressants, and salicylates.

73.D ★ ★ ★ ★

This is viral encephalitis. Cerebrospinal fluid examination obtained by a lumbar puncture is the most appropriate option. It usually shows a raised protein and lymphocyte count with a normal glucose concentration but can be normal.

A This is unlikely to help in the diagnosis.

B AND E The history is not suggestive of an abscess, space-occupying lesion, or stroke. Although imaging of the brain may aid the diagnosis, it is not the choice that will 'produce the definitive diagnosis'.

C Whilst an EEG may show sharp wave activity in one or both temporal lobes of brains with viral encephalitis, it would be used diagnostically less often than a lumbar puncture.

Extended Matching Questions

1. J ★

This was previously known as a pseudo-seizure. The man would still be drowsy 20min after a generalized seizure (post-ictal) and would most likely have bitten the lateral edge of his tongue.

2. K ★

Often caused by anti-hypertensives, a postural drop should be sought in the examination using lying/sitting and standing blood pressure readings. Metformin does not cause hypoglycaemia.

3. A ★

Exertional syncope and chest pain together with the narrow pulse pressure are due to a narrowing of the left ventricular outflow tract. An ejection systolic murmur radiating to the carotids increasing with squatting and decreasing with standing distinguishes it from the murmur associated with hypertrophic cardiomyopathy (HOCM).

4. M ★

This is a classical description of a simple faint followed by some hypoxic 'jerks', which can be mistaken for epilepsy. However, the preceding symptoms and recovery afterwards are typical of a vasovagal syncope.

5. E ★

Against the background of personality change, this man is most likely to have collapsed secondary to a brain tumour. Micturition syncope would not result in an extended change in consciousness level.

6. G ★★★

Broca's area (Figure 8.8) is the area responsible for the production of speech. Although this man understands what is being said to him (Wernicke's area is intact), he cannot generate words fluently, which leads to expressive dysphasia.

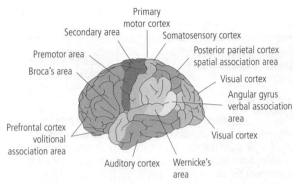

Figure 8.8

7. B ★★★

This woman has vocal symptoms typically experienced in multiple sclerosis. It is caused by ataxic muscles: dysarthria with scanning, staccato speech.

8. I ★★★

Bulbar palsy affects cranial nerves VII, IX, X, and XII causing a weakness/paralysis of the muscles involved in the articulation of speech. This is often associated with motor neurone disease, although this can also cause a pseudo-bulbar palsy – 'pseudo' because the palatal muscles are not directly affected but rendered hypertonic by an upper motor neurone lesion: the muscles become spastic and the speech harsh and strained.

9. N ★★★

This woman has fluent aphasia due to damage to Wernicke's area (see Figure 8.8): she phonates and articulates words fluently (Broca's area is intact) but these are largely meaningless – a receptive dysphasia.

10. J ★★★

These symptoms arise from fatiguing muscles in myaesthenia gravis. As she uses her muscles, the demands placed on an already depleted number of working post-synaptic acetylcholine receptor sites increases, such that interference of neuromuscular transmission starts to cause functional problems.

11. F ★

This man is a newly diagnosed diabetic in diabetic ketoacidosis. Sudden collapses need cardiac, neurological, and endocrine assessment, so a full neurological examination (L) and an ECG (B) will also be necessary. Depending on the history, a blood alcohol level (E) may be useful, as might a CT head scan (H) and, in the future, an EEG (J). However, rather than a cardiac or neurological cause, the gradual history is more suggestive of an endocrine problem.

12. K ★

Chronic kidney disease and a postural drop in blood pressure are suggestive of anaemia. Given the sudden nature of the collapse, an ECG (B), pulse oximetry (O), a full neurological examination (L), and blood glucose levels (F) would all be useful in the immediate assessment but would be less likely to get to the root of the problem.

13. C ★

This man has a classical history for Stokes–Adams attacks: syncope due to transient ventricular fibrillation or asystole. This might be captured on a 24h Holter monitor rather than a one-off ECG (B). The twitching may suggest a neurological cause, but the short-lived nature of the attacks and the late age of onset would make a neurological assessment (L), a CT head (H) and an EEG (J) the wrong path of investigation to go down.

14. A ★

This story is very suspicious of an anaphylactic reaction to the iodine contrast. The best way to determine whether it is or not is to treat it: if the patient improves, then the diagnosis is correct. Although the patient may also have chest pathology and is complaining of shortness of breath, there is no time to be wasted waiting for a chest X-ray (G). Pulse oximetry (O) would be sensible without getting to the root of the problem. The sudden nature of the breathlessness brings a pulmonary embolus and treatment with low-molecular-weight heparin (Q) into play, but the lack of pain counts against this. A pneumothorax and needle decompression (P) is also possible (and should be excluded by examination of the chest), but is less likely than a contrast reaction.

15.1 ★

Episodic breathlessness and collapse in a young person with a family history is suggestive of a cardiac cause: specifically hypertrophic cardiomyopathy. Although an ECG (B) might give some useful information, and a 24h ECG (C) may also be indicated, an echocardiogram would be more conclusive: asymmetrical septal hypertrophy would be strongly supportive of the diagnosis. A chest X-ray (G), a full blood count (K), and pulse oximetry (O) would all be part of the general work-up.

16.C ★★★

The pain is unilateral and usually affects the same side. Acute attacks can be treated with 100% oxygen or sumatriptan.

17.F ★★★

This is typical for a migrainous headache, which can occur with or, as in this example, without an aura.

18.K ★★★

An intense, stabbing pain lasting a few seconds has been triggered following stimulation of the affected area. The patient probably warrants an MRI to rule out secondary causes.

19.E ★★★

Early features are often non-specific, with meningism (neck stiffness, photophobia, and Kernig's sign), rash, and reduced consciousness being much later signs.

20.H ★★★

These are typical symptoms of raised intracranial pressure. Although evidence of papilloedema should be sought, it only occurs in 50% of cases and this woman will need a CT head scan.

CHAPTER 9

RHEUMATOLOGY

For many, rheumatology revision conjures up lists of acronyms and abbreviations pertaining to diminishingly rare, almost mythical syndromes. Then there are the seemingly overlapping symptoms of a range of similar-sounding conditions that are invariably treated by some form of steroid. The reality is that joint disease is common and debilitating but often treatable, and is therefore a core area for all those studying clinical medicine.

Even without a hefty knowledge of the area, it should be possible to ask the right questions in order to offer a concise summary of symptoms when taking a history and carrying out an examination:

- Is there any pain?

- How many joints are affected?

- Which joints?

- Is there swelling?

- Is there erythema?

- Is there loss of function?

- How is their gait?

- Is there any morning stiffness?

- Is there systemic upset?

- Are there extra-articular symptoms?

- Are there any related diseases?

- What is the patient's drug history?

In summary:

Mr R has an acute monoarthritis of the metacarpo-phalangeal joint of his right great toe. It is red, swollen, and exquisitely tender to touch, such that he cannot weight bear. He is afebrile.

There is a whitish nodule on his left ear. He has hypertension and takes bendroflumethiazide 2.5mg PO once daily.

The challenge then is to have the knowledge and confidence to suggest diagnoses and management plans. Whilst it may take years to be able to separate gout from pseudo-gout, it is within the scope of this chapter to aim to provide some of that knowledge and confidence by focusing on a number of the key bread-and-butter areas.

Whether in general practice, the Emergency Department or the wards, back pain is so common that, as well as mastering a slick examination, it is vital to develop a good feel for the red and yellow flags. As the population ages and junior doctors spend more time on wards for older adults, a sound understanding of the impact and treatment of osteoarthritis is essential. A good grasp of the crystal arthropathies and rheumatoid arthritis should equally be within our armoury.

Although part of every assessment, it is the extra-articular features that take rheumatology from rheumatoid arthritis and beyond to the connective tissue diseases. Having established a feel for the joint itself, the next step is to go further and complete the picture by being sensitive to changes in nails, skin, and other entire organ systems.

In this way, the rheumatologist is a general physician with a keen eye for detail and the ability to make unifying diagnoses. Although patients with a vasculitis are few and far between, they offer fascinating physiological insights and – as well as being fertile areas for examination questions – should engender in us the ability to meet a patient and ask appropriately: is there a rheumatological cause for these symptoms? ∎

RHEUMATOLOGY
SINGLE BEST ANSWERS

1. A 29-year-old woman has had tender swollen wrists for 2 weeks. This happened a year ago when two of her fingers were swollen for a short period but improved without treatment. She has also noticed a red rash across her face recently, despite the weather being largely cloudy. Which *single* autoantibody is most consistent with the diagnosis? ★

A Anti-acetylcholine receptor

B Anti-dsDNA

C Anti-mitochondrial

D Anti-Scl-70

E Anti-smooth muscle

2. A 22-year-old man has been struggling to get out of bed in the morning for the past few months. As the day progresses, he feels his stiffness loosening, but by the evening, he has severe back pain. He has been otherwise fit and well, smokes ten cigarettes a day and consumes 30 units of alcohol a week. Which *single* examination finding is most likely to support the diagnosis? ★

A Impaired sensation over L5–S1 dermatome

B Pain on straight leg raise

C Raised brown plaques on soles

D Saddle anaesthesia

E Tender sacroiliac joints

3. A 68-year-old man has had progressively worsening lower back pain over the last month. He had previously been mobilizing with a frame but this morning felt too weak to get out of bed. He has not passed urine for over 12h. He receives a 3-monthly injection of goserelin for carcinoma of the prostate. Flexion at the hip is weak, especially on the right. Reflexes are brisk at the right knee and ankle with an upgoing plantar. Sensation from the right mid-thigh distally is dulled. Which is the *single* most appropriate course of action? ★

A CT head scan

B MRI of the spine

C Ultrasound scan of the bladder

D X-ray of the lumbar spine

E X-ray of the pelvis

4. A 26-year-old man has been suffering with a stiff back for the past year. The pain is very low down and especially bad first thing in the morning. He is a keen sportsman and has noticed that the pain eases the more activity he does. Which *single* arrow in the image in Figure 9.1 is most likely to indicate the anatomical origin of symptoms? ★

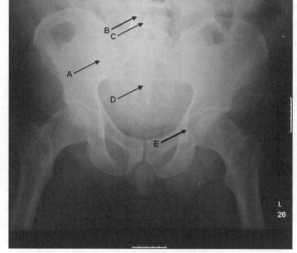

Figure 9.1

5. A 42-year-old woman has painful red lesions over the extensor aspect of both her legs and thighs. The lesions have appeared over the last few weeks. She also has a non-productive cough and pain and stiffness of her ankles. A chest X-ray is performed (Figure 9.2).

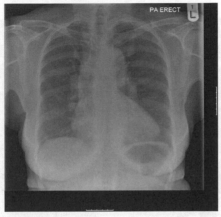

Figure 9.2

```
T 37°C, HR 75bpm, BP 140/80mmHg, SaO₂ 96% on
air.
```

Which *single* pair of investigations would be most likely to support the diagnosis? ★

A Angiotensin-converting enzyme (ACE) levels + serum calcium

B Anti-nuclear antibodies + anti-dsDNA antibodies

C Creatine kinase + muscle biopsy

D Early morning urine + sputum samples

E Rheumatoid factor + erthyrocyte sedimentation rate (ESR)

6. A 62-year-old man has pain in his left knee. It is particularly bad after long days on his feet, but is not especially stiff in the mornings. He has otherwise been fit and well. An X-ray is arranged (Figure 9.3). Which is the *single* most appropriate initial treatment for his pain? ★

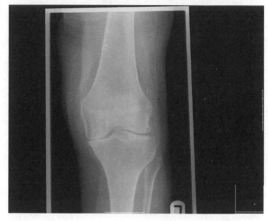

Figure 9.3

A Celecoxib 100mg PO twice daily
B Diclofenac 50mg PO three times daily
C Glucosamine 1.5g PO once daily
D Paracetamol PO 1g four times daily
E Tramadol PO 50mg four times daily

7. A 72-year-old woman has been started on a new medication for her rheumatoid arthritis. The drug has only been licensed for use over the last 2 months and is given as a monthly injection. Within 2 weeks of starting the new drug treatment, the woman develops widespread urticaria. She feels well but makes an appointment to see her GP, by which time the reaction is starting to settle. Which is the *single* most appropriate initial management? ★

A Contact the National Patient Safety Agency (NPSA) with details of the reaction

B Discuss the reaction with the relevant drug company

C Inform the Medicines and Healthcare Products Regulatory Agency (MHRA) about the nature of the reaction to the drug

D Refer her urgently back to her rheumatologist

E Wait and see whether she reacts to the next injection as this reaction is settling

8. A 29-year-old woman has had painful fingers in cold weather for as long as she can remember. The tips change colour, turning from white to blue and then to red. Which is the *single* most appropriate explanation for this woman's symptoms? ★

A Aneurysms and thrombosis in medium-sized arteries

B Autoantibodies against platelet membranes

C Connective tissue weakness causing capillary dilatation

D Hyperactive sympathetic system causing vasoconstriction

E Inflammation of arteries and veins due to an unknown cause

9. A 48-year-old man has had an increasing pain in his right buttock over the past 6 months. He feels it travel all the way down the back of his right thigh as far as the knee. The pain is worsened by coughing and bending forward. The doctor thinks it might be sciatica and refers him for an MRI. Which *single* detail from the history suggests that his pain is *not* due to sciatica? ★

A He does not feel pain in his calf or ankle

B He has had it for 6 months

C The pain is worsened by bending forward

D The pain is worsened by coughing

E The pain starts in his buttock

10. A 38-year-old woman has had pain in her lower back for the past 2 weeks. She cannot relate it to any trauma and has noticed no pattern in how it affects her. It has forced her to miss 2 weeks of work, just after she had returned following 3 months off with wrist pains. She is using codeine 60mg PO four times daily and citalopram 40mg PO once at night. There is no evidence of soft-tissue or skeletal injury and there is a full range of lumbar flexion and extension both forwards and laterally. Which is the *single* most important consideration when monitoring her symptoms? ★

A She is already on a high-dose analgesia regimen

B She is at risk of developing chronic pain

C She is at risk of missing significant time at work

D She is liable to suffer an acute depressive episode

E Her symptoms may be linked to a previous wrist injury

11. A 52-year-old woman is being treated palliatively but has intractable pain. She has systemic sclerosis and has been told by her team of specialists that she has reached the end stages of the disease. She asks the on-call junior doctor to relieve her pain once and for all and suggests adding large amounts of potassium to her IV fluids. The palliative care registrar had earlier pronounced her fully competent. Which is the *single* most appropriate next step? ★ ★

A Contact her next of kin before making a decision either way

B Give potassium as requested as it would be in her best interests to die

C Give potassium as requested as she is competent

D Refuse as active euthanasia is illegal

E Refuse as it would be in her best medical interests to live

12. A 20-year-old man has suddenly developed a swollen right knee. He noticed it for the first time on waking this morning when he felt pain on attempting to weight bear. He recalls no injury to the knee and has not experienced this before. He is otherwise well. The knee is warm, tender, and swollen with an obvious effusion palpable. A diagnostic joint aspiration is carried out. Which *single* organism is most likely to be isolated on culturing the aspirate? ★ ★

A *Escherichia coli*

B *Neisseria gonorrhoeae*

C *Pseudomonas aeruginosa*

D *Staphylococcus aureus*

E *Streptococcus pneumoniae*

13. A 51-year-old woman is having increasing difficulty swallowing and has noticed that the skin on her hands and feet is getting increasingly tight. Although she has previously enjoyed winter holidays, she now finds her hands get very cold, even on not particularly cold days. Which *single* autoantibody is most consistent with the diagnosis? ★ ★ ★

A Anti-centromere

B Anti-dsDNA

C Anti-Ro

D Anti-Scl-70

E Rheumatoid factor

14. A 44-year-old woman has felt lethargic with generalized joint pains for the past 48h. She feels generally unwell. This is the third episode in the last year, despite continued treatment with azathioprine 150mg PO once daily.

```
T 37.7°C, HR 85bpm, BP 115/80mmHg.
```

She has multiple mouth ulcers and non-tender cervical lymphadenopathy. Which would be the *single* most useful investigation to monitor disease activity? ★ ★ ★

A Complement

B Creatine kinase

C CRP

D Joint aspiration

E Rheumatoid factor

15. A 55-year-old man has a swollen left foot. He does not remember any recent trauma or other provoking factors. He takes omeprazole 20mg PO once daily for a previous duodenal ulcer, smokes ten cigarettes a day and drinks 40 units of alcohol a week.

```
T 37.1°C, HR 82bpm, BP 142/75mmHg.
```

The metatarsophalangeal joint of the big toe is hot, erythematous, and exquisitely tender. Which is the *single* most appropriate treatment for this man's symptoms? ★ ★ ★

A Allopurinol 100mg PO once daily

B Colchicine 500µg PO four times daily

C Indomethacin 50mg PO once daily

D Morphine sulphate 10mg/5mL PO PRN

E Naproxen 500mg PO twice daily

16. A 55-year-old woman has swollen painful joints. The pain is present all the time but increases on movement and is worse by the end of the day. Her knees are swollen bilaterally and crepitus can be felt on passive movement. Which *single* examination finding would be most likely to support the diagnosis? ★ ★ ★

A Hyperextension at the proximal interphalangeal joints

B Onycholysis

C Soft-tissue swelling

D Squared thumb

E Thoracic kyphosis

17. A 75-year-old woman has felt lethargic for the past year. She has noticed stiffness and pain in her neck and across her shoulders, particularly in the morning. She also feels she has lost weight in this time. Which *single* investigation is most likely to support the diagnosis? ★ ★ ★

A Calcium

B Erythrocyte sedimentation rate (ESR)

C Neck and shoulder X-rays

D Peripheral blood film

E Thyroid function tests

18. A 47-year-old man has had a painful right wrist for the past 3 months. It began gradually but is now so bad that he is finding it difficult to open bottle tops or turn on taps. His left wrist has also started to twinge. Both are particularly bad in the morning, remaining stiff for the first 3 or 4h of the day. He is otherwise well, except for a persistent itchy rash on the extensor surfaces of his arms and back. Which *single* further finding would most support the likely diagnosis? ★ ★ ★

A Early diastolic heart murmur

B Nodules on elbows

C Onycholysis

D Squared thumbs

E Whitish nodule on pinna of ear

19. A 33-year-old man has excruciating pain in his lower back. It came on suddenly 2 days ago and is constant. It radiates into his buttock and on movement travels quickly down the back of his right leg and into his calf and foot. He can raise his right leg straight off the bed to an angle of 20° before the pain is reproduced. Which *single* examination finding will confirm the diagnosis? ★ ★ ★

A Dullness to percussion in lower abdomen

B Hypertonia in right leg

C Reduced perineal sensation

D Reduced sensation in plantar aspect of right foot

E Reduced sensation below the knee

20. A 30-year-old woman has felt increasingly lethargic over the past week. She has also noticed that several painful joints have started to swell. She has suffered with episodes similar to this recurrently for the last 2–3 years. She has raised patches on her cheeks and ears.

Urine dipstick: protein 3+.

Anti-nuclear antibody: positive.

Which *single* further symptom would be most supportive of the likely diagnosis? ★ ★ ★

A Mouth ulcers

B Recurrent sexually transmitted infections

C Rigors

D Sore throat

E Upper limb muscle weakness

EXTENDED MATCHING QUESTIONS

Causes of skin conditions

For each scenario, choose the *single* most likely
dermatological condition from the list of options
below. Each option may be used once, more than
once, or not at all. ★

A Acanthosis nigricans

B Dermatitis herpetiformis

C Erythema chronicum migrans

D Erythema marginatum

E Erythema multiforme

F Erythema nodosum

G Lipodermatosclerosis

H Necrobiosis lipoidica

I Pyoderma gangrenosum

J Scabies

K Varicella-zoster virus

L Vitiligo

1. A 55-year-old man has been unwell for the last 2 days. He has generalized myalgia, a persistent headache, feels feverish and lethargic, and has a worsening rash on his torso. He thought his tiredness was to be expected having just returned from a rural walking holiday. The circular rash has an indurated dark red central area with a surrounding paler red-coloured area.

2. A 25-year-old woman has had a rash on her thighs and shins over the last week. She has no relevant past medical history and is recovering well 3 weeks after being diagnosed with glandular fever, which improved with symptomatic treatment only. The lesions are tender, smooth, shiny nodules. They are purple coloured and between 1 and 3cm in diameter.

3. A 48-year-old woman has had 'bruising' over her shins for the last few weeks. She thought they were improving, but recently they changed into yellow-coloured lesions. She accidentally knocked her leg on a door a week ago and soon after she developed an ulcer over one of the yellow lesions.

4. A 50-year-old woman has had some lesions on her legs for the last 2 months. Initially she thought that she had been bitten by an insect, but they did not disappear and are now much larger and more painful. The skin is now ulcerated and has developed a purple border. She takes infliximab for rheumatoid arthritis.

5. A 37-year-old woman has been suffering from worsening diarrhoea and weight loss. She is increasingly tired and is becoming withdrawn from her friends and family. Over the last month, she has started to suffer from itchy groups of blisters on both her elbows and forearms, which appeared after a burning and stinging sensation.

Causes of swollen joints

For each case of a swollen joint, choose the *single* most likely diagnosis from the list of options below. Each option may be used once, more than once, or not at all. ★

A Ankylosing spondylitis

B Cellulitis

C Gout

D Osteoarthritis

E Pseudo-gout

F Psoriatic arthritis

G Reactive arthritis

H Rheumatoid arthritis

I Septic arthritis

J Systemic lupus erythematosus

6. A 76-year-old man has a severely painful left ankle. It has come on rapidly over the last 3 days such that he can no longer put weight on it. He has hypertension and says he has been started on a new tablet within the last 3 months. His foot is very swollen and erythematous.

7. A 78-year-old woman has noticed her left knee become increasingly swollen over the last 2 weeks. She has had pain in the joint for many years now. She takes alendronate 70mg PO weekly and Calcichew D3 tablets PO at night. The joint is swollen and fluctuant with a positive bulge test. It is held in fixed flexion at 20°.

8. A 38-year-old man has extreme pain in his left foot. It has progressed rapidly over the past 48h such that he is now struggling to stand. He says he has suffered this type of pain before and confesses to regular IV drug use. His foot is swollen and very inflamed, with erythema spreading proximally from the toes to the medial malleolus.

9. A 74-year-old woman has a large swelling in her left knee. It came on suddenly and grew rapidly in size over a 12h period. She is clammy and rather anxious. The knee is swollen and fluctuant. It is held in flexion at 20°. She is noted to have a urine output of <15mL/h.

10. A 30-year-old woman has a painful and swollen right ankle. It has developed gradually over the last week or so. She has suffered flare-ups of the same joint at regular intervals over the last 18 months. The first attack occurred within a month of a urinary tract infection, but otherwise she has remained well.

Single Best Answers

1. B ★   OHCM 8th edn → p556

This woman has systemic lupus erythematosus (SLE) associated with a malar rash. There are a number of autoantibodies that are detected in this disease including rheumatoid factor (RhF), anti-Ro, anti-ribonucleoprotein, and anti-Smith antibodies. Although anti-dsDNA antibodies are the most specific antibody in SLE, only about 60% of cases will be positive, whilst more than 95% of cases will be positive for anti-nuclear antibodies.

A These antibodies are produced in myaesthenia gravis.

C Anti-mitochondrial antibodies are produced in primary biliary cirrhosis.

D Anti-Scl-70 antibodies are produced in diffuse systemic sclerosis.

E Autoimmune hepatitis involves anti-smooth muscle antibodies.

2. E ★   OHCM 8th edn → p552

Non-traumatic back pain in a young person is always concerning, but persistent back stiffness in a young man is highly suspicious for ankylosing spondylitis.

A This describes a common peroneal nerve lesion: clearly unilateral and most likely after trauma to the lateral aspect of the knee.

B This describes pain on hip flexion and extension that are suggestive of sciatic nerve root irritation.

C The brown plaques are keratoderma blenorrhagica, which occurs with mouth ulcers in a reactive arthritis, i.e. a sterile arthritis affecting the lower limbs within a month of a urethritis.

D These are worrying features that should raise the alarm for a potential cord compression, most commonly post-traumatic or due to metastatic disease.

3. B ★   OHCM 8th edn → p544

This man is displaying the signs of acute cord compression – upper motor neurone signs below the lesion with urinary retention. Whilst there are other causes of compression (e.g. myeloma, disc protrusion, spinal abscess), given this man's concurrent malignancy, it is most likely to be due to spinal metastasis. Once detected by MRI, the metastasis may be suitable for shrinkage by radiotherapy.

A plain X-ray of the lumbar spine (D) may support clinical suspicions, but in an emergency such as this, there should be no delay in seeking the imaging most likely to seal the diagnosis.

4. A ★

Arrow A is pointing to the sacroiliac joints. Although a plain X-ray may be normal in early ankylosing spondylitis, it is the sacroiliac joints that are first affected – usually the lower half of the joints on the iliac side. For a better image of sacroiliitis, MRI is preferable.

B   This is the lumbar vertebral body.

C   This is the lumbar spinous process.

D   This is the sacral spinous process.

E   This is the sacroischial joint.

5. A ★

This is a presentation of sarcoidosis, as suggested by the skin lesions – erythema nodosum – the polyarthralgia, and the bilateral hilar lymphadenopathy on the chest X-ray. Diagnosis would be supported by a raised ESR, deranged liver function tests, high levels of serum ACE, and hypercalcaemia.

B   These are raised in systemic lupus erythematosus (SLE)

C   The muscle enzymes creatine kinase and alanine transaminase are raised in dermatomyositis: diagnosis is confirmed by muscle biopsy.

D   These are used if tuberculosis is suspected.

E   Rheumatoid factor is positive in 70% of patients with raised inflammatory markers (ESR and C-reactive protein).

6. D ★

The X-ray shows the classical findings of osteoarthritis: loss of joint space, subchondral bone cysts, and osteophytes. The first-line treatment is regular paracetamol with topical non-steroidal anti-inflammatory drugs (NSAIDs) for knees and hands. Should this provide insufficient pain relief, oral NSAIDs, COX-2 inhibitors, and opioids could then be considered. As shown in Figure 9.4, these

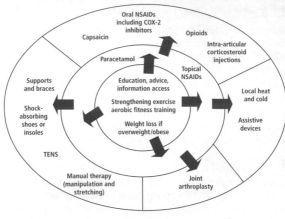

Figure 9.4

'relatively safe pharmaceutical options' are the next stage after the core treatments (in the central circle) have been considered.

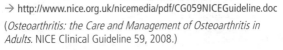

→ http://www.nice.org.uk/nicemedia/pdf/CG059NICEGuideline.doc

(*Osteoarthritis: the Care and Management of Osteoarthritis in Adults.* NICE Clinical Guideline 59, 2008.)

7. C ★

Only limited information is available from clinical trials on the safety of new medicines. The MHRA rely on spontaneous reports of all suspected reactions (including those not thought to be serious) via the 'yellow card' system. These can be found in the back of the British National Formulary (BNF) or completed on line.

8. D ★   OHCM 8th edn → p722

This woman has been experiencing the peripheral ischaemia that is characteristic of Raynaud's syndrome. Vasospasm is brought on by cold weather or stress and may be primary (idiopathic Raynaud's disease) or secondary (to connective tissue/haematological disorders: Raynaud's phenomenon).

A This occurs in polyarteritis nodosum.

B These are produced in idiopathic thrombocytopaenic purpura.

C This is hereditary haemorrhagic telangiectasia (Osler–Weber–Rendu syndrome).

E This is Buerger's disease.

9. A ★

The pain from sciatica (i.e. irritation to the sciatic nerve: L4, L5, and S1) radiates into the buttock, down the back of the thigh and – crucially – below the knee into the calf and ankle. It may be that this man is suffering from nerve root pain (which features in C and D) and warrants an MRI of his lumbar spine, but the roots involved are likely to be L2 and L3 rather than any of the sciatic roots.

10. B ★

All options are reasonable to differing degrees. However, crucial to this case are the 'yellow flags' for the development of chronic pain: depression, time off work, and extended rest. These are some of the psychosocial factors that are known to put an individual at risk of developing long-term disability. It is therefore essential to see the bigger picture in such a case and to understand that the presence of this collection of problems is predictive of serious long-term impairment: whilst each immediate problem needs to be addressed, more important is holistic attention over time.

→ http://archive.student.bmj.com/issues/03/04/education/97.php

→ http://cks.library.nhs.uk/back_pain_low_and_sciatica

11. D ★★

As the Lillian Boyes case showed (in which her doctor was charged with attempted murder having injected her with two ampoules of potassium chloride: he remains the only doctor ever to have been convicted in the UK of a 'mercy killing'), no matter how compassionate the action of the doctor, actively helping a patient to die remains illegal in the UK, regardless of whether the patient has capacity to ask for that help.

12. B ★★   OHCM 8th edn → p546

In a young person (aged 19–25 years), this is the most common pathogen responsible for a septic joint. This may be related to the nascent sexual activity common to this group. In older adults, *S. aureus* is the commonest cause.

13. A ★★★   OHCM 8th edn → p554

This woman has limited systemic sclerosis, which includes the diagnosis of CREST (calcinosis, Raynaud's syndrome, (o)esophageal dysmotility, sclerodactyly, and telangiectasia) with anti-centromere antibodies detected in up to 30% of cases. She has dysphagia, sclerodactyly, and secondary Raynaud's phenomenon. Skin involvement is limited to the face, hands, and feet. Other changes consistent with this diagnosis are telangiectasia and oesophageal dysmotility.

B This occurs in 60–75% of cases of systemic lupus erythematosus (SLE).

C This occurs in 30% of SLE cases and 75% of primary Sjögren's syndrome cases.

D This occurs in 50% of diffuse systemic sclerosis.

E This occurs in <100% of Sjogren's syndrome and Felty's syndrome cases and 70% of rheumatoid arthritis.

14. A ★ ★ ★   OHCM 8th edn → p556

The scenario describes a flare-up of systemic lupus erythematosus (SLE): as well as monitoring urine for blood and protein, and determining CRP, erythrocyte sedimentation rate (ESR) and blood pressure, the best way to monitor disease activity is via antibody titres and complement levels (they would be low during a flare-up as they are consumed).

B This is used to support a diagnosis of dermatomyositis.

C This is a key marker of any acute inflammation or infection and is therefore useful here, but not specific.

D This is the critical step in the management of an acutely hot – and therefore potentially infected – joint.

E Rheumatoid factor is positive in ~70% of rheumatoid arthritis sufferers; a high titre with a high ESR is found in severe disease.

15. B ★ ★ ★

An 'exquisitely tender' single joint should always raise the suspicion of gout, particularly in someone with a high alcohol intake. Treatment is by high-dose, fast-acting strong non-steroidal anti-inflammatory drugs (NSAIDs) (such as indomethacin, C) *unless* contraindicated – as in this case where the patient has had peptic ulcer disease. Although it is slower acting, colchicine is next in line (caution needs to be taken in those with renal impairment). Allopurinol (A) should not be started in an acute attack, although it should be continued in those already using it. Opioids (D) are useful as adjuncts in pain control.

Jordan KM, Cameron JS, Snaith M, *et al.* (2007). British Society for Rheumatology and British Health Professionals in Rheumatology Guideline for the Management of Gout. *Rheumatology (Oxford)* 46:1372–1374.

→ http://rheumatology.oxfordjournals.org/cgi/content/full/46/8/1372

16. D ★★★ OHCM 8th edn → p546

A story of background joint pain that worsens with activity is strongly suggestive of osteoarthritis. Post-menopausal women are prone to generalized disease suffering damage to the distal interphalangeal joint of the hands and the knees. It is also known as 'nodal osteoarthritis' as they are more likely to develop Heberden's nodes ('lumps' at the distal interphalangeal joint), as well as deformity of the thumbs.

A This is found in rheumatoid arthritis, which normally causes pain and swelling of the small joints of the hands and feet and is worse in the morning.

B This is seen in psoriatic arthritis; joint pain usually follows the onset of psoriasis but not always. There are five patterns of psoriatic arthritis but it would be unlikely for any of them to comprise the distribution of joints affected in this case.

C This is a sign of a crystal arthropathy, which is more likely to affect one single joint for a short time (an acute monoarthropathy).

E This is found in ankylosing spondylitis, which usually presents in younger men with the gradual onset of lower back stiffness that is worse in the mornings.

17. B ★★★ OHCM 8th edn → p559

Despite being one of the most common reasons for long-term steroid use in the community, there is widespread disagreement as to what polymyalgia rheumatica (PMR) is and how it should be diagnosed. A 2008 report summarized a consensus process to identify a potential classification process for PMR. It listed the following current criteria as being in use:

- Age >50 years
- Bilateral aching of neck, shoulders, and pelvic girdle
- Morning stiffness >1h
- Duration of symptoms >1month
- ESR >40mm/h
- Depression and/or weight loss
- Other diagnoses excluded
- Rapid response to prednisolone (<20mg/day).

The aim is to develop an internationally recognized classification criteria with the next step being an international prospective study.

A A test for calcium would be carried out if either sarcoidosis or a malignancy was suspected. Both are unlikely here.

C This would be important to exclude both cervical spondylosis and osteoporosis and should therefore happen before the diagnosis of PMR can be pronounced.

D This woman's symptoms could fit with a haematological malignancy but these tests would only be indicated if basic blood tests showed abnormalities of the cell lineages.

E Again, these would be essential at the start of the investigation process but are unlikely to prove diagnostic.

Dasgupta B, Salvarani C, Schirmer M, *et al.* (2008). Developing classification criteria for polymyalgia rheumatica: comparison of views from an expert panel and wider survey. *J Rheumatol* 35:270–277.

→ http://jrheum.org/content/35/2/270.abstract

18. C ★ ★ ★ OHCM 8th edn → p552

An important skill to develop is the ability to classify joint pain and to begin to suggest a diagnosis. This man has an asymmetrical oligoarthritis (suggestive of either a crystal, reactive, or psoriatic arthritis) with morning stiffness and loss of function (typical of an inflammatory process). As with any joint complaint, it is important to perform a full extra-articular examination. Nail changes would be strongly supportive of the diagnosis in this case, as they occur in 80% of psoriatic arthritides. Varying patterns of arthritis occur in 10–40% of psoriasis sufferers.

A This is seen in rheumatoid arthritis, which is more likely to cause a polyarthritis.

B This is a potential extra-articular finding in ankylosing spondylitis, indicative of aortic regurgitation.

D A feature of osteoarthritis, due to bony enlargement and remodelling of the carpometacarpal joint.

E A description of the tophi that usually only appear in chronic sufferers of gout.

19. D ★ ★ ★

This is classic sciatica involving impingement of the sciatic nerve at the level of S1. Pain is felt in the distribution of the sciatic nerve in the thigh and below the knee. The history and positive straight leg raise confirm this diagnosis.

A Urinary retention (along with loss of the cremasteric reflex, elicited by stroking the superomedial part of the thigh) would suggest compression of the L1–L2 nerve root.

B Together with hyper-reflexia, this is a feature of a right-sided upper motor neurone lesion.

C This is a feature of cauda equina syndrome, caused by compression of the cauda equina below L2.

E Together with absent ankle reflexes, this is a feature of subacute combined degeneration of the cord, due to vitamin B_{12} deficiency.

Koes BW, Van Tulde MW, and Peul WC (2007). Diagnosis and treatment of sciatica. *BMJ* **334**:1313–1317.

→ http://www.bmj.com/cgi/content/extract/334/7607/1313

20. A ★ ★ ★   OHCM 8th edn → p556

Flare-ups of systemic lupus erythematosus (SLE) are different for all patients but most commonly include: lethargy, joint pain and oedema, mouth ulcers, and proteinuria. They may need to be managed in an inpatient setting for the administration of IV fluid and steroid therapy.

B AND D These are driving at a reactive arthritis, but neither would explain the rash, the proteinuria, or the fact that the patient is anti-nuclear antibody positive.

C This would be possible if this were a septic arthritis, but this normally affects a single joint and with no autoimmune background.

E This is playing on the skin rash and the immunology and is suggestive of a dermatomyositis: again, painful joints and renal dysfunction are uncommon in this condition, which would be more likely to test positive for extractable nuclear antigens (specifically anti-Jo) than anti-nuclear antibodies.

Extended Matching Questions

1. C ★

Erythema chronicum migrans is the rash sometimes seen in Lyme disease, caused by the spirochaete *Borrelia burgdorferi*, which is transmitted via the bite from an *Ixodes* tick. The classic 'bullseye'-looking rash is only seen in ~10% of cases.

2. F ★

Erythema nodosum is associated in this case with Epstein–Barr virus, but in up to 50% of cases, no cause is identified. It occurs as a result of inflammation of subcutaneous fat.

3. H ★

Necrobiosis lipoidica is a necrotizing skin condition usually occurring in people with diabetes.

4. I ★

Pyoderma gangrenosum is of unknown aetiology but is thought to be due to neutrophil dysfunction. It is also associated with inflammatory bowel disease and a number of haematological disorders.

5. B ★

Dermatitis herpetiformis is often found in combination with coeliac diease: 80% of people will see their gastrointestinal and dermatitis symptoms improve with a gluten-free diet, although sometimes dapsone is required.

6. C ★

Gout occurs when uric acid crystals precipitate on joint cartilage, tendons, and the surrounding tissues. Uric acid is produced during the metabolism of purines, either from the diet or generated from cell breakdown. It may have been precipitated by the introduction of a thiazide diuretic, which competes with the same transporter as uric acid.

7. D ★

The proximity and friction of the bones has led to the development of a haemarthrosis.

8. B ★

This deep infection of the skin and subcutaneous tissues involves mainly *Streptococcus* and will need to be treated with systemic antibiotics.

9. I ★

This woman is in danger of becoming very unwell very quickly. She is showing a system inflammatory response that has already started to affect her renal function. She may need her knee joint to be washed out by a surgeon, as well as IV antibiotics and fluid support.

10. G ★

Typically affecting the lower limbs, reactive arthritis occurs within a month of a urethritis and can become chronic or relapsing, as in this case.

CHAPTER 10
SURGERY

S tarting a surgical job can feel like learning a completely new language. It may be the first time seeing patients in acute severe pain with a variety of lumps and bumps and a past history of previously unheard of complex operations. It can be easy to get hung up on whether the distended large bowel loop on the X-ray is a caecal or sigmoid volvulus, or whether the strangulated hernia is a femoral or inguinal hernia.

Ultimately, however, the most important point is that, as a junior doctor, it is being able to recognize that the patient is acutely unwell and likely to require an operation that will save lives.

Ironically, a surgical rotation involves little time in the operating theatre: mostly it will be spent dealing with problems during the peri-operative period. This will often start a week or two before the patient is even admitted in the shape of a pre-assessment clinic. These are a good opportunity to see stable patients with interesting pathology and good clinical signs and to establish how well they look before the majority of their large bowel or their stomach is removed.

The pre-operative preparation of the patient goes beyond bloods and a cursory chat, and will require one to be on the lookout for previously undiagnosed cardiorespiratory or rheumatological conditions, among others, that might affect the patient getting to or staying safely asleep under anaesthesia. Liaising with the anaesthetist about possible sources of difficulty well in advance of the planned procedure will ensure that operations do not get cancelled (and keep our neck off the block…).

The acute abdomen will take centre stage during surgical takes. A thorough history and sound anatomical knowledge will establish the time scale of the illness, as well as the likely organs involved. Accurate and careful palpation of the abdomen will determine guarding or percussion tenderness, and simple bedside observations and tests can greatly aid the diagnosis.

Surgical specialties have a heavy reliance on imaging – IV urogram, ultrasound, erect chest X-ray, CT/MRI scan – each providing different information for the symptoms displayed. The theory behind selecting the right medium can be learnt, but the ability to interpret it may take a good deal longer. It is essential, too, to become accustomed to the myriad of surgical tubes – two- and three-way urinary catheters, central venous pressure (CVP) lines, naogastric and nasojejunal tubes, IV lines and post-operative drains – each one giving different information on how the patient (and the doctor) is coping with the stresses of surgery.

Post-operatively, analgesia and a step-wise approach to progression using the World Health Organization analgesic ladder enable us to offer the patient the most comfortable and speedy recovery. Patient-controlled analgesia and epidurals are becoming more commonplace, and pain teams will often review patients daily, providing good learning opportunities and points of reference if difficulties arise.

This chapter emphasizes the fact that the time between the knife breaking the skin and the wound being closed is a tiny fraction of the whole process of 'surgery'. Pre-operative preparation, consent, knowledge of anaesthesia and post-operative management of pain, fluids, and complications will be where our skills are employed – and tested. ■

SINGLE BEST ANSWERS

1. A 48-year-old man is found to have an expansile mass in his abdomen. He undergoes an ultrasound examination and is found to have an abdominal aortic aneurysm (AAA), which is 4.5cm in diameter. He is told that the aneurysm can enlarge and asks for advice about reducing his risk of rupture. He is currently taking metformin for type 2 diabetes. His body mass index (BMI) is 33kg/m².

T 36.6°C, HR 85bpm, BP 135/90mmHg.

Which is the *single* most appropriate piece of advice? ★

A Close blood glucose monitoring

B CT scan every 6 months

C Lose weight

D Reduce blood pressure

E Ultrasound scans every 3 months

2. A 72 year man collapses at home. He has had 4h of back pain. Prior to this episode he has been fit and well.

HR 120bpm, BP 90/70mmHg.

There is an expansile mass palpable in his abdomen. Which is the *single* most appropriate course of action? ★

A Arrange consent for immediate laparotomy

B Ask surgical registrar to assess when available

C CT scan of the abdomen

D Insert urinary catheter

E Ultrasound scan of the abdomen

3. A 75-year-old man has had a sudden onset central abdominal pain for 30min. He is confused and a collateral history is taken from his wife. He smokes 20 cigarettes per day and drinks 30 units of alcohol per week. He opens his bowels every 3 days and takes bendroflumethiazide 2.5mg PO once daily for hypertension.

```
T 36.8°C, HR 110bpm, BP 90/50mmHg, BM
7.5mmol/L.
```

Which is the *single* most likely diagnosis? ★

A Acute pancreatitis

B Perforated duodenal ulcer

C Perforated diverticula

D Ruptured abdominal aortic aneurysm (AAA)

E Ureteric colic

4. A 23-year-old man has had right iliac fossa pain for the last 24h. He has passed urine on eight occasions already today and is complaining of pain each time he goes. He opened his bowels today and has not had any diarrhoea, although he vomited earlier in the day. He has taken analgesia at home without much effect.

```
T 37.4C, HR 88bpm, BP 130/75mmHg.

CRP 30mg/L, WCC 15 × 10⁹/L, INR 1.6.

Bilirubin 10µmol/L, ALP 555U/L, AST 88IU/L,
GGT 40IU/L.
```

Which is the *single* most likely explanation for the blood results? ★

A Gallstones

B Pancreatitis

C Paracetamol overdose

D Sepsis

E Viral hepatitis

5. A 29-year-old woman has had abdominal pain for 3 days. It began around the umbilicus but is now worse on the right side of her abdomen. She has a poor appetite and intermittent nausea. Her periods are regular but heavy and she is currently mid-cycle. Her abdomen is tender to light palpation and percussion in the right iliac fossa.

```
T 37.4°C, HR 105bpm, BP 95/65mmHg.

Urinary β-human chorionic gonadotrophin
(β-hCG): negative
```

Which is the *single* most likely diagnosis? ★

A Acute appendicitis

B Ectopic pregnancy

C Endometriosis

D Ovulation pain

E Pelvic inflammatory disease

6. A 31-year-old woman has pain in her upper abdomen. It has been constant for 4h and radiates to her back. She feels nauseated but has not vomited. She recalls a similar episode 3 months previously, but she did not see a doctor at that time. She drinks 20 units of alcohol a week. She cannot get comfortable and her abdomen is tender to deep palpation in the right upper quadrant.

```
T 36.9°C, HR 95bpm, BP 130/90mmHg.
```

Which is the *single* most likely diagnosis? ★

A Biliary colic

B Chronic pancreatitis

C Hepatitis C

D Peptic ulcer disease

E Renal colic

7. A 44-year-old woman has generalized abdominal pain. It has been intermittent but is getting progressively more intense. She is feeling shivery and nauseous. She recalls a similar episode 3 months ago but that passed after a few days. She has recently been advised to amend her diet as her cholesterol levels are raised.

T 38.2°C, HR 110bpm, BP 95/65 mmHg.

Which is the *single* most likely examination finding to confirm the diagnosis? ★

A Epigastric pain, even on light palpation

B Pain and discoloration around the umbilicus and in the flanks

C Pain more in the right iliac fossa than in the left iliac fossa when the left is pressed

D Pain on palpation of the loins

E Pain on palpation of the right upper quadrant (RUQ) that interrupts deep inspiration

8. A 72-year-old woman has cramps in her buttocks after walking for 20m. The pain eases once she rests but comes on again at that fixed distance. She has ischaemic heart disease and type 2 diabetes. The junior doctor performs an examination of her lower limb arterial system including peripheral pulses. Which is the *single* most important additional examination to perform? ★

A Auscultation of the carotid arteries

B Auscultation of the heart

C Lower limb venous system

D Musculoskeletal examination of the lower limbs

E Palpation of the abdomen

9. A 75-year-old woman has had a painful left leg for 24h. The entire leg is swollen and red. She has 24h care and requires help to transfer from bed to chair following a stroke 3 years ago. She has chronic obstructive pulmonary disease (COPD) and uses home oxygen.

```
T 36.2°C, HR 88bpm, BP 155/90mmHg, SaO₂ 92%
on air.
```

Which is the *single* most likely diagnosis? ★

A Cellulitis

B Deep vein thrombosis (DVT)

C Lymphoedema

D Ruptured Baker's cyst

E Superficial thrombophlebosis

10. A 55-year-old woman has had a scaly, itchy rash around her right nipple for 3 weeks. She has been using a moisturiser but has not seen any improvement. She has not felt a lump in her breasts or had any discharge from the nipples. There is no family history of breast cancer and a mammogram last year was normal. Which is the *single* most appropriate next step? ★

A Hydrocortisone cream 1% twice daily

B Reassure and ask to come back in 2 months if it is still present

C Patch allergy testing

D Routine referral to a dermatologist

E Urgent referral to the breast unit

11. A 75-year-old lady has had 3 days of intermittent abdominal pain with vomiting. She had an abdominal hysterectomy 15 years previously. Her abdomen is distended with tinkling bowel sounds. There is a tender lump palpable in the right groin.

```
T 37.5°C, HR 110bpm, BP 110/80 mmHg.
```

Which is the *single* most likely diagnosis? ★

A Band adhesions

B Obstructed femoral hernia

C Lymphoma

D Pancreatic cancer

E Ulcerative colitis

12. A 19-year-old woman has a 2cm × 2cm mobile, non-tender, soft lump with smooth edges in her right breast. She takes the combined oral contraceptive pill. Her mother had breast cancer aged 48. She is referred and undergoes standard quadruple assessment at the local breast unit. Which is the *single* most appropriate management? ★

A Aspirate the lump and send the contents for cytology

B Core biopsy of the lump

C Leave the lump and no need for follow-up

D Leave the lump, but if it is still there in 2 months time, remove it surgically

E Surgical excision of the lump

13. A 62-year-old man is sweating and shivering 5 days after he had a lump in his groin resected. The on-call junior doctor is bleeped to the ward to review the observations chart (Figure 10.1). Which *single* process is most likely to explain the pattern seen on the chart? ★

A Abscess

B Fistula

C Haematoma

D Haemorrhage

E Sinus

14. An 88-year-old woman has had severe pain in her left leg for the past week. It came on suddenly while at rest. She has carcinoma of the bronchus with cererbral metastases and smokes 20 cigarettes a day.

```
HR 90bpm, BP 165/90mmHg
```

The leg is dark blue and mottled up to the mid-calf with fixed staining of the toes. It is cold with no pulses palpable distal to the popliteal. The surgeon explains that the correct management option is amputation. Which *single* factor is most likely to have influenced the surgeon's opinion? ★

A Age >80 years

B Continues to smoke

C Limb is non-viable

D Metastatic disease

E Patient does not have capacity

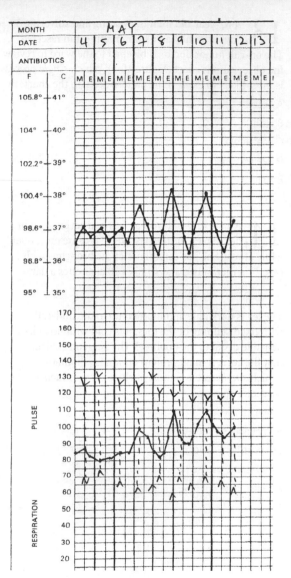

Figure 10.1

15. A 28-year-old man has had 3 days of abdominal pain. He is vomiting and does not want to eat. He feels the need to belch regularly and has not had his bowels open in 5 days. He suffers with acid reflux and had a laparotomy following a stab wound 3 years previously. He has a distended abdomen that is diffusely tender with high pitched bowel sounds. An abdominal X-ray is performed (Figure 10.2).

```
T 36.9°C, HR 100bpm, BP 115/80mmHg.
```

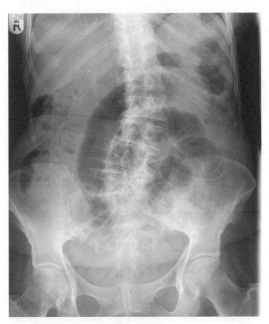

Figure 10.2

Which would be the *single* most appropriate next step in management? ★

A CT scan of the abdomen

B Insert nasogastric tube

C Regular high-dose laxatives

D Urgent colonoscopy

E Urgent laparotomy

16. A 32-year-old man has had severe pain whilst defecating over the last 2 months. The pain starts as he passes the stool but continues long after he has finished. He has seen small amounts of bright red blood on the tissue paper and is now nervous of opening his bowels as a result of the pain. A digital rectal examination is too painful to be carried out.

T 36.2°C, HR 70bpm, BP 128/75mmHg.

Which is the *single* most likely diagnosis? ★

A Anal fissure

B Haemorrhoids

C Perianal abscess

D Proctalgia fugax

E Rectal carcinoma

17. A 42-year-old man has developed acute pain over an inguinal hernia. He is vomiting and unable to tolerate oral analgesia. He is prescribed IM morphine. Which is the *single* safest area of the gluteal muscle in which to administer the injection? ★

A Central

B Inferolateral

C Inferomedial

D Superolateral

E Superomedial

18. A 53-year-old woman has had a swelling and aching sensation in her left groin for the past 6 months. She had some varicose veins removed from her right leg 5 years ago. The fluctuant swelling is below and lateral to the pubic tubercle and does not disappear on lying down. There is no cough impulse detected. Which is the *single* most likely cause of the groin swelling? ★

A Femoral hernia

B Inguinal hernia

C Lipoma

D Lymph node

E Saphena varix

19. A 68-year-old woman has had central abdominal pain for the last 12h. She feels more bloated than usual and although she has vomited on four occasions, this has made her feel better. She opened her bowels today with a normal soft stool. There is a Kocher scar on her abdomen, which is soft but slightly distended, and there are only occasional bowel sounds heard. Blood tests are normal. Which is the *single* most likely diagnosis? ★

A Gallstone ileus

B Large bowel obstruction

C Paralytic ileus

D Pseudo-obstruction

E Small bowel obstruction

20. A 55-year-old man has a painful right calf. It has come on suddenly and is making it difficult for him to walk. He is in such pain that he has come to the Emergency Department out of hours. The entire right leg is swollen, with the calf more than 5cm larger than the left. There is pitting oedema to the knee with tenderness locally over the mid-calf. Which is the *single* most appropriate management? ★

A Defer treatment until after a Doppler ultrasound scan

B Measure D-dimer

C Start heparin

D Start warfarin

E Start warfarin + heparin

21. A 76-year-old man is given IV fluids and catheterized during conservative treatment of an attack of acute pancreatitis. On the second day, he feels much better and the catheter is removed at 8am. That evening, the on-call junior doctor is called because the man has abdominal pain and distension.

```
T 36.6°C, HR 90bpm, BP 140/80mmHg.
```

Which is the *single* most appropriate next step in management? ★

A Abdominal ultrasound scan

B Abdominal X-ray

C Catheterize the patient

D Insert nasogastric tube

E Urgent amylase

22. A 55-year-old woman has had abdominal pain for a week. She has had a total abdominal hysterectomy and an appendicectomy in the past 5 years. An abdominal X-ray is performed (Figure 10.3).

`T 37.1°C, HR 115bpm, BP 140/90 mmHg.`

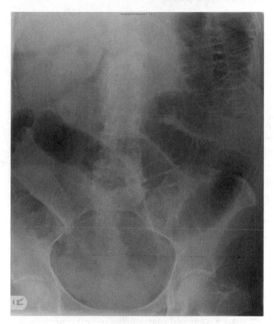

Figure 10.3

Which *single* pair of details from the history would be most likely to support the diagnosis? ★

A Diarrhoea + recent foreign travel

B Dizziness + melaena

C Fluctuating bowel habit + weight loss

D Intermittent constipation + rectal bleeding

E Vomiting + bowels not open for several days

23. A 25-year-old man has gradually worsening scrotal pain over a 3-day period. It started as a dull ache but is now excruciating. His pain is partially relieved by elevation of the testes. The cremasteric reflex is absent. Which is the *single* most likely diagnosis? ★

A Acute epididymo-orchitis

B Indirect inguinal hernia

C Strangulated inguinal hernia

D Testicular torsion

E Testicular tumour

24. A 55-year-old man with severe abdominal pain undergoes a laparotomy. He is found to have a badly devascularized transverse colon. Which *single* arterial supply is most likely to have been compromised? ★

A Ascending colic artery

B Ileocolic artery

C Middle colic artery

D Right colic artery

E Superior rectal artery

25. A 28-year-old man undergoes an emergency laparotomy following a gunshot wound to his abdomen. The anaesthetist requires a rapidly acting agent in order to be able to intubate the non-starved patient safely. Which is the *single* most appropriate choice? ★

A Bupivacaine

B Dantrolene

C Lidocaine

D Propofol

E Suxamethonium

26. An 18-year-old man is brought to the Emergency Department having fallen off his bicycle. He was clipped on his right side, with his left side landing on the kerb. He has bruising to his left chest, flank, and thigh. His abdomen is tender in the left hypochondrium.

```
HR 120bpm, BP 105/80mmHg, RR 22/min, SaO₂
97% on air.
```

Which is the *single* most likely diagnosis? ★

A Colonic perforation

B Haemothorax

C Liver capsule rupture

D Renal haematoma

E Ruptured spleen

27. A 72-year-old man has had severe pain in his lower abdomen for the past 12h. He is nauseous and unable to walk.

```
T 37.2°C, HR 100bpm, BP 90/60mmHg.
```

There is a lump in his right groin that neither the patient nor doctor can reduce. Which is the *single* additional feature that should prompt the most urgent attention? ★

A Bowels not opened for the past 4 days

B Lump has previously always been irreducible but painless

C Lump is warm and tender to touch

D Patient has had three previous laparotomies

E Pain radiates down into scrotum

28. A 30-year-old man has had a swelling in his scrotum for several weeks. He says it disappears when lying down and that occasionally he has an aching feeling in his groin. There is a soft, irregular lump palpable in the left testicle. It is non-tender and does not transilluminate. It is not possible to get above it and there is no cough impulse present. Which is the *single* most likely diagnosis? ★

A Hydrocele

B Inguinal hernia

C Spermatocoele

D Testicular tumour

E Varicocoele

29. An 82-year-old woman has become increasingly drowsy through the course of an evening. Two days previously, she underwent emergency repair of an incarcerated femoral hernia. The on-call junior doctor is contacted by the ward who relay the woman's latest observations over the phone:

```
T 38.2°C, HR 110bpm, BP 90/70mmHg, SaO₂ 94%
on air, urine output 25mL/h.
```

Which is the *single* feature that is most of concern? ★

A Increasing drowsiness

B Low oxygen saturation and no oxygen therapy

C Low urine output

D Pulse rate higher than systolic blood pressure

E Raised temperature 48h after surgery

30. A 62-year-old man has had epigastric and central abdominal pain over the last 4 days. He feels bloated and has been vomiting dark-coloured fluid for the last 12h. His bowels have not opened for 3 days although he is still passing flatus. Which *single* further feature in the history would be most supportive of the likely diagnosis? ★

A Drinks 40 units of alcohol per week

B Eats a lot of takeaway foods

C Previous open cholecystectomy

D Recent foreign travel

E Regularly takes naproxen for back pain

31. A 74-year-old man has been troubled by pain in his calves for many years. The walking distance at which it comes on has dropped from 50m to 10m, despite him giving up smoking, losing weight and lowering his blood pressure. His family doctor is considering starting a new medication. Which is the *single* most appropriate class of medication? ★

A β-Blocker

B Calcium channel inhibitor

C Diuretic

D Inotropic sympathomimetic

E Peripheral vasodilator

32. A 33-year-old man is undergoing an elective hernia repair. The anaesthetist uses the same agent for induction and maintenance. As he injects it, he tells the patient that it will sting a little around the injection site. Which *single* agent has the anaesthetist most likely used? ★

A Desflurane

B Midazolam

C Propofol

D Suxamethonium

E Thiopental

33. A 53-year-old man is attending a pre-operative assessment before an elective cholecystectomy. He had an inferior myocardial infarction 3 years ago but otherwise has had no health problems. He is taking aspirin 75mg PO once daily, simvastatin 40mg PO once at night, perindopril 4mg PO once daily, and atenolol 50mg PO once daily. Which is the *single* most appropriate piece of advice regarding his medications during the peri-operative period? ★

A All his medications need to be stopped the week before the planned operation

B All his medications should be continued but omitted on the morning of the operation

C Subcutaneous heparin injections should replace the aspirin for 5 days before the operation; the other medications can be continued

D The aspirin should be changed for clopidogrel a week before the planned operation

E The aspirin should be stopped 7 days before the operation but all his other medications continued as normal

34. A 36-year-old man has had pain around his anus and fresh rectal bleeding for 24h. He opens his bowels every 3 days and passes hard pellet-like stools. He has had small amounts of rectal bleeding previously and over recent weeks felt 'something come down' as his bowels opened, which he then pushes back inside. He has a thrombosed external haemorrhoid but no necrotic tissue. Which is the *single* most appropriate management? ★

A Banding of haemorrhoid

B High-fibre diet

C Emergency open haemorrhoidectomy

D Emergency stapled haemorrhoidectomy

E Ice pack therapy

35. A 55-year-old man has severe central abdominal pain that radiates into his back. It started 2h ago and, although it initially settled, it returned after his lunch and he has vomited twice. His pain is reduced but not eliminated by IV morphine. He has mild exercise-induced asthma and has had an epigastric hernia for years.

```
T 36.3°C, HR 85bpm, BP 140/70mmHg.

Abdomen: soft, central tenderness, scanty
bowel sounds.
```

An abdominal X-ray shows a few small bowel loops on the right side of the abdomen. Which *single* additional history supports the diagnosis? ★

A His bowels have not opened for 3 days

B The epigastric hernia has not got bigger recently

C The pain is better sitting forward

D There has been no haematemesis

E There is a family history of colorectal cancer

36. A 45-year-old woman has had severe abdominal pain for the past 48h. It radiates through to her back and can only partially be relieved by bending forwards. She has vomited several times. She is otherwise well and does not drink alcohol.

```
T 37.6°C, HR 120bpm, BP 95/45mmHg.
```

Her abdomen is tense and generally tender, especially at the epigastrium. Which *single* further factor would most support the likely diagnosis? ★

A 10kg weight loss in past month

B Familial hyperlipidaemia

C On oral contraceptive pill

D Recent foreign travel

E Recent total abdominal hysterectomy

37. A 67-year-old man has a sudden onset of epigastric pain that woke him up 4h ago. He has never had pain as severe as this before: it moves into both flanks, although it seems to improve if he sits forward. He has vomited four times but just feels nauseous now. He takes perindopril 4mg once daily for hypertension. He drinks 6 units of alcohol per week.

```
T 36.6°C, HR 86bpm, BP 135/75mmHg.
```

His abdomen is soft but tender particularly over the upper and central abdomen. Which is the *single* most likely diagnosis? ★

A Acute appendicitis

B Acute pancreatitis

C Mesenteric ischaemia

D Perforated duodenal ulcer

E Upper small bowel obstruction

38. A 20-year-old man has extreme pain in his right calf after walking only short distances over the past few weeks. It eases quickly with rest and came on suddenly. He is a non-smoker and a keen athlete. His family doctor refers him for an MRI scan of his calf. Which *single* process is most likely to be responsible for his symptoms? ★

A Autoimmune inflammation of vascular walls

B Entrapment of vessel

C Inflammation of artery

D Impingement of nerve

E Stenosis of artery

39. A 36-year-old woman has an infected insect bite and has been feverish for a week. The Emergency Department doctor refers the patient to the surgical on-call team. The surgical registrar is on the way to the operating theatre, but tells the surgical junior doctor that the patient does not have a surgical problem and that he should discharge her with antibiotics and no follow-up. The area of cellulitis covers an area about 8cm × 8cm and has surrounding induration. The junior doctor is unsure whether there is an abscess present. Which is the *single* most appropriate next step? ★

A Arrange an outpatient ultrasound scan and give her a week of oral antibiotics

B Call your Registrar to see the patient when she is out of the theatre

C Discharge her with a course of antibiotics and no outpatient follow-up

D Give her oral antibiotics and ask her to return if things do not improve

E Use a needle and syringe and try and aspirate pus from the inflamed area

40. A 38-year-old woman is undergoing a mastectomy and latissimus dorsi reconstruction. She has been given a non-depolarizing neuromuscular blocking agent intra-operatively. Following completion of the operation, the anaesthetist needs to reverse this block. Which is the *single* most appropriate choice? ★

A Atracurium

B Glycopyrronium

C Neostigmine

D Suxamethonium

E Thiopental

41. A 24-year-old woman has had abdominal pain for the last 48h. It has been associated with nausea but no vomiting. Her last menstrual period was normal and finished 3 days ago. She has had no vaginal discharge and is not sexually active. She has had a recent persistent coryzal illness.

```
T 36.6°C, HR 63bpm, BP 125/75mmHg.

Urine dipstick: trace blood.
```

Her abdomen is soft but tender in the right iliac fossa, with no guarding or rebound tenderness. Which *single* additional finding is most likely to support the diagnosis? ★

A Cervical excitation

B Pause in inspiration on palpation of the right upper quadrant

C Right renal angle tenderness

D Soft stool on digital rectal examination

E Tender lymph nodes palpable in the neck

42. A 40-year-old woman has had a small sebaceous cyst on her back removed. The doctor wants to use 1% lidocaine as a local anaesthetic before closing the wound (maximum dose is 3mg/kg). The patient weighs 50kg. Which is the *single* maximum amount of 1% lidocaine that can be administered? ★

A 1.5ml

B 3ml

C 5ml

D 15ml

E 30ml

43. A 66-year-old woman has pain in her right hip 24h after having varicose veins stripped. The junior doctor is called to the ward. As he is reviewing the history, he realizes that he failed to make an entry in the notes during the morning ward round. It is now mid-afternoon. Which is the *single* most appropriate action? ★

A Find whoever led the morning round and ask them to make an entry

B Ignore the omission and move on to the next consultation

C Write the notes in now but mark the entry 'in retrospect'

D Write the notes in now with the current time

E Write: 'patient not seen on morning ward round'

44. A 70-year-old man had right iliac fossa pain for 10 days and underwent an open appendicectomy of a gangrenous appendix. Two days post-operatively, he is taking sips of fluids but feels bloated, nauseous, and sweaty.

```
T 36.2°C, HR 90bpm, BP 140/80mmHg,
RR 30/min.
```

Which is the *single* most appropriate next step? ★

A CT pulmonary angiogram + low-molecular-weight heparin

B ECG + cardiac enzymes

C Erect chest X-ray + abdominal X-ray

D Nasogastric tube + IV fluids

E Urinary catheter + furosemide 40mg IV

45. A 28-year-old woman has had pain under her right ribs for the last 12h since eating a lunch of chicken and chips. It radiates to her back and is associated with three or four bouts of vomiting. Although she has had this type of pain before, it has never been as bad as on this occasion. She had a caesarean section 3 years ago and takes the progestogen-only pill each day.

```
T 36.2°C, HR 80bpm, BP 130/66mmHg.
```

Her abdomen is soft but tender in the right upper quadrant in the mid-clavicular line on inspiration. Which is the *single* most appropriate initial imaging? ★

A Abdominal CT scan

B Endoscopic retrograde cholangiopancreatography (ERCP)

C Hepatobiliary iminodiacetic acid (HIDA) scan

D Magnetic resonance choleangiopancreatography (MRCP)

E Ultrasound scan of gallbladder

46. An 82-year-old man is seen in the Emergency Department with an incarcerated inguinal hernia. The surgical team deem him to have the capacity to decide the course of treatment and he consents to an urgent laparotomy. While he is awaiting a theatre slot, his pain increases and he becomes more unwell. He tells nursing staff that he no longer wants the operation and would like to withdraw his consent. Which is the *single* most appropriate course of action? ★

A Ask his next of kin to persuade him to have the operation

B Proceed to theatre as consent cannot be revoked

C Proceed to theatre under a section of the Mental Health Act 2007

D Reassess his capacity, given the change in his condition

E Respect his wishes as he has already been shown to have capacity

47. A 77-year-old man has had loose bloody bowel motions for the last 3 months. He has mixed Alzheimer's and vascular dementia with a mini mental state examination (MMSE) score of 14/30. The surgical team plan to investigate his symptoms with a colonoscopy. When seeking his consent, it is clear that he does not understand the explanations, cannot retain information, and cannot weigh up the risks and benefits. Which would constitute appropriate consent in this case? ★

A Verbal consent from the man

B Verbal consent from the man's next of kin

C Written consent by a doctor as proxy

D Written consent from the man

E Written consent from the man's next of kin

48.

A 62-year-old man has developed pain in his upper abdomen, which radiates into his back and loin. He returned from the High-Dependency Unit to a general surgical ward 3 days after a complex bowel resection. He is on a sliding scale insulin infusion for his type 1 diabetes.

```
T 38.4°C, HR 110bpm, BP 110/60mmHg, SaO₂ 96%
on air.
```

```
Urine dipstick: nothing abnormal detected.
```

```
Ultrasound scan of liver: no gallstones
seen.
```

He is tender in the right upper quadrant. Which is the *single* most likely explanation for these new symptoms? ★ ★

A Basal pneumonia

B Cholecystitis

C Liver abscess

D Pyelonephritis

E Renal stone

49.

A 21-year-old woman has had right iliac fossa pain, which started during the previous evening following her dinner. She vomited twice but now she just feels nauseous and is not hungry. She has passed eight to ten loose stools over the last 12h and has also found that she needs to pass urine more often than usual.

```
T 37.6°C, HR 90bpm, BP 130/75mmHg.
```

```
Urine dipstick: blood 1+, leukocytes 1+.
```

Which is the *single* most likely diagnosis? ★ ★

A Appendicitis

B Gastroenteritis

C Mesenteric adenitis

D Pelvic inflammatory disease

E Urinary tract infection

50. A registrar-led surgical ward round is in progress. The next patient has had a femoral-popliteal bypass but is in a side room because he is positive for *Clostridium difficile* toxin. In the side room, the doctor handles the patient's observation chart and then his drug chart. He does not have any physical contact with the patient before he moves on to the next patient. Which is the *single* most appropriate step before seeing the next patient? ★ ★

A Nothing – he did not touch the patient

B Nothing, unless he examines the next patient

C Put on a pair of gloves before examining the next patient

D Wash his hands with alcohol gel

E Wash his hands with soap and water

51. A 66-year-old man has passed blood with his stools for the last 6 weeks. Which is the *single* clinical feature that would be most suggestive of a carcinoma rather than haemorrhoids? ★ ★

A Anaemia

B Change in bowel habit

C Fresh rectal bleeding

D Itching around the anus

E Rectal mucous discharge

52. A 76-year-old woman is to undergo an elective hemi-colectomy for a caecal carcinoma. She has type 2 diabetes and has had previous arterial ulcers in the left leg (most recent ankle brachial pressure index (ABPI) 0.4). The junior doctor is asked to prescribe compression stockings as prophylaxis for venous thromboembolic disease (VTE). Which is the *single* most appropriate course of action? ★ ★

A Elevate legs with no compression

B High-pressure compression

C Keep legs dependent with no compression

D Low-pressure compression

E Low- or high-pressure compression at night only

53. A 33-year-old woman is a front seat passenger in a head on collision with another car. She sustains multiple long bone fractures and a splenic tear. During a laparotomy, she undergoes a splenectomy and fixation of her fractures. She is transferred to the Intensive Therapy Unit for initial post-operative management. Which is the *single* most appropriate step to take before discharge? ★ ★

A No specific prophylaxis or treatment is recommended once she has left the hospital

B The patient should be booked in for an influenza vaccination at the start of the winter months

C The patient should receive *Haemophilus influenzae* type B (HiB), pneumococcal, and meningitis C vaccines and take regular penicillin on discharge

D The patient should have a 2-week course of penicillin at home to take should she become unwell

E Vaccines are not indicated but the patient may require immunoglobulin treatment if she becomes unwell in the future

54. A 65-year-old woman has had left-sided abdominal pain, been off her food, and felt tired for the last 3 days. She has passed three or four loose stools each day and urine frequently. Her bowels usually open twice weekly, often followed by a few days of loose stools. Any pain that she has previously had settles after spending a few days in bed.

`T 37.8°C, HR 92bpm, BP 155/82mmHg.`

Her abdomen is soft but slightly distended and tender in the left iliac fossa. Which is the *single* most likely diagnosis? ★ ★

A Coeliac disease

B Colonic carcinoma

C Diverticulitis

D Irritable bowel syndrome

E Viral gastroenteritis

55. A 66-year-old woman has had diarrhoea associated with pain in the left side of her abdomen over the last 3 days. Normally, she opens her bowels once or twice a week, but over the last 12h, she has passed very loose stools with a large amount of mucus and bright red blood.

`T 37.7°C, HR 86bpm, BP 138/76mmHg.`

Her abdomen is soft but distended and tender in the left iliac fossa. She is admitted and treated with antibiotics and returns 6 weeks later for a colonoscopy. Which is the *single* most likely finding on colonoscopy? ★ ★

A Friable sigmoid colon mucosa that bleeds on contact

B Large ulcerated lesion in the ascending colon

C Mucosal projections through the circular muscle of the colon

D Multiple pedunculated polyps in the distal colon

E Patchy ulcerated fissures throughout the colon

56. A 58-year-old woman has had left-sided abdominal pain and been off her food for the last week. Initially, she passed loose stools with mucus and small amounts of blood but her bowels have not opened for the last 48h. Since a teenager, she has always had a tendency to be constipated but can also be affected by episodes of loose stools over a number of days and abdominal pain relieved by passing flatus.

```
T 37.9°C, HR 90bpm, BP 142/82mmHg.

Hb 11.8g/dL, WCC 14.2 × 10⁹/L,
platelets 340 × 10⁹/L.
```

Her abdomen is soft but tender in the left iliac fossa. Which is the *single* most appropriate management? ★ ★

A Blood transfusion + laparotomy

B Colonoscopy + water-soluble enema contrast

C High-fibre diet + laxatives

D Nasogastric tube + IV fluids

E Nil by mouth + IV antibiotics

57. A 58-year-old man has felt feverish and has had a distended upper abdomen for the last 2 days. He has only recently left hospital, prior to which he recalls severe abdominal pain and vomiting. He drinks 40 units of alcohol per week.

```
T 38.2°C, HR 90bpm, BP 156/90mmHg.
```

His abdomen is soft but there is a 10cm × 8cm mass in the upper abdomen. Which is the *single* most likely cause for the abdominal mass? ★ ★

A Ascites

B Gastric volvulus

C Hepatomegaly

D Liver abscess

E Pancreatic pseudocyst

58. A 64-year-old man has had pain in his left lower leg for the last 4 days. He says he has lost feeling in the lower part of it over the last day or two. He has hypertension, type 2 diabetes, and schizophrenia. The limb is very pale and no pulses are palpable. The on-call surgical team explain to the man that at this stage the best option would be a below-knee amputation of the limb. The man refuses. Which is the *single* most appropriate next step? ★ ★

A Assess the man's capacity to make such a decision

B As the man has a mental illness, operate in his best interests

C Operate having detained the man under a section of the Mental Health Act 2007

D Respect the man's wishes and do as he wants

E Seek consent for the surgery from his next of kin

59. A 44-year-old man has severe right-sided abdominal pain, which moves down into his groin. The pain started suddenly and comes and goes in waves. He vomited twice when the pain started and his bowels have not opened today. He admits to eating a poor diet with regular take-away meals and drinks 20 units of alcohol per week usually all at the weekend. He is taking oral non-steroidal anti-inflammatory drugs (NSAIDs) for a soft-tissue injury. Which is the *single* most useful piece of advice for this man to prevent further presentations? ★ ★

A Cut down on alcohol binges

B Drink 2–3L fluid per day

C Follow a low-fat diet

D Only take NSAIDs after meals

E Use regular laxatives and aim for two soft stools per day

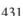

60. A 62-year-old man has been passing small amounts of blood with his bowel movements for 2 months. He is not sure whether it is mixed with the stool but the blood is bright red in colour and he thinks it is getting less. He has always been troubled by constipation but he has not noticed any change in his bowels recently. He has osteoarthritis and takes regular diclofenac for symptomatic relief. He has no family history of bowel cancer. Which is the *single* most appropriate management? ★ ★ ★

A Add omeprazole 40mg PO once daily

B Commence regular lactulose 20ml PO twice daily

C Routine referral to surgical outpatients clinic

D Send a full blood count and review if he is anaemic

E Urgent 2-week referral to surgical outpatients clinic

61. A 60-year-old man with a rectal carcinoma underwent a low anterior resection 4 days ago. He has now become unwell and complains of chest pain. He has chronic obstructive pulmonary disease (COPD) and takes long-term oral steroids but has no history of cardiac disease.

```
T 37.5°C, HR 95bpm, BP 125/74mmHg,
SaO₂ 92% on 28% O₂.
```

An ECG is performed and shows tall P waves in the inferior leads. His urine output is 30–40ml/h. Which is the *single* most likely cause of his deterioration? ★ ★ ★

A Anastomotic leak

B Aspiration pneumonia

C Basal atelectasis

D Myocardial infarction

E Pulmonary embolism

62. A 42-year-old man has started passing small amounts of fresh blood with his bowel motions over the last 4 weeks. He is opening his bowels three times daily, whereas before he opened them only once daily, but this is not associated with any other change in his stools. He has not noticed any tiredness, weight loss, or change in his appetite. His abdomen is soft and non-tender. A digital rectal examination reveals soft stool with no blood or mucus. Which is the *single* most appropriate next step? ★ ★ ★

A Arrange to review in 2 months

B Arrange to review in 2 weeks

C Reassure and ask to return if things do not improve

D Routine referral to surgical outpatients clinic

E Urgent referral to surgical outpatients clinic

63. A 44-year-old woman is having a laparotomy for adhesional small bowel obstruction. She had an open cholecystectomy 18 years ago, but otherwise has been in good health and has no other medical problems. The operation goes well and the abdomen is closed in layers. The skin in the midline is closed with metal clips. Which is the *single* earliest day after her operation that the clips could start to be taken out? ★ ★ ★

A 2 days

B 4 days

C 6 days

D 8 days

E 10 days

64. An 85-year-old woman has had lower abdominal pain for 1 week. She has been vomiting and not had her bowels open for 10 days. She lives alone and has vascular dementia. Her abdomen is distended and diffusely tender with tinkling bowel sounds. The surgical registrar explains to the woman that she needs emergency surgery: she flatly refuses to give her consent. The surgeon notes that she is unable to comprehend and retain information about her clinical situation or to weigh up the risks and benefits of the proposed treatment. Which would be the *single* most appropriate course of action? ★ ★ ★

A Ask a member of the woman's family to persuade her that surgery would be in her best interests

B Ask a psychiatrist to admit the woman under the Mental Health Act 2007 so that he can legally proceed to surgery

C Proceed to surgery if the surgeon feels it would be in the woman's best interests

D Respect the woman's wishes

E Seek consent from the woman's next of kin

65. An 81-year-old man has metastatic prostatic carcinoma. He is taking 30mg of modified release morphine orally twice daily for pain with three 10mg doses of morphine liquid for breakthrough pain over a 24h period. He is rapidly deteriorating and the on-call registrar feels that the best strategy now would be to commence a diamorphine syringe driver. The junior doctor has been asked to write the prescription. Which is the *single* most appropriate 24h dose of subcutaneous diamorphine? ★ ★ ★

A 30mg

B 45mg

C 90mg

D 135mg

E 180mg

66. A 32-year-old man is knocked off his bicycle at 25mph, landing heavily on his left side, and has pain in his left shoulder. He was wearing a helmet and did not lose consciousness. His Glasgow Coma Scale (GCS) score is 15/15. He has some bruising and tenderness over the left eight and ninth ribs posteriorly and tenderness over the left clavicle. The trauma series of X-rays show no abnormalities. A left shoulder X-ray shows an undisplaced fracture of the clavicle. Which is the *single* most appropriate next step? ★ ★ ★

A Admit and observe for 24h before discharge

B CT scan of the abdomen

C Discharge home with analgesia and a sling

D MRI of the left shoulder

E Facial X-rays

$67.$ An 81-year-old woman has had central abdominal pain over the last 24h. She usually has difficulty opening her bowels and has been passing minimal flatus for the past 3 days. Her abdomen is distended with a tympanic percussion note. An abdominal X-ray is performed (Figure 10.4).

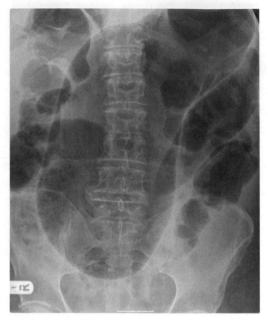

Figure 10.4

```
T 36.7°C, HR 88bpm, BP 155/86mmHg.
Hb 12.6g/dL, WCC 8.5 × 10⁹/L.
Venous blood gas: pH 7.44, base excess -0.7.
```

Which is the *single* most appropriate initial management? ★ ★ ★

A Barium enema

B CT scan of the abdomen

C Flexible sigmoidoscopy

D Laparotomy

E Laxative therapy

68. A 58-year-old man has had rapidly worsening pain near his rectum for 4 days. He has had normal bowel movements and has passed no blood.

`T 37.8°C, HR 90bpm, BP 125/80mmHg.`

His abdomen is soft and non-tender. The medial side of his right buttock is erythematous, indurated, and warm and tender, but with no obvious focus. A digital rectal examination reveals no external sites of bleeding and an empty rectum with no blood but a thickened right lateral wall. Which *single* additional feature in the history would be most concerning? ★ ★ ★

A He has a family history of colorectal cancer

B He has previously had haemorrhoids

C He has recently completed a course of antibiotics

D He has type 2 diabetes

E He is nauseous and has vomited

69. A 74-year-old woman has undergone a femoral hernia repair. She takes metformin for type 2 diabetes and stopped her aspirin a week ago. She is commenced on enoxaparin 40mg SC and has three doses of antibiotic prophylaxis peri-operatively. She makes a slow post-operative recovery and on day 8, despite regularly receiving low-molecular-weight heparin (LMWH), develops a tender right calf. An ultrasound scan shows the presence of a deep vein thrombosis (DVT). Which *single* pair of investigations should be performed? ★ ★ ★

A Activated partial thromboplastin time (APTT) + international normalized ratio (INR)

B Factor V Leiden + factor VII

C Fibrinogen + haemoglobin

D Platelets + potassium

E Protein S + protein C

70. A 77-year-old woman has had severe pain in her left hand for 3h. It came on suddenly and is associated with numbness and tingling. She has had two previous myocardial infarctions and takes digoxin 62.5mcg PO once daily for an irregular heart rhythm. Her left hand is cold and white with a capillary refill time of <2s. Sensation is decreased from the wrist distally, but power is unaffected. Which would be the *single* most appropriate treatment? ★ ★ ★

A Amputation

B Angioplasty

C Bypass

D Embolectomy

E Heparinization

71. A 66-year-old man has had central abdominal pain for the past 4 weeks. It radiates through to his back and is associated with nausea. He has not felt hungry during this time and has lost more than 5kg. His abdomen is tender in the epigastrium.

```
Bilirubin 146µmol/L, ALP 766IU/L,
AST 32IU/L, GGT 480IU/L.
```

Which is the *single* most appropriate next step? ★ ★ ★

A CT scan of the abdomen

B Endoscopic retrograde cholangiopancreatography (ERCP)

C Hepatobiliary iminodiacetic acid scan (HIDA)

D Magnetic resonance cholangiopancreatography (MRCP)

E Ultrasound scan of the liver

72. A 74-year-old woman has had lower abdominal pain and vomiting for 5 days. Her bowels have not opened in this time and she feels extremely bloated. She is in a considerable amount of pain. She takes levothyroxine 100mcg PO once daily. She smokes 20 cigarettes a day and drinks 15 units of alcohol a week. An abdominal X-ray is performed (Figure 10.5).

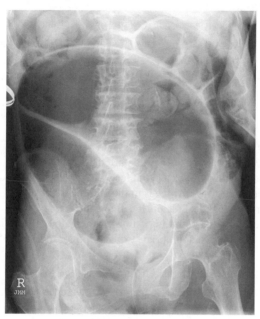

Figure 10.5

T 36.4°C, HR 90bpm, BP 128/80mmHg.

Which is the *single* most likely diagnosis? ★ ★ ★

A Incarcerated umbilical hernia

B Gallstone ileus

C Perforated duodenal ulcer

D Severe constipation

E Sigmoid volvulus

73. A 64-year-old woman has had loose stools, rectal bleeding, and weight loss for the last 6 months. The day after a colonoscopy, she has an episode of chest pain while getting washed and dressed.

```
T 36.6°C, HR 105bpm, BP 125/80mmHg,
SaO₂ 93% on 2L O₂.
```

Which is the *single* most appropriate initial management? ★ ★ ★

A CT pulmonary angiogram (CT-PA)

B D-dimer

C Erect chest X-ray

D Therapeutic dose of low-molecular-weight heparin (LMWH)

E Ventilation/perfusion (VQ) scan

74. A 28-year-old man has had a painful swelling for 2 weeks. He was started on a course of flucloxacillin 1 week ago but feels things have worsened since then. The swelling is in the midline in the upper part of the gluteal region. It is fluctuant, 2cm × 2cm in size and the surrounding skin is erythematous. Which is the *single* most appropriate explanation for the cause of this lump? ★ ★ ★

A An in-growing hair characteristically is the cause

B Chronic constipation is recognized to increase the incidence

C High alcohol consumption typically is linked with these

D Poor anal hygiene is characteristically to blame

E Poor diabetic control is recognised to increase the incidence

75. A 60-year-old woman has come to pre-assessment clinic to discuss the surgical repair of her para-umbilical hernia. She is accompanied by her husband. He is very keen that the operation goes ahead and does most of the talking. The patient herself appears rather anxious and does not say much.

The surgeon running the clinic explains the risks and benefits of the surgery with a view to gaining the patient's written consent to proceed to theatre. Which is the *single* most appropriate way for the surgeon to gain consent for the operation? ★ ★ ★

A Ask the husband to give written consent as he has been the main point of contact

B Ask the patient to give written consent as she has been given a full explanation

C Ask to talk to the patient on her own before addressing consent

D Postpone gaining written consent until the morning of surgery

E Verbal consent is sufficient if a full explanation has been given

76. A 77-year-old man has a rectal adenocarcinoma and has had his consent taken for an anterior resection. The surgeon has left instructions in the medical notes for the patient to be given bowel preparation the day before the operation. The nursing staff call the junior doctor to prescribe the medication for the patient. Which is the *single* most appropriate preparation to prescribe? ★ ★ ★

A Docusate sodium 200mg PO twice daily

B Lactulose 50ml PO twice daily

C Macrogol (polyethylene glycol 3350) 1 sachet PO twice daily

D Senna 4 tablets PO twice daily

E Sodium picosulphate 10mg 1 sachet PO twice daily

77. A 25-year-old woman has noticed a lump in her neck. She is worried about it as she also thinks she has lost some weight recently. The mass is fluctuant and moves superiorly when she swallows and protrudes her tongue. Which is the *single* most likely anatomical site of the lump? ★ ★ ★

A Arising from the jugular lymph sac

B Inferior to the angle of the mandible

C Upper third of the sternocleidomastoid

D Midline below the hyoid bone

E Superior to the carotid bifurcation

78. A 68-year-old woman has had central abdominal pain for 3 days. Over the last 12h, the pain has become more intense and she has vomited four times. She has not opened her bowels for 2 days. She has type 2 diabetes and takes aspirin 75mg once daily and gliclazide 80mg twice daily.

```
T 36.4°C, HR 90bpm, BP 128/80mmHg.
```

An abdominal X-ray is performed (Figure 10.6). Her abdomen is distended with a tympanic percussion note.

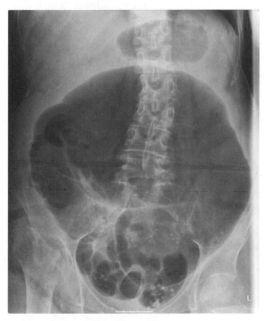

Figure 10.6

Which is the *single* most likely diagnosis? ★ ★ ★

A Absolute constipation

B Caecal volvulus

C Incarcerated epigastric hernia

D Perforated gastric ulcer

E Small bowel obstruction

79. A 47-year-old man has a sudden onset of upper abdominal pain that radiates into his back. He has vomited six or seven times but now just feels nauseous. His bowels opened normally today and he has no urinary symptoms. He drinks 30 units of alcohol a week.

```
T 36.6°C, HR 86bpm, BP 165/75mmHg.
```

His abdomen is soft but tender, particularly in the epigastric region. The junior doctor is asked to formally grade the severity of this man's condition. Which *single* investigation will be most useful? ★ ★ ★

A Amylase

B Creatinine

C C-reactive protein

D Lipase

E Urea

80. A 22-year-old woman has an emergency bowel resection for a superior mesenteric artery thrombosis. Which *single* diagnostic test is most likely to identify the cause? ★ ★ ★ ★

A Anti-phospholipid antibodies

B Anti-thrombin

C Factor V Leiden

D Protein C

E Protein S

81. A 55-year-old man undergoes a laparoscopic anterior resection. His operation is uneventful and he has a fentanyl/bupivacaine epidural post-operatively for pain relief with good effect. He is given a low-molecular-weight heparin (LMWH) subcutaneously as thromboprophylaxis. On day 2 post-operatively, he is starting to tolerate oral fluids and eat. The decision is taken to stop the epidural. Which is the *single* earliest time at which the epidural can be safely removed after the dose of LMWH? ★ ★ ★ ★

A Immediately

B 2h

C 6h

D 10h

E 24h

82. A 44-year-old woman has chronic pain due to an intra-abdominal malignancy. She currently takes morphine modified release (MR) 30mg twice daily and morphine liquid 10mg as required for breakthrough pain (max. every 4h). Over the last month, the pain has gradually worsened such that she now needs to take 10mg of the morphine liquid regularly every 4h. Which is the *single* most appropriate change to her morphine regime? ★ ★ ★ ★

A MR 30mg twice daily; liquid 20mg every 4h as required

B MR 30mg twice daily; liquid 20mg every 1h as required

C MR 30mg twice daily; liquid 40mg every 4h as required

D MR 60mg twice daily; liquid 10mg every 4h as required

E MR 60mg twice daily; liquid 20mg every 4h as required

83. A 43-year-old man has abdominal pain following an endoscopic retrograde cholangiopancreatography (ERCP) and sphincterotomy 2 days ago for a gallstone obstructing his common bile duct. He now has severe pain, which is worse in his right upper quadrant and radiates down into his flank, associated with nausea and vomiting twice this morning.

```
T 37.5°C, HR 90bpm, BP 115/75mmHg.
```

```
Sodium 135mmol/L, potassium 3.5mmol/L,
creatinine 90μmol/L, amylase 78U/dL.
```

His abdomen is tender with guarding throughout the right side. Which *single* investigation is most likely to confirm the diagnosis? ★ ★ ★ ★

A Abdominal ultrasound scan

B Abdominal X-ray

C CT scan of the abdomen

D IV urogram (IVU)

E Magnetic resonance cholangiopancreatography (MRCP)

84. A 38-year-old man attends the pre-operative assessment clinic a week before his inguinal hernia repair. He has no past medical history and takes no medications. He smokes ten cigarettes a day and drinks 25 units of alcohol a week.

```
T 37°C, HR 75bpm, BP 130/70mmHg.
```

The nursing staff asks the junior doctor which pre-operative tests need to be done. Which *single* test below is recommended pre-operatively? ★ ★ ★ ★

A Chest X-ray

B Clotting screen

C ECG

D Full blood count

E No tests required

85. A 34-year-old woman has had a laparoscopic appendicectomy. The surgeon has resected a moderately inflamed but not gangrenous appendix. The abdominal wounds are closed layer by layer. The junior doctor has assisted on a number of laparoscopic operations and the consultant asks him to close the skin using non-absorbable sutures. Which is the *single* most appropriate choice? ★ ★ ★ ★

A Dexon®

B Ethilon®

C Monocryl®

D PDS®

E Vicryl®

86. A 69-year-old woman underwent a femoral artery aneurysm repair 4 days ago. She has become unwell over the last 48h with a cough productive of green sputum.

```
T 38.5°C, HR 88bpm, BP 145/86mmHg.

Sodium 139mmol/L, potassium 4.1mmol/L,
creatinine 88μmol/L.
```

Blood cultures grow a multi-resistant *Staphylococcus aureus* in both bottles. She is started on vancomycin 1g IV twice daily. A trough level is taken before the third dose and found to be 20.4mg/L (trough level range <15mg/L). Which is the *single* most appropriate next step? ★ ★ ★ ★

A It is on the borderline of normal limits, so give the fourth dose of 1g

B No need to repeat the level; give the fourth dose at 750mg

C Omit the fourth dose and change the dosing regime to 1g once daily

D Repeat the level and change the dosing regime to 1g every 18h

E Repeat the level and give the fourth dose at 750mg when in range

EXTENDED MATCHING QUESTIONS

Surface anatomy

For each scenario, choose the *single* most likely anatomical location from the list of options below. Each option may be used once, more than once, or not at all. ★

A At the level of a horizontal line from left to right anterior superior iliac spine

B At the level of the umbilicus

C Between L1 and L4 posteriorly

D Between T9 and L1 posteriorly

E Between the anterior superior iliac spine and the pubic tubercle

F Halfway along a line from the midline just superior to the umbilicus

G In the right subcostal margin in the midclavicular line

H Just inferior and lateral to the pubic tubercle

I Just superior and medial to the pubic tubercle

J Just superior to the midpoint of a line between the anterior superior iliac spine and pubis

K Midway between the xiphisternum and the pubis

L Two-thirds of the way along a line from the umbilicus to the anterior superior iliac spine

M Over the ninth to the eleventh ribs

1. A 44-year-old man has been brought in to the Emergency Department following a motor vehicle collision. His Glasgow Coma Score (GCS) score is 8 and he has a rigid abdomen. Soon after he arrives, he goes into ventricular fibrillation (VF). Cardiopulmonary resuscitation (CPR) is commenced and one of the doctors wants to take a blood sample from the femoral artery.

2. A 33-year-old woman has had right-sided abdominal pain for the last 12h associated with three episodes of vomiting. She is examined and the doctor thinks she might have appendicitis because she is maximally tender over McBurney's point.

3. A 73-year-old woman has had central abdominal pain and vomiting for the last 12h. She has noticed a lump in her groin, which she thinks appeared at the same time as the symptoms started. The doctor examining her thinks she might have a strangulated femoral hernia.

4. A 28-year-old woman has had back ache and felt feverish for the last 3 days. Her urine dipstick shows nitrites, leukocytes, and blood, and the doctor thinks she might have pyelonephritis. The patient is sitting up and the doctor wants to palpate over the kidneys to assess for any tenderness.

5. A 32-year-old man returned from a month long trip to Nigeria. He took no anti-malarial prophylaxis while abroad and now feels feverish and tired and has generalized arthralgia. The doctor thinks he might have malaria and wants to palpate over the spleen to rule out any enlargement.

Causes of hernia

For each scenario, choose the *single* most likely hernia from the list of options below. Each option may be used once, more than once, or not at all. ★

A Direct inguinal

B Divarication

C Epigastric

D Femoral

E Incisional

F Indirect inguinal

G Littré's

H Obturator

I Paraumbilical

J Richter's

K Spigelian

L Umbilical

6. A 44-year-old woman has a swelling in her groin. She has been aware of it in the past, but it usually disappears by itself. Over the last 6h, she has felt bloated and has vomited four times. Her bowels opened this morning, but she has not passed any flatus in the last few hours. The lump is below and lateral to the pubic tubercle.

7. A 51-year-old man has a painful lump in his groin. This cannot be reduced back into the abdomen and he is taken to the operating theatre for it to be repaired. In the hernia sac is a Meckel's diverticulum.

8. A 56-year-old woman has a lump on her abdominal wall just inferior to the umbilicus. The swelling is not easy to palpate, but can be localized to the left lateral border of the rectus abdominis muscle.

9. A 27-year-old man has a lump in his right groin. Although he has been aware of it for 6 months, it was not until today that it became bigger than usual. The lump is reducible and with pressure over an area about 1.5cm above the femoral pulsation in the right groin, it does not reappear.

10. A 48-year-old man has a lump in his anterior abdominal wall. He has noticed it increasingly over the last few years when he tries to sit up from his bed in the morning. The lump is seen in the midline when the man lifts his head from the bed or coughs.

Diagnosis of rectal bleeds

For each of the following patients with rectal bleeding, choose the *single* most likely diagnosis from the list of options below. Each option may be used once, more than once, or not at all. ★

A Anal cancer

B Anal fissure

C Angiodysplasia

D Caecal cancer

E *Clostridium difficile* colitis

F Crohn's disease

G Diverticulitis

H Haemorrhoids

I Ischaemic colitis

J Perianal haematoma

K Sigmoid cancer

L Ulcerative colitis

11. A 55-year-old man has noticed bright red blood in the toilet each time he passes a stool for the last couple of months. It often seems to coat the faeces and on occasions drips into the pan as he stands. He has felt an intermittent itch around the anus but has otherwise been well.

12. A 60-year-old man has felt his bowels to be incompletely empty, even straight after defaecating, for the past 6 weeks. He has been intermittently constipated during this period. When he has opened his bowels, it has been loose, with blood and mucus mixed in with it.

13. A 40-year-old man has had abdominal cramps and increasingly loose bowel motions over the past few days. Latterly, these motions have contained streaks of blood and mucus. He has lost his appetite and feels feverish and generally unwell. He has experienced these episodes before and suffers from fluctuating weight.

14. A 64-year-old woman has had 3 days of generalized abdominal pain with the most tenderness on the left side. It has been intermittent and relieved by defaecation. She has latterly had a day of very loose motions, the last heavily blood-stained. She is nauseous and feels unwell.

15. A 55-year-old man has noticed his toilet paper intermittently stained with blood after wiping. Defaecation itself has become very painful, as though he were passing a very sharp object. He is left with a residual uncomfortable itch around his back passage.

Causes of rectal bleeding

For each rectal bleed, choose the *single* most likely pathophysiological source from the list of options below. Each option may be used once, more than once, or not at all. ★ ★ ★ ★

A Friable submucosal veins in the ascending colon

B Malignant growth in the caecal epithelium

C Malignant growth in the rectal epithelium

D Split in the squamous lining of the lower anal canal

E Swollen, inflamed anal blood vessels

F Tract between the anal canal and the perianal skin

G Transmural inflammation involving the terminal ileum

H Ulcerated rectal mucosa with pseudopolyps

I Vasa rectae in the submucosa

16. A 72-year-old man has had a sudden, painless loss of blood. The blood is dark red and mixed in with the stool. He has always been slightly constipated and has gained a small amount of weight recently following a recent admission for left-sided abdominal pain that settled with antibiotics.
Haemoglobin 11.5g/dL.

17. A 77-year-old woman has passed small amounts of blood over the last 2 months. She gets the urge to open her bowels, but is left feeling like she has not passed everything when she has finished. Her stools are harder than before, making opening her bowels painful, and she has tried a local anaesthetic cream with little effect.

18. A 28-year-old man has recently noticed small amounts of fresh blood after opening his bowels. He has a poor diet and only opens his bowels three times a week with hard, pellet-like stools. He has never experienced this before. His father was recently diagnosed with a colonic adenocarcinoma.

19. A 72-year-old man has passed a large amount of fresh blood rectally. This was painless and has never happened before. He opens his bowels once daily and his stools are normally soft. He takes metformin for type 2 diabetes. A CT angiogram identifies the cause of the bleeding.

20. A 26-year-old man has had diarrhoea and has felt feverish since returning from his holiday a week ago. He is opening his bowels four to six times daily and passing stools with mucus and blood, but often gets little warning he needs to go. Nobody else in the family is unwell. His older brother is being treated for irritable bowel syndrome.
Haemoglobin 9.5g/dL.

Single Best Answers

1. D ★   OHCM 8th edn → pp656–657

The risk of rupture of an AAA 4.0–5.0cm in diameter is 1% per year. There is no formal surveillance programme in place nationally. The UK Small Aneurysm Trial randomized 1090 patients with an AAA of 4–5.5cm in diameter to surveillance or an operation. There was no statistical benefit in offering patients early surgery.

Aneurysms obey the Law of Laplace, namely, that as a vessel increases in radius the inward force on the vessel decreases and the aneurysm continues to expand until it ruptures. However, stopping smoking and controlling hypertension is the best way to reduce the rate at which this occurs.

The UK Small Aneurysm Trial Participants (1998). Mortality results for randomized controlled trial of early elective surgery or ultrasonographic surveillance for small abdominal aortic aneurysms. *Lancet* **352**:1649–1655.

→ http://www.thelancet.com/journals/lancet/article/PIIS0140-6736(98)10137-X/fulltext

2. A ★   OHCM 8th edn → pp656–657

It is likely that this man has ruptured an abdominal aortic aneurysm. Although the junior doctor cannot know this for sure, he needs to be able to deal with uncertainty, manage risk, and take the safest option available: this means that he does not waste time with unnecessary investigations (C and E), does not pass the buck or miss the urgency of the situation (B), and does not get distracted by details (D). If he can appreciate the bigger picture and sees that this man is shocked (enough to collapse) with a palpable source of bleeding, then he should have the confidence to summon whoever can take consent from the patient for immediate surgery. Once senior doctors are aware of the emergency, he can concentrate on stabilizing the patient by securing good IV access, sending bloods and cross-matching >10U, fluid resuscitating, inserting a catheter, and performing an ECG.

A key point here is that it is much safer for the junior to over-react in potentially serious clinical situations. There is no harm done if the registrar races to see this man but is not convinced of the diagnosis and feels the patient is stable enough for a CT scan rather than an immediate laparotomy. Harm is done if the junior doctor downplays a situation and does not escalate it fast enough because of his own doubts, fears of being proved wrong or overly cautious by seniors, or simply because he has failed to appreciate the gravity of the situation.

3. D ★   OHCM 8th edn → pp656–657

In an elderly man presenting with sudden abdominal pain, shock, and confusion, the most important diagnosis that must be excluded is an AAA. Imaging should not delay the treatment, which is an operation. Mortality is 70–95%.

4. D ★

This young man later underwent an open appendicectomy for a pus-filled appendix. The deranged liver function tests and clotting are a result of the sepsis. The other options could not account for the urinary symptoms and deranged blood results.

5. A ★   OHCM 8th edn → pp610–611

This is as classical a presentation of appendicitis as you could wish for: the migratory nature of the pain (as visceral pain becomes local peritonism), the nausea, the low-grade fever, and tachycardia (Alvarado score >7). In female patients, the chief differential diagnosis is an ectopic pregnancy, but this is virtually excluded by a negative pregnancy test. Neither C nor E is likely to cause such rapidly developing clinical pictures, but E at least would remain an important differential if laparoscopy revealed a benign-looking appendix. Other supporting evidence for an acute appendix would be a raised WCC comprising 75% neutrophils.

→ http://www.rcsed.ac.uk/journal/svol1_1/10100006.html

6. A ★   OHCM 8th edn → pp636–637

The clues here are: this is a recurrent problem; constant pain with nausea lasting <6h, radiates to back; and correct demographic. Pain from the intermittent obstruction of the biliary tree by gallstones can present with a variety of clinical signs, but tends to include an inability to keep still, a tachycardia, and tenderness in the upper abdomen with no guarding.

B Sufferers of chronic pancreatitis normally live with a degree of pain, which occasionally flares up; they would be unlikely to present for the first time with two separate episodes of very short-lived pain.

C Hepatitis C is unlikely; if acute it is often asymptomatic and if chronic it is likely to present with a range of associated chronic symptoms.

D Whilst peptic ulcer disease is a good differential diagnosis, it is more likely to present with ongoing pain that occasionally flares up rather than two distinct episodes of pain as in this case.

E Renal colic is unlikely given the lack of urinary symptoms.

7. E ★   OHCM 8th edn → pp636–637

The history is suggestive of biliary disease: a woman in her 40s with high cholesterol who has had similar previous episodes. She also has a fever, rigors, and mild hypotension so this is an attack of acute cholecystitis. Examination of her abdomen would reveal epigastric or RUQ pain. On palpation of the RUQ, she is likely to pause whilst trying to take a deep breath in. This is known as Murphy's sign, which is said to be 97% sensitive for cholecystitis.

A This is suggestive of acute pancreatitis.

B These are Cullen's sign (periumbilical discoloration) and Grey Turner's sign (flanks), also seen (rarely) in acute pancreatitis.

C This is Rovsing's sign, which is supportive of an appendicitis.

D This is found in renal or ureteric inflammation (pyelonephritis or calculus disease).

Singer AJ, McCracken G, Henry MC, Thode HC, and Cabahug JC (1996). Correlation among clinical, laboratory, and hepatobiliary scanning findings in patients with suspected acute cholecystitis. *Ann Emerg Med* 28:267–272.

8. E ★

This woman has intermittent claudication caused by arterial disease. The most serious consequence of this would be an abdominal aortic aneurysm, hence the need to palpate the abdomen. All other options would be helpful in completing the picture but it is E that is the one that simply cannot be missed.

→ http://www.sign.ac.uk/pdf/qrg89.pdf

9. B ★   OHCM 8th edn → pp580–581

Lower limb paralysis and her severe lung disease put her at a moderate to high risk of DVT and makes this the most likely diagnosis.

A This is unlikely as she is afebrile and systemically well.

C There is no history of malignancy or lymph node biopsies to suggest this.

D AND E Neither ruptured cysts nor thrombophlebosis cause such widespread oedema.

10. E ★

Urgent referral should be made in the case of unilateral eczematous skin or nipple change that does not respond to topical treatment. In this case Paget's disease of the breast needs to be ruled out.

→ http://www.nice.org.uk/guidance/CG27

11. B ★

This woman has features of bowel obstruction. The key to the cause is the tenderness of the groin lump. If it were non-tender, this would be less likely to be the cause of her symptoms.

A If there were no lump, then, given the surgical history, band adhesions would be the most likely cause of obstruction.

C Lymphomas can present with enlarged 'rubbery' inguinal lymph nodes, but these are more likely to be painless and non-tender and associated with a range of other symptoms (e.g. malaise, night sweats, low grade fever).

D Pancreatic cancer is unlikely to present in this way (it is usually either painless jaundice, epigastric pain and anorexia, or acute pancreatitis, depending on the part of pancreas affected) or to spread to inguinal lymph nodes.

E Attacks of ulcerative colitis usually present with bloody diarrhoea and abdominal pain rather than bowel obstruction and are not typical for this age group.

12. C ★   OHCM 8th edn → p605

This is a fibroadenoma: commonly found in teenagers with an increased incidence in those on the oral contraceptive pill. It should only be removed if it causes pain or discomfort. It 'never' becomes malignant but occasionally a lobular carcinoma can involve a fibroadenoma.

13. A ★

The chart shows a temperature that varies from normal or below normal to well above normal. The fact that this variation happens in a 'swinging' pattern is classically suggestive of a collection of pus. If such a finding leads to the suspicion of an abscess, then the normal course of events is to try and find its location: in this case, this is likely to be fairly straightforward given the recent surgery, but some imaging will be required along with a prolonged course of antibiotics and drainage of the pus.

14. C ★   OHCM 8th edn → pp658–659

The length of symptoms and the clinical findings suggest that this woman's leg has suffered irreversible ischaemia. In cases such as this where blood has stagnated in the arterial tree and clotted (hence the fixed dark blue staining), any attempt to revascularize the limb could be dangerous as it risks a 'reperfusion injury'.

All other options are inappropriate. Neither the patient's age (A) nor smoking habits (B) should influence management, whilst the fact she has cancer (D) is a risk for the development of the ischaemia in the first place but should not drive how it is treated. In scenarios where patients are said to have cerebral disease, it is tempting to assume they do not have capacity (E): this is clearly a mistake. In this case, even if the patient was shown to not have capacity, this would not change the surgeon's opinion, as amputation of the limb would remain in her best interests.

Tailor J, Parkinson M, and Handa A (2008). Acute limb ischaemia. *Student BMJ* 1:80–81.

→ http://archive.student.bmj.com/issues/08/02/education/080.php

15. B ★   OHCM 8th edn → p612

This man has a bowel obstruction. His history is very suggestive and is qualified by an X-ray showing dilated loops of the small bowel. Given his surgical history, the most likely cause is band adhesions. The aim in managing the condition is to relieve pressure on the bowel: partial small bowel obstruction is therefore managed conservatively by passing a nasogastric tube and rehydrating with IV fluids. In most cases, surgery will not be necessary; indeed, the goal is to avoid surgery for fear of producing more adhesions and a cycle of recurrent pain and obstruction.

There is no need for imaging (A) in simple adhesional small bowel obstruction, but in large bowel obstruction a colonoscopy (D) (or gastrograffin enema) may be useful in visualizing a mechanical cause for the blockage. Large bowel obstruction is also likely to need surgery sooner (E), particularly with gross dilatation of the caecum. Laxatives (C) would not be helpful in this situation, although in large bowel obstruction, enemas can be used with discretion.

16. A ★   OHCM 8th edn → p632

This is a typical description of an anal fissure and can initiate a cycle of: pain – fear to pass stool – constipation – pain.

B Haemorrhoids do cause the passage of bright red blood but they are not painful unless they thrombose and become enclosed by the anal sphincter causing distal venous engorgement.

C A DRE may well be too painful to carry out, but there is likely to be swelling and erythema evident around the perineum, which would also be generally tender to the touch.

D This is an idiopathic cause of an intense stabbing pain deep in the rectum due to cramping of either the pubococcygeus or levator ani muscles. Pain can be brought on by defaecation, but this can also relieve it and there is no associated blood loss.

E This is a relatively rare malignancy that can present in a young man with bleeding but also with a range of other symptoms. It is not impossible given this scenario, but certainly is not the most likely cause here.

17. D ★

The 'upper outer quadrant' is the 'safe area' avoiding the sciatic nerve and the surrounding vasculature.

18. A ★

This woman has an incarcerated femoral hernia and a cough impulse is not always present due to the small size of the femoral canal. The anatomy of the femoral canal is that the anterior border is the inguinal ligament, the posterior border is the pectineal ligament, the medial border is the lacunar ligament and the lateral border is the femoral vein.

B Classically, an inguinal hernia would be superior and medial to the pubic tubercle.

C This would be more firm and situated just below the surface of the skin

D An enlarged inguinal lymph node would not be fluctuant.

E This is a dilatation of the saphenous vein at its junction with the femoral vein but would disappear on lying down.

19. E ★

This is a small bowel obstruction secondary to adhesions from the previous open cholecystectomy procedure (which left the Kocher scar). This means a gallstone (A) cannot be the cause of the obstruction. Paralytic ileus (C) is more likely to occur in the acute recovery phase following surgery and pseudo-obstruction (D) is like mechanical bowel obstruction with no cause found and usually involves the large bowel (B).

20. E ★   OHCM 8th edn → pp580–581

This is a common dilemma in the Emergency Department and requires the doctor to be able to use the Wells score for DVT probability accurately. This man scores 4 and is thus in the high probability for DVT group; as such, it is advised that he is started on both heparin and warfarin with a view to stopping the heparin once his international normalized ratio (INR) is >2 for 2 days.

A If the probability is high enough to warrant a scan, then treatment should be instigated in the interim.

B This is the right course of action if the probability is low (score 0); if the D-dimer is normal, DVT is excluded; if it is raised, treat as intermediate probability.

C Heparin alone should be started for the intermediate group (score 1–2) with a view to adding in warfarin if a Doppler ultrasound scan is positive.

D This should not be prescribed alone as is initially pro-thrombotic.

Dewar C and Corretge M (2008). Interrater reliability of the Wells score as part of the assessment of DVT in the emergency department: agreement between consultant and nurse practitioner. *Emerg Med J* **25**:407–410.

→ http://emj.bmj.com/cgi/content/abstract/25/7/407

21.C ★

This man is in acute urinary retention and needs a catheter re-sited. Giving an α-receptor blocker at the same time would be useful as it helps increase the chances of his bladder functioning normally the next time the catheter is removed.

As a sideline, when is the best time to remove a catheter ('TWOC' – trial without catheter)? As most management decisions stem from ward rounds, catheters tend to be removed at various points through the morning. However, research suggests that a better time would be midnight for inpatients and 6am for those in their own home.

→ http://www.nursingtimes.net/ntclinical/procedure_to_undertake_a_trial_without_catheter.html

22.E ★

From the X-ray and the history of previous abdominal surgery, this woman is likely to have bowel obstruction due to band adhesions.

A These indicate gastroenteritis.

B This is an upper gastrointestinal bleed

C These indicate a colorectal malignancy.

D This is either acute diverticulitis *or* inflammatory bowel disease.

23.D ★   OHCM 8th edn → p654

The rapid progression of symptoms is concerning. Such severe pain that can be alleviated by positioning of the scrotum (Prehn's sign)

should always raise the suspicion of torsion and prompt urgent surgical review. A tumour (E) is unlikely to present this acutely, nor is a stable hernia – a strangulated hernia (C) is more likely to present with the symptoms of bowel obstruction. The main differential in these circumstances is usually A (indeed they can occur together): this is the most common cause of acute scrotal pain and presents with severe pain and a red, warm, and oedematous testicle. The most sensitive physical finding for separating the two is the cremasteric reflex (stroking the superior medial thigh causes elevation of the ipsilateral testicle): in patients with torsion, it is absent; in those with epididymo-orchitis, it is present.

David JE, Yale SH, and Goldman IL (2003). Urology: scrotal pain. *Clin Med Res* 1:159–160.

→ http://www.pubmedcentral.nih.gov/articlerender. fcgi?artid=1069041

24. C ★

The middle colic artery (and the left colic artery, a branch of the inferior mesenteric artery) supply the transverse colon.

25. E ★   OHCM 8th edn → pp574–575

As this man is having emergency surgery, he has not been able to empty his stomach unlike elective patients who have been prepared by remaining 'nil by mouth'. To prevent aspiration of gastric contents into his respiratory tract, 'rapid sequence induction' must be carried out using a fast-acting depolarizing neuromuscular blocking agent.

A AND C These are agents used for local or regional anaesthesia.

D Propofol is used at induction and maintenance of elective cases.

B Dantrolene is actually a treatment for malignant hyperpyrexia, which is a rare complication of suxamethonium use.

26. E ★   OHCM 8th edn → p582

Rupture of the spleen is the most common intra-abdominal injury following blunt trauma. It should be suspected in all those who present after such an event with a tachycardia and abdominal pain.

A This is more common following penetrating trauma of the abdomen but does happen, particularly in those with inflammatory bowel disease.

B This is possible in such a scenario but unlikely given his oxygen saturations and respiratory rate.

C This is more likely following a penetrating trauma.

D This does occur in blunt trauma as the 12th rib compresses against the lumbar spine but would present with frank haematuria.

27.B ★   OHCM 8th edn → pp614–615

Something has happened to this man's groin lump. The sudden onset of severe pain is concerning in itself, but the worst-case scenario would be strangulation (i.e. ischaemia of the bowel within the hernial sac). Whilst A and D suggest that the hernia is causing or may go on to cause obstruction of the bowel, and C and E are non-specific findings, it is B that is most concerning. If a hernia that has always been irreducible suddenly becomes the source of severe pain, then strangulation has to be suspected with an urgent trip to theatre essential.

28.E ★

A varicocoele is a largely asymptomatic and slowly developing testicular lump. It occurs via the same mechanism that leads to varicose veins in the legs. On examination, it can be revealed by asking the patient to stand or strain (anything to increase intra-abdominal pressure). It does not transilluminate and on palpation feels like a twisted mass (classically a 'bag of worms'). If idiopathic, 98% occur in the left testicle due to the venous drainage system (the left testicle drains via the renal vein, the right drains directly into the inferior vena cava). If a right varicocoele is diagnosed, then there may be concern for a pelvic or intra-abdominal malignancy.

A Hydrocoeles are normally painless, although they can become uncomfortable if large. They are said to transilluminate: that is, light shone through one will be visible from the other side.

B A hernia should have a cough impulse.

C Spermatoceles are small cystic masses that are separate from the testicle so can be 'got above' and they transilluminate.

D A tumour would feel hard and rough to palpation and would probably be associated with lymph node enlargement. It should also be possible to get above a tumour.

29.D ★

The figures relayed to the doctor are represented by the image shown in Figure 10.7 and are known colloquially as showing the 'Portsmouth sign'. The fact that the blood pressure markers ('seagulls') are being rapidly engulfed by the rising pulse rate ('cliffs')

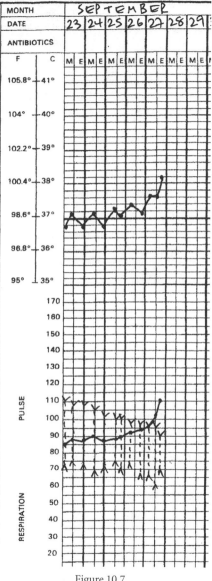

Figure 10.7

is a poor prognostic sign. It suggests deteriorating output and thus end organ instability and is demanding of urgent attention. Whilst all options should be of some concern, it is D that would be the hardest to reverse.

30. C ★

This is adhesional small bowel obstruction following previous surgery. Treatment would be conservative with 'drip (IV fluids) and suck (NG tube)' before a CT scan and a laparotomy to divide the adhesions.

A This is linked to peptic ulcer disease and pancreatitis.

B This is suggestive of biliary tract pain.

D This would cue a gastroenteritis.

E This is a risk factor for peptic ulcer disease.

31. E ★

The drug suggested for use in intermittent claudication is cilostazol, a selective cyclic AMP phosphodiesterase inhibitor that acts as an arterial vasodilator and has antiplatelet activity.

A This would increase peripheral vasoconstriction.

B This refers to drugs such as nifedipine that promote coronary vasodilatation, thus reducing myocardial oxygen consumption.

C A diuretic is indicated in heart failure and hypertension.

D Examples of this are dobutamine and dopamine; they increase contractility of the heart with little effect on rate.

→ http://www.sign.ac.uk/pdf/qrg89.pdf

32. C ★   OHCM 8th edn → pp574–575

Of the options listed, propofol would be most likely to be used as an IV infusion from induction through to maintenance. A and E can be used as induction, whilst D is used for rapid sequence induction and B for sedation purposes.

33. E ★

Aspirin needs to be stopped 5–7 days before the operation to prevent complications with haemostasis peri-operatively such as haematoma formation. The rest of the medications can be continued and taken on the morning of the operation with a sip of water.

34. E ★   OHCM 8th edn → pp634–635

Conservative treatment with ice packs, analgesia, and topical lidocaine or glyceryl trinitrate ointment is the treatment of choice.

Emergency intervention in a patient with thrombosed external haemorrhoids can lead to anal stenosis or damage to the sphincter complex as a result of disruption of the normal anatomy by oedema.

General measures directed at avoiding constipation (eating lots of fibre, drinking good volumes of water, avoiding codeine-based analgesics, and toileting regularly) are often enough to treat small, non-prolapsing haemorrhoids but would not be able to deal with the extreme pain of this acute situation.

35. C ★

This is acute pancreatitis secondary to gallstones. The pain often radiates to the back and is relieved to some degree by sitting forward.

A His bowel frequency does not add to this diagnosis.

B Although it is good to know that his hernia is no bigger, epigastric hernias rarely strangulate and this is not the cause of such acute severe pain.

D This is useful but the pain is more typical of acute pancreatitis than a gastric ulcer.

E Malignancy is not a likely cause and therefore does not add to the diagnosis.

36. B ★   OHCM 8th edn → pp638–639

The first thing to note is that this woman is hypotensive and tachycardic: with these vital signs, acute epigastric pain that radiates through to the back, is relieved by sitting forward, and is associated with nausea is highly suggestive of pancreatitis – even in those who do not drink alcohol. In someone presenting like this, it is vital to screen for other possible triggers: have they had gallstones before? Has anyone in their family had them? Do they have high cholesterol/triglycerides (hyperlipidaemia may be responsible for 1–7% of all cases of acute pancreatitis)? If the answer is yes to any of these, then basic pancreatitis bloods should be sent and an ultrasound scan of the liver requested.

A This is suggestive of a malignant process; if pancreatic, it would present with painless jaundice.

C Cholestasis is known to occur in pregnancy, which also increases the risk of developing gallstones. This is not the case with the oral contraceptive pill, as its levels of oestrogen are negligible.

D This may have been the cause of a gastroenteritis, which would be likely to cause diarrhoea as well as vomiting and a less serious clinical picture than the one depicted here.

E Recent surgery raises the possibility of adhesional bowel obstruction, which would present with abdominal distension and pain, vomiting, and reduced bowel movements.

Gan SI, Edwards AL, Symonds CJ, and Beck PL (2006). Hypertriglyceridaemia-induced pancreatitis: a case-based review. *World J Gastroenterol* **12**:7197–7202.

→ http://www.wjgnet.com/1007-9327/12/7197.pdf

37. B ★

This is most likely to be acute pancreatitis, possibly due to gallstones. The sudden onset of the pain, which can radiate into the flanks and/or back, is a very different presentation to that experienced with appendicitis (A) or small bowel obstruction (E). He would be more unwell if he had infarcted his bowel (C) and he has no risk factors for a duodenal ulcer (D).

38. B ★

The symptoms described sound like the pain of intermittent claudication that is caused by atherosclerotic limb ischaemia. However, in a young person with no risk factors, there is likely to be another pathology at play. The most likely of these is something relatively benign such as popliteal artery entrapment syndrome in which malformation of the gastrocnemius muscles leads to vascular compromise (either congenital or acquired – as can happen due to overgrowth in some athletes). This in itself is rare and not important: what is important is the lateral thinking that is required when dealing with common symptoms occurring in uncommon patient groups. It would be all too easy to tell this man to lose weight, improve his diet, and lower his blood pressure whilst missing what may be a very treatable cause of his problems.

A Vasculitis can cause ischaemia to limbs, i.e. Churg–Strauss syndrome, but very rarely.

C This refers to Buerger's disease (thrombophlebitis obliterans) that afflicts young heavy smokers; inflammation and thrombosis of the arteries can lead to gangrene.

D This is a reasonable differential in this demographic, but would cause compromise in the distribution of the 'trapped' nerve.

E A healthy non-smoker is unlikely to suffer from atherosclerosis, but in the right population, intermittent claudication is almost always due to the ischaemia caused by a damaged peripheral arterial system.

39. B ★

Recognizing and working within the limits of your competence is hugely important and ultimately not only protects the patient but also the junior doctor. When the Emergency Department is busy, it would be tempting to try and aspirate the area (E) or just give her antibiotics and ask her to come back if things worsen (D). However, if you are not sure about the diagnosis, you must ask the patient to wait for a senior doctor review.

→ http://www.gmc-uk.org/guidance/good_medical_practice/ GMC_GMP.pdf

40. C ★   OHCM 8th edn → pp574–575

In order to reverse the block, the anaesthetist has to select an agent that will increase the amount of acetylcysteine at the neuromuscular junction. The anticholinesterase neostigmine will do just this but has to be given with glycopyrronium (B) to minimize its muscarinic side effects (such as a build up of secretions). Atracurium (A) and suxamethonium (D) are both agents that block the neuromuscular junction, whilst thiopental (E) is used in induction.

41. E ★

The causes of abdominal pain in a young woman are numerous. Although pain that localizes to the right iliac fossa should raise the alarm for a potential appendicitis, this woman has not vomited, is afebrile, and has no guarding or rebound tenderness (and none of the examination findings listed are specific to appendicitis). Mesenteric adenitis should be considered if other causes have been excluded (or deemed very unlikely) in the setting of a recent coryzal illness and palpable lymph nodes.

A This finding is suggestive of an ectopic pregnancy.

B This is Murphy's sign of acute cholecystitis.

C This is suggestive of pyelonephritis.

D This is most likely to be a normal finding consistent with many diagnoses!

42. D ★

1% lidocaine means there is 1g of lidocaine in 100ml or 10mg/ml. The maximum dose the woman can have is 150mg, which equates to 15ml.

43. C ★

In busy jobs this can happen. If the notes aren't readily available as the post-take surgical team are motoring from ward to ward, then even the speediest junior doctor is going to have trouble keeping up. Often the best approach in the absence of notes is to have a clear sheet of paper to hand and to record the consultation ready to go into the notes when they surface. If, however, as in this case where a record of the consultation simply wasn't made anywhere, then common practice is to admit as much by marking the entry relating to the consultation as 'retrospect', including the time to which it refers and the time at which it is eventually being written.

44. D ★

This man has a post-operative ileus and needs to be treated by the 'drip and suck' regimen with IV fluids to rest the bowel and a nasogastric tube to decompress the stomach (which in this case is splinting his diaphragm and making it difficult for him to breathe).

45. E ★   OHCM 8th edn → pp636–637

A simple ultrasound scan will detect gallstones, which are most likely the cause of this woman's discomfort. She can be booked for an elective cholecystectomy in a few weeks time. HIDA (C) detects cystic duct obstruction, whilst ERCP (B) and MRCP (D) are used for diagnostic evaluation of the pancreaticobiliary duct systems.

46. D ★

An individual's capacity to make a decision may fluctuate or be temporarily affected by factors such as pain, fear, confusion, or the effects of medication. To respond to this, the surgical team in this case need to understand that assessment of capacity must be time- and decision-specific.

→ http://www.gmc-uk.org/guidance/ethical_guidance/consent_guidance/Consent_guidance.pdf

(see p36: Re MB (Adult, medical treatment) [1997] 38 BMLR 175 CA. *Capacity to refuse treatment*.)

47. C ★

The man is shown to not have capacity and neither he nor his next of kin can give informed consent. The team need to sign a form stating this, with one of them acting as proxy consent giver explaining why the procedure is necessary.

48. B ★ ★

Not, perhaps, a particularly common scenario, but a useful reminder that acute cholecystitis can occur in the absence

of gallstones. This man has all the risk factors for such an
occurrence – diabetes, time on the High-Dependency Unit, and
a recent serious illness.

A A basal pneumonia would be highly likely in such a scenario but
does not fit the findings.

C The normal ultrasound scan makes an infective mass in the liver
unlikely.

D AND E The clear urine counts against any renal pathology.

49. A ★ ★   OHCM 8th edn → pp610–611

Appendicitis is the commonest cause of an acute abdomen. However,
it does not always present with typical migratory periumbilical to right
iliac fossa pain. The position of the appendix determines the symptoms
and signs produced and this can mimic other diagnoses.

This woman has right iliac fossa pain, nausea, vomiting, and
a tachycardia: although the history does not sound 'classical'
(indeed, it is a reasonable history for gastroenteritis), in patients
with right iliac fossa tenderness it is always important to think of
appendicitis. An Alvarado score can then be calculated and the
opinion of a surgeon sought if indicated.

50. E ★ ★

Despite not touching the patient, the doctor must clean his hands
with soap and water because *C. difficile* is spread by spores and
cannot be 'washed' off with alcohol gel.

51. B ★ ★

Although many of these can be associated with both conditions
including a severe anaemia as a result of haemorrhoids, a change
of bowel habit should alert you to other pathologies and warrants
further investigation.

52. A ★ ★

There are very few contraindications to compression stockings but it
is important to think before prescribing them to everyone. The two
categories to be wary of are unstable cardiac failure and peripheral
arterial disease. Those with no evidence of acute heart failure and an
ABPI >0.8 are safe to use high-pressure compression (indicated as
therapy for ulcers of vascular aetiology rather than VTE prophylaxis).
Those with an ABPI >0.5 but <0.8 should use low-pressure
compression (into which category come most anti-VTE disease
stockings or bandages), whilst those with an ABPI <0.5 or evidence
of acute heart failure should be managed with leg elevation and no
compression.

Bryant R and Nix D (2007). *Acute and Chronic Wounds: Current Management* Concepts, 3rd edn. Mosby, St Louis.

53. C ★★

The patient should have the HiB, pneumococcal, and meningococcal C vaccines following the operation (this should ideally happen 14 days before surgery but is obviously not possible in emergency cases such as this). The pneumococcal vaccine should be repeated every 3–5 years. In addition to this, she should be commenced on penicillin V 500mg twice daily as a continual prophylaxis against encapsulated bacteria.

Bridgen M (2001). Detection, education and management of the asplenic or hyposplenic patient. *Am Fam Physician* 63:499–506.

→ http://www.aafp.org/afp/20010201/499.html

54. C ★★   OHCM 8th edn → pp630–631

This is an acute attack of diverticulitis affecting the sigmoid colon. The patient describes previous episodes of painful diverticulosis with alternating constipation and diarrhoea and pain in the left iliac fossa. Such a chronic history may be common to both coeliac disease and irritable bowel syndrome (but clearly not gastroenteritis), but the acute presentation is not typical for either. If this altered bowel habit were to continue for 6 weeks, this woman would warrant urgent referral to surgical outpatients for suspected cancer.

55. C ★★   OHCM 8th edn → pp630–631

This woman had an acute attack of diverticulitis. This was treated with IV analgesia, IV antibiotics, and a period of no oral intake. A colonoscopy is not carried out during the acute phase due to the risk of perforation but would show the mucosa herniating through the colonic wall where the anterior and posterior branches of the marginal artery enter.

A This is ulcerative colitis.

B This is carcinoma.

D This is polyposis.

E This is Crohn's disease.

56. E ★★   OHCM 8th edn → pp630–631

This woman has had an acute attack of diverticulitis. This should be initially treated 'conservatively' – nil by mouth, IV analgesia, and IV antibiotics. A CT scan would be useful and would most likely show fat stranding and the diverticulae in the colon and rule out perforation and abscess. A colonoscopy should not be carried out acutely due to the risk of perforation.

57. E ★★ OHCM 8th edn → p638

This man has an excessive alcohol intake and a recent admission for pancreatitis. This all points towards the diagnosis being a pseudocyst where fluid pools in the lesser sac, the cavity posterior to the stomach and adjoining omenta.

Ascites (A) causes a generalized abdominal fullness rather than a localized mass, whilst a liver abscess (D) is unlikely to be felt as a mass at all. This man may indeed have hepatomegaly (C) but this is likely to be chronic and would not explain his acute medical problems. Gastric volvulus (B) is more likely to present with vomiting and upper abdominal pain.

58. A ★★

The fact that a person has a mental illness does not mean they automatically lack capacity. Those who are shown to have capacity can make decisions to refuse treatment even if those decisions appear irrational to the doctor or may place the patient's health or their life at risk.

C This can only be done if he is deemed not to have capacity and then it can be carried out in his best interests.

D This depends whether he has capacity or not.

E His next of kin cannot give consent on his behalf.

→ http://www.gmc-uk.org/guidance/ethical_guidance/consent_guidance/Consent_guidance.pdf

(Re C (Adult, refusal of treatment) [1994] 1 All ER 819. In *Consent: Patients and Doctors Making Decisions Together*, p35. General Medical Council guidance, 2008.).

59. B ★★ OHCM 8th edn → pp640–641

This is a classical presentation of a renal stone. Good preventative advice would be to drink plenty of fluids and avoid certain foods depending on the stone's biochemical make-up; for example, oxalate levels are increased by chocolate, spinach, tea, and rhubarb.

A This advice applies to alcoholic gastritis.

C This is for biliary colic.

D This is for gastritis secondary to NSAIDs.

E This is for constipation.

60. E ★★★

In those over the age of 60 years, a history of fresh rectal bleeding of more than 6 weeks duration should not be attributed to diclofenac or haemorrhoids. Regardless of whether there is any change in bowel habit, an urgent referral should be made to be seen within 2 weeks in a surgical outpatient clinic. Guidance states that, when referring, all that is required is an abdominal and a rectal examination and a full blood count, so as to not delay specialist assessment.

→ http://www.nice.org.uk/nicemedia/pdf/CG027quickrefguide.pdf

(*Referral Guidelines for Suspected Cancer*. NICE Clinical Guideline 27, 2005.)

61. A ★★★

He has two risk factors that increase the likelihood of an anastomotic leak – a low anastomosis (risk is increased the lower the anastomosis) and he also takes long-term steroids. This is the most likely diagnosis and we should remember that *any change in physiology after a bowel resection is due to a leak until proven otherwise.* This man will need a CT scan with contrast to make the diagnosis.

B There is nothing to suggest that this man has aspirated.

C This generally occurs within 48h, but is unlikely to cause chest pain.

D The ECG changes are P pulmonale consistent with right atrial hypertrophy due to chronic lung disease and not a myocardial infarction.

E This is too soon for a post-operative pulmonary embolism. In a study of patients in the 40–60 years age range, it is suggested that the mean time to diagnosis was 11 days, although in patients under 40 years of age, the mean time was 3 days.

Hope WW, Demeter BL, Newcomb WL, *et al.* (2007). Postoperative pulmonary embolism: timing, diagnosis, treatment, and outcome. *Am J Surg* **194**:814–818; discussion 818–819.

62. B ★★★

Anyone aged 40 years and older who reports rectal bleeding with a change of bowel habit towards looser stools and/or increased stool frequency persisting for 6 weeks or more should be urgently referred. The history in this case – although suspicious of a sinister cause – is only of 4 weeks' duration. Pending a review at 6 weeks, a full blood count should be taken to detect any anaemia present ready for urgent referral to surgical outpatients if things do not settle.

→ http://www.nice.org.uk/nicemedia/pdf/CG027quickrefguide.pdf
(*Referral Guidelines for Suspected Cancer*. NICE Clinical Guideline 27, 2005.)

63.D ★ ★ ★

Metal clips can start to come out between 7 and 10 days after the operation. This depends very much on the pre-morbid fitness of the patient, which may have an impact on wound healing. This includes factors such as increasing age, malignancy, smoking, and steroid use.

64.C ★ ★ ★

As displayed by the surgeon's notes, this lady lacks capacity to make an informed decision. In other words, she cannot understand information relevant to that decision, she cannot retain it, she cannot weigh it up as part of the process to make a decision, and she is unable to communicate any decision.

Any act done to this woman or decision made on her behalf must be done or made in her best interests. If, after considered discussion with the patient and/or relatives/carers/attorneys, the surgeon feels that to proceed to theatre would be in her best interests (and this decision is not based on her age, appearance, or behaviour), then there can be said to be 'sufficient compliance' with the Mental Capacity Act 2005.

A It may be reasonable for the woman's family to talk through the options with her, but as she lacks capacity this would not be decisive.

B If the surgeon acts as outlined above, he would be acting appropriately under the Mental Capacity Act 2005 and no intervention from a psychiatrist would be needed.

D It would be wrong for the surgeon to accept a decision from a patient whom it has been demonstrated is unable to make decisions: however, if the surgeon were to decide that conservative management rather than surgery was in her best interests, that is another matter.

E An adult cannot make decisions on another adult's behalf (unless they have been granted Lasting Power of Attorney).

→ http://www.opsi.gov.uk/acts/acts2005/ukpga_20050009_en_1
(The Mental Capacity Act 2005.)

65.A ★ ★ ★

In the palliative care setting, syringe drivers are given subcutaneously. The total daily dose of oral morphine is converted into a dose of subcutaneous diamorphine by dividing this by 3.

Diamorphine is used in preference to morphine because of its greater solubility when compared with morphine. This means that larger doses can be put into the syringe driver should they be required.

66. B ★ ★ ★

The pain in the left shoulder could be attributed to the fractured clavicle. However, taking into account the mechanism of injury and bruising to the left posterior ribs, a splenic injury should be ruled out. The most appropriate way of doing this is with a CT scan of the abdomen.

67. C ★ ★ ★

This is a sigmoid volvulus, and the treatment of choice if there is no evidence of ischaemic bowel is the placement of a rectal flatus tube under sigmoidoscopic guidance. This is effective in 70–90% of cases with a further 5% being reversed by barium enema (A). Blood-stained effluent and devitalized mucosa on sigmoidoscopy and a leucocytosis or pyrexia would suggest a laparotomy (D) is needed.

68. D ★ ★ ★

The scenario describes what sounds like some kind of perianal abscess. Whilst E suggests systemic upset and the need for treatment, it is the association of diabetes and perianal infection that would be most concerning. This is because of the strong link between diabetes and the very serious necrotizing infections that can arise as complications of perianal abscesses. Fournier's gangrene is a polymicrobial necrotizing fasciitis of the genital, perianal, or perineal areas. The classical symptoms are severe pain, swelling, and fever. It most often affects those with systemic disease: 32–60% of those who get Fournier's gangrene have diabetes. It is a surgical emergency requiring prompt treatment in the form of antibiotics and appropriate drainage, as well as wide debridement.

Whilst A and B would be red herrings in this scenario, non-resolution after a course of antibiotics (C) would be concerning as it suggests that this may be more than just a standard case of cellulitis.

→ http://www.cambridgemedicine.org/cammed/article/ viewArticle/116/149

69. D ★ ★ ★

Development of a DVT while on heparin should prompt investigation of heparin-induced thrombocytopenia (HIT). This is more common with unfractionated heparin, but it can develop, although less commonly, with prolonged LMWH therapy. Most commonly this is after 5–10 days. Although the platelet count drops, this disorder is pro-thrombotic, with venous thromboembolism being about four times as common as arterial.

Heparin can also inhibit aldosterone secretion and hence cause hyperkalaemia. Patients with diabetes mellitus, chronic renal failure, acidosis, and raised potassium, or who are taking potassium-sparing drugs seem to be more susceptible. The Committee on Safety of Medicines (CSM) recommends baseline and regular measurement of potassium should be made in those at risk or those receiving therapy for more than 7 days.

70.D ★★★

This woman has suffered an acute vascular event causing ischaemia of her left hand. The two main causes of limb ischaemia are embolic (30%) and thrombotic (60%). This woman has three features that make an embolus the likely cause: sudden onset of symptoms (hours), upper limb affected (thromboses rarely occur in the upper limbs), and a fibrillating heart. Examination reveals a white hand, which suggests that the occlusion is recent as there has not been time for the arterial tree to come out of spasm and allow deoxygenated blood into the tissues turning them purple. Sensory deficit means the limb is in danger and in need of emergency surgery.

All other options are used to treat thrombotic ischaemia. Heparin (E) is used pending investigations prior to reperfusion therapies such as bypass (C) or angioplasty (B) with amputation (A) clearly a last resort for an irreversibly ischaemic limb.

→ http://student.bmj.com/issues/08/02/education/080.php

71.B ★★★ OHCM 8th edn → p756

Whilst all options would provide useful information regarding this man's pancreatic tumour, it is only the ERCP that would allow immediate treatment of his severe obstructive jaundice (ALP>AST) in the form of stenting.

72.E ★★★ OHCM 8th edn → pp612–613

The history of progressive distension is suggestive of some form of bowel obstruction. The obstruction in this case is a product of severe constipation (D): the faecally and gas-loaded segment of bowel twists on its mesenteric pedicle creating a closed loop. The result is a single grossly dilated loop of bowel seen on X-ray as showing the 'coffee bean' sign. It reaches up towards the xiphisternum and has oedematous walls, seen as thick white boundaries replacing the usual haustra.

A AND B These may cause intestinal obstruction, but would be unlikely to create the closed loop seen here.

C This is more likely to present with sudden pain and rapid haemodynamic decompensation, with the tell-tale finding of subphrenic air seen on an erect chest X-ray.

73. D ★ ★ ★

The history is suspicious of bowel cancer. Further to this, the woman has had an episode of chest pain associated with low oxygen saturations and tachycardia. A pulmonary embolism (PE) is top of the differentials. She should be given therapeutic LMWH and the investigations booked to confirm the diagnosis. These depend on local policy but will be either a VQ scan (E) or CT-PA (A). A D-dimer test (B) is sensitive but not specific for PE. Negative D-dimers do not exclude a PE in a patient who is deemed to be at high risk.

74. A ★ ★ ★

Although not proven, the commonest cause for pilonidal abscesses is thought to be an in-growing hair. *Pilo* means hair and *nidal* means nest.

75. C ★ ★ ★

A patient's consent to a particular treatment may not be valid if it is given under pressure or duress exerted by another person.

A Her husband cannot consent on her behalf.

B Before accepting a patient's consent, you must consider whether they have been given the information they want or need, and how well they understand the details and implications of what is proposed. This is more important than how their consent is expressed or recorded.

D Although consent might be obtained like this in practice, in this situation it could leave the woman (who may not want the operation) in a situation where she feels she cannot now avoid it.

E An operation requires written consent unless it is conducted in an emergency and then the verbal consent given must be recorded in the notes.

→ http://www.gmc-uk.org/guidance/ethical_guidance/ consent_guidance/Consent_guidance.pdf

(Re T (Adult) [1992] 4 All ER 649. In *Consent: Patients and Doctors Making Decisions Together*, p39. General Medical Council guidance, 2008.).

76. E ★★★

This is available in combination with magnesium oxide (in the commercially available Picolax). Pre-operative bowel preparation often differs between surgeons. Those who use Picolax believe that the bowel should be emptied before the operation whilst others believe that the use of this preparation instead of a phosphate enema increases the risk of an anastomotic leak due to the spill of bowel contents. The others are all useful in the gradual softening of stool and are thus more often employed as laxatives rather than in bowel preparation.

77. D ★★★ OHCM 8th edn → p600

A fluctuant mass that rises on swallowing and protrusion of the tongue is a thyroglossal cyst. These grow in the midline between the isthmus of the thyroid and the hyoid bone. They are normally asymptomatic but can cause anxieties, as in this case and so are resected surgically.

A This is the usual position of cystic hygromas.

B This is a submandibular salivary stone.

C This is a branchial cyst.

E This indicates carotid body tumours.

78. B ★★★ OHCM 8th edn → p613

Caecal volvulus commonly presents with large bowel obstruction and a classical 'comma-shaped' shadow in the mid-abdomen. Treatment involves colonoscopic decompression or a right hemi-colectomy if the colon is ischaemic.

A This is more of a description than a diagnosis: if this woman is not opening her bowels or passing flatus, then she can be said to have absolute constipation as a feature of her caecal volvulus.

C This could present with bowel obstruction, but there would be a tender, irreducible abdominal mass on examination and different X-ray findings depending on the level of the obstruction.

D The pain would be more sudden and likely to cause haemodynamic compromise. An erect chest X-ray may show free subphrenic air.

E Vomiting would be an expected feature in the history with high-pitched bowel sounds on examination. An X-ray would show dilated loops of small bowel centrally.

79. E ★★★ OHCM 8th edn → p613

This man presents with the symptoms of acute pancreatitis. The junior doctor is being asked to assess the severity of his presentation based on the modified Glasgow criteria.
This score is then used as a prognostic guide. Of the options given, only E is needed to compile the Glasgow score. A score of 3 or more within 48h of onset of symptoms suggests a severe attack and may well require High-Dependency Unit/Intensive Therapy Unit support.

Renal failure and dyspnoea, which can develop into adult respiratory distress syndrome (ARDS) can occur in severe diseases. Although amylase (A) confirms the diagnosis of pancreatitis, it is not a good marker of severity and can be normal in severe pancreatitis.

Beckingham I and Bornman P (2001). ABC of diseases of liver, pancreas, and biliary system: acute pancreatitis. *BMJ* **322**:595–598.

→ http://www.bmj.com/cgi/content/short/322/7286/595

80. A ★★★★

Together with homocysteine, these increase the risk of arterial thrombosis. The other diagnostic tests are predictive of an increased risk of venous thrombosis.

81. D ★★★★

The placement or removal of an epidural catheter should be 10–12h after the last dose of LMWH thromboprophylaxis. If the patient is receiving a treatment dose of LMWH, this time should be extended to 24h. Following removal, subsequent LMWH should be given no sooner than 4h. These precautions reduce the chances of developing spinal haematomas.

82. E ★★★★ OHCM 8th edn → pp534–535

If the as-required morphine liquid is being used as regularly as this for as long as this, then the regime needs to be rethought. To do this, the amount of as-required liquid (10mg/4h = 60mg) taken daily should be added to the amount of MR (60mg) to give a total daily dose (TDD=120mg). The new dose of MR can be calculated by dividing the new TDD by 2 (=60mg). The new as-required liquid dose can be calculated by dividing the new TDD by 6 (=20mg).

83. C ★★★★

Although post-ERCP pancreatitis is common, this man's amylase is normal and pain distribution is not typical. He has in fact perforated his duodenum following the sphincterotomy. A CT scan would be the best modality as it would show a collection and free air in the retroperitoneal space. He has guarding as a result of the peritoneal inflammation caused by the retroperitoneal collection.

84. E ★ ★ ★ ★

NICE recommendations are available for recommended preoperative tests. This man is an American Society of Anaesthiologists (ASA) grade 1 or a 'normal healthy patient'. The surgery he is awaiting is graded as grade 2 (intermediate). The recommendations suggest that no tests are required, although if the patient has any urinary symptoms, a urine dipstick could be considered.

→ http://www.nice.org.uk/nicemedia/pdf/CG3NICEguideline.pdf

(*Pre-operative Tests: the Use of Routine Pre-operative Tests for Elective Surgery*. NICE Clinical Guideline 3, 2003.)

85. B ★ ★ ★ ★

This is a polyamide monofilament and can be used to close skin wounds but must be removed. All of the others are absorbable.

A AND E These are synthetic braided materials that are more suited to closing subcutaneous fat.

C AND D These are reasonable alternatives to non-absorbable materials for both transcutaneous and subcuticular sutures.

86. E ★ ★ ★ ★

The level should be repeated 12h later, when normal renal function should be in range. Vancomycin has linear kinetics so a proportional reduction in dose should yield similar results in the level. A dose of 750mg twice daily will ensure an adequate trough level that will be an effective bacteriocidal agent. Vancomycin activity is time dependent, with the antimicrobial activity depending on the length of time the vancomycin is above the minimum inhibitory concentration of the organism.

Extended Matching Questions

1. J ★

This is the location of the femoral artery.

2. L ★

This is the most common location of the base of the appendix attachment to the caecum.

3. H ★

Inguinal hernias are superior and medial to the pubic tubercle – the location of the external inguinal ring.

4. C ★

This is the normal position of erect kidneys. The right kidney lies 1cm lower than the left.

5. M ★

This is the expected location of the spleen on the right.

General feedback on 1–5:
A is an aortic bifurcation at L4; B is the T10 dermatome; E is the inguinal ligament; G is the position of the gall bladder; H indicates the position for palpation of a femoral hernia; I is the superficial inguinal ring; and D, F, K are non-specific surface landmarks.

6. D ★

These are found in the femoral canal, which is an anatomical weakness just below the inguinal ligament. Half of these hernias present with obstructed contents and require emergency surgical treatment.

7. G ★

This is named after a 17th century anatomist and involves a hernia with a sac containing a Meckel's diverticulum. They are understandably rare, but when they do occur are more common on the right and in men.

8. K ★

These are hernias that protrude through the Spigelian fascia – the aponeurosis between the semilunar line and rectus abdominis below the arcuate line. Although these are rare, it is important to be aware of them, because they are small and are at high risk of strangulation.

9. F ★

Although the classification of many inguinal hernias is often only revealed intra-operatively, the anatomical description in the question will allow the differentiation in this case. The landmark is the internal or deep inguinal ring, which is the point where an 'indirect' hernia enters the inguinal canal.

10. B ★

The rectus abdominis muscles should meet in the midline at the linea alba. If this does not happen, for example in obese patients, lifting their head off the bed or coughing will cause a dome-like protrusion to appear. This is not strictly a true hernia.

11.H ★

It can be difficult to differentiate external anal symptoms from those originating from within the large bowel. Good clues are bright red blood seen on toilet paper and itching.

12.K ★

This man's main complaint is tenesmus, commonly a signal of serious pathology. If found in conjunction with rectal bleeding, it warrants urgent investigation.

13.L ★

If someone reports recurrent episodes of rectal bleeding and fluctuating weight with systemic symptoms, it is likely they are suffering from a chronic inflammatory condition. The presence of fever and pain suggests that this is an infective bout of colitis that will need antibiotic as well as steroid treatment.

14.G ★

Left-sided pain relieved by opening the bowels suggests the presence of diverticula. Rectal bleeding makes this an attack of diverticulitis that will need monitoring for signs of infection and may require antibiotic treatment.

15.B ★

As with the first case, this man has symptoms that suggest an external cause for his bleeding. He has also sharp pain on passing stools, which is suggestive of a fissure.

16.I ★★★★

Sudden and painless bleeding is typical of diverticular disease and often resolves with bed rest, but may require a transfusion.

17.C ★★★★

This lady has a rectal carcinoma where almost half of all colorectal cancers are located and is the reason for a rectal examination in everyone with rectal bleeding. The mass is giving her tenesmus – a feeling of incomplete defaecation.

18.E ★★★★

This young man has haemorrhoids secondary to his poor diet and resultant hard, pellet-like stools.

19.A ★★★★

This is angiodysplasia and usually presents as fresh rectal bleeding in the elderly. A mesenteric angiogram can aid identification of the bleeding lesion and allow therapeutic embolization.

20.H ★★★★

This man is having an attack of ulcerative colitis and is now anaemic. Crohn's disease would be unlikely to present with bloody diarrhoea.

CHAPTER 11
CLINICAL CHEMISTRY

With so many tests available and increasingly fast laboratory processors, there is a growing temptation to request large numbers of blood tests on each and every patient. What we should remember is that they should be used as an adjunct to the history and clinical examination. Results should reinforce the likely diagnosis and rule out our differentials, rather than be used to make the diagnosis *de novo*.

What makes things easier is to know how serum biochemistry and homeostasis are regulated and then to consider a number of questions:

- Which hormones are involved in the control of this electrolyte?

- What happens when these are increased or decreased?

- Does the patient have any renal or hepatic impairment?

- Are they taking any drugs that might be affecting serum electrolyte levels?

- Have they taken an overdose?

- Is the patient dehydrated/hypovolaemic/hypoxic?

It can seem daunting at first when results come back unexpectedly out of range. They must be considered in combination with the patient's clinical status: if the numbers just don't fit, then repeat the test – they may not be right.

However, there are a few 'unmissable' electrolyte derangements that need to be dealt with immediately. Once detected they should trigger the following thoughts:

Deranged serum level	Issues to consider	Check
Sodium	Patient dehydrated? Oedematous?	Urine sodium Urine osmolality
Potassium	In keeping with clinical picture or repeat sample?	Urea and electrolytes (U&E), 12-lead ECG
Calcium	Is the albumin normal?	U&E, phosphate and alkaline phosphatase

Interpreting serum values is important, but to prevent iatrogenic derangement, careful use and prescription of IV fluids is also needed. Does a patient who looks hypovolaemic, has a low blood pressure, and is tachycardic need crystalloids, colloids, or blood? Are they elderly or do they have cardiac failure and therefore require cautious replacement? Do they have liver failure? Might they benefit from CVP monitoring? This chapter will help consideration of the whole picture before putting pen to paper and prescribing 4L of fluids a day for an elderly man with left ventricular failure.

Another test that is incredibly useful is blood gases. There are occasions when an arterial sample is needed, but otherwise the majority of information can be gleaned from a venous sample. It is one of the most useful tools available and invaluable in an emergency, particularly when there is little history available or the patient is very unwell. Hydration status, oxygenation (arterial blood gases), acid–base balance, and response to the treatment being given can be easily followed using this test. This is another unmissable area that needs to be comprehensively understood for the examination room and emergency room alike. ■

CLINICAL CHEMISTRY
SINGLE BEST ANSWERS

1. A 28-year-old woman has been short of breath for 12h and is feeling generally unwell. An arterial blood gas is taken:

pH 7.50, pCO₂ 3.2kPa, pO₂ 8.8kPa, base excess -0.2mmol/L, bicarbonate (HCO₃⁻) 18.0mmol/L.

Which is the *single* most likely diagnosis? ★

A Diabetic ketoacidosis

B Methanol overdose

C Panic attack

D Pulmonary embolus

E Severe vomiting

2. A 66-year-old woman has had pain in her left thigh for the past 6 months. She is slightly unsteady on her feet and has begun to limp.

Hb 11.1g/dL, WCC 5.5 × 10⁹/L, platelets 230 × 10⁹/L.

Calcium 2.55mmol/L, phosphate 10mmol/L, ALP 455IU/L.

Which is the *single* most likely cause of this woman's symptoms? ★

A Chronic myeloid leukaemia

B Lymphoma

C Osteomalacia

D Osteoporosis

E Paget's disease

$3.$ An 82-year-old woman has had pain in her lower abdomen and blood in her stools for the past week. She takes furosemide 20mg PO once daily and ramipril 5mg PO once daily. She remains nil by mouth pending a CT scan of her abdomen and in the meantime is started on IV fluid therapy:

- Saline 0.9% 1L + 20mmol KCl/4h
- Dextrose 5% 1L/6h
- Dextrose 5% 1L/8h.

The surgical registrar is later concerned by the fluid regimen. Which *single* pair of examination features are most likely to cause her concern? ★

A Decreased Glasgow Coma Scale (GCS) score + decreased muscle tone

B Decreased urine output + decreased skin turgor

C Dry mucous membranes + generalized wheeze in chest

D Polyuria + polydipsia

E Raised JVP + peripheral oedema

4. A 50-year-old man has vomited blood. He has had an urgent endoscopy and band ligation of oesophageal varices and is recovering in hospital. He is receiving IV fluid therapy:

- Saline 0.9% 1L/8h
- Dextrose 5% 1L/8h
- Saline 0.9% 1L + 20mmol KCl/8h.

The medical registrar crosses out the above regimen and explains to the junior doctor he has made a mistake. Which is the *single* most likely explanation of the junior doctor's mistake? ★

A The patient is likely to be hypokalaemic and needs more potassium

B The patient already has raised total body sodium and needs dextrose instead

C The patient has suffered losses and needs more rapid replacement

D The patient is likely to be hypoglycaemic and needs more sugar infused

E The patient is likely to be oedematous and should be fluid restricted

5. A 72-year-old woman is being treated for a urinary tract infection. The laboratory ring the ward with some urgent blood results:

Sodium 140mmol/L, potassium 6.8mmol/L, creatinine 95μmol/L, urea 4.2mmol/L.

Which is the *single* most appropriate next step? ★

A Calcium chloride 10% 10ml IV

B Calcium resonium 15g PO three times daily

C Dextrose/insulin infusion

D ECG and repeat sample

E Intravenous normal saline 1L/4h

6. A 66-year-old man has noticed a strange tingling around his mouth for the past few weeks. It was very subtle at first but has become increasingly apparent. He also feels tired, unmotivated, and low in mood. He has type 1 diabetes and uses regular non-steroidal anti-inflammatory drugs (NSAIDs) for osteoarthritis and gout. Which *single* examination finding is most likely to support the diagnosis? ★

A Carotid bruit

B Neck goitre

C Nystagmus

D Parotid gland swelling

E Twitching facial muscles

7. A 62-year-old man is recovering after an emergency hemi-colectomy for a ruptured appendix abscess. On the second day after surgery, the registrar asks for potassium to be added to the man's IV fluid therapy.

```
Day 2 fluid balance:
```
- In: 3100ml
  - Hartmann's IV 3000mL
  - Water PO 100mL
- Out: 3450mL
  - Urine 1400mL
  - Stoma 1800mL
  - Abdominal drain 180mL
  - Vomit 50mL

Which is the *single* most likely reason the registrar has made this request? ★

A Due to excessive blood loss

B Due to high output from the stoma

C Prophylaxis against further vomiting

D Standard after every colectomy

E Standard if fluid regimen is Hartmann's

8. A 46-year-old woman has had 3 days of upper abdominal pain with nausea, especially after eating fatty foods. She is asked to remain nil by mouth while awaiting an ultrasound scan and is given IV fluid therapy:

- Saline 0.9% 1L + 20mmol KCl/8h
- Saline 0.9% 1L/8h
- Saline 0.9% 1L + 20mmol KCl/8h

The surgical registrar later says that she has not had the right fluid regimen. Which is the *single* most likely reason for the registrar's opinion? ★

A Not enough glucose

B Not enough fluid volume

C Too much fluid volume

D Too much potassium

E Too much sodium

9. A 64-year-old man has felt unwell for the past 5 days. He has been nauseous and has had sweats and shakes at night. He has hypertension and had a metallic mitral valve replacement 2 years ago.

T 37.9°C, HR 110bpm, BP 85/60mmHg.

He is clammy and cold peripherally. His abdomen is tender in the right upper quadrant. The on-call junior doctor wants to start IV antibiotics immediately. Which is the *single* most appropriate next step? ★

A Give a STAT dose of IV gentamicin prior to any further action

B Only start broad-spectrum IV antibiotics if T>38°C

C Start empirical treatment with broad-spectrum IV antibiotics

D Start empirical treatment with broad-spectrum oral antibiotics

E Take multiple blood cultures prior to starting any antibiotics

10. A 72-year-old woman has had muscle cramps for the last hour. She feels dizzy and weak. She has been taking furosemide 80mg IV twice daily for an exacerbation of congestive cardiac failure.

```
T 35.6°C, HR 120bpm, BP 100/75 mmHg.
```

She has decreased tone in all four limbs. Which *single* management option would be most likely to improve this woman's symptoms? ★

A Digoxin 500mcg IV STAT

B Potassium chloride 10mmol/h IV

C Quinine sulphate 300mg PO once every night

D Sotalol 80mg PO twice a day

E Spironolactone 30mg PO once a day

11. A 76-year-old man has become increasingly confused over a 24h period. In the 4 or 5 days prior to this, he has felt lethargic and weak but had a very powerful thirst. He is well known to the palliative care team at the hospital for the management of his multiple myeloma. Which would be the *single* most important step in management? ★ ★

A Bendroflumethiazide 2.5mg PO once daily

B Calcium gluconate 10% 10mL IV over 2min

C Dexamethasone 8mg PO twice daily

D Dextrose 10% 200mL IV STAT

E Pamidronate 30mg IV over 3h

12. A 67-year-old woman is confused and cannot relate her full history. An arterial blood gas sample is taken (on room air):

pH 7.27, pCO$_2$ 3.2kPa, pO$_2$ 12.2kPa.

Bicarbonate (HCO$_3^-$)15mmol/L, sodium 136mmol/L, potassium 3.6mmol/L, chloride 110mmol/L.

Which is the *single* most probable cause of the blood gas results? ★ ★

A Acute renal failure

B Alcohol overdose

C Diarrhoea

D Salicylate poisoning

E Severe vomiting

13. A 22-year-old man has felt generally unwell for the last 24h. An arterial blood gas sample is taken (on room air):

pH 7.25, pCO$_2$ 2.2kPa, pO$_2$ 11.8kPa.

Bicarbonate (HCO$_3^-$)10mmol/L, sodium 140mmol/L, potassium 4.4mmol/L, chloride 110mmol/L.

Which is the *single* most probable cause of the blood gas results? ★ ★

A Burns

B Diabetic ketoacidosis

C Diarrhoea

D Renal tubular acidosis

E Severe vomiting

14. An 80-year-old woman has been housebound for years and has fallen and fractured her left hip. Previously, she had a slow, distinctive waddling gait and severe bone pain, and used two sticks to help her get about. Which is the *single* most likely explanation for her problems? ★ ★

A Arrested bone development

B Increased bone turnover

C Multiple bone cysts

D Normal amount of bone but low mineral content

E Reduced cortical bone density

15. A 32-year-old man is started on a course of chemotherapy for acute lymphoblastic leukaemia. Two days after his first dose of chemotherapy, he becomes unwell and is admitted to hospital following a seizure.

```
T 37.2°C, HR 85bpm, BP 140/75mmHg.
```

Which *single* biochemical finding is most consistent with the diagnosis? ★ ★ ★

A Hypercalcaemia

B Hyperuricaemia

C Hypokalaemia

D Hypomagnesaemia

E Hypophosphataemia

16. A 59-year-old woman has had a bone mineral density scan. It has been 3 years since she went through the menopause and she is otherwise well. She is concerned as her mother fractured her hip in her late 60s and there is a strong family history of coeliac disease. Her BMI is 21kg/m².

T-score: −2.6.

The family doctor advises her to start taking bone protection therapy. Which *single* factor should most have influenced the doctor's decision? ★ ★ ★

A Purely on strength of T-score

B T-score + family history of coeliac disease

C T-score + low BMI

D T-score + maternal history of a fracture at <75 years

E T-score + untreated premature menopause

EXTENDED MATCHING QUESTIONS

Management of osteoporosis

For each scenario outlined, choose the *single* most appropriate next management step from the list of options below. Each option may be used once, more than once, or not at all. ★

A Alendronate

B Calcitriol

C Dual energy X-ray absorptiometry (DEXA) scan

D Home modifications + hip protectors

E Hormone-replacement therapy

F Quit smoking + reduce alcohol intake

G Raloxifene

H Strontium ranelate

I Teriparatide

J Vitamin D

1. An 82-year-old woman has had a fall at home. A plain X-ray of her hips confirms a fracture of the left femoral neck.

2. A 70-year-old woman visits her doctor for an annual review of her rheumatoid arthritis. She asks him whether she should be taking any medicine to protect her bones.

3. A 68-year-old woman has had pain in her right leg for the past 24h. She recalls a stumble down some stairs since when she has been limping. An X-ray of her pelvis shows an intra-capsular fracture of the right femoral head.

4. An 80-year-old woman has had a sore throat for the past week. She visits her family doctor for the first time in many years. She smokes three cigarettes a day and drinks ten units of alcohol a week. Her BMI is 18kg/m^2.

5. A 59-year-old woman has had back pain for the past 2 weeks. She went through the menopause at the age of 39 for which she received no treatment. A plain X-ray of her lumbar spine confirms a wedge fracture at L4/L5.

Causes of hyponatraemia

For each patient with hyponatraemia, choose the *single* most likely cause from the list of options below. Each option may be used once, more than once, or not at all. ★

A Addison's disease

B Cardiac failure

C Dermal losses

D Drip arm used

E Diuretic excess

F Glucocorticoid insufficiency

G Nephrotic syndrome

H Liver cirrhosis + ascites

I Severe hypothyroidism

J Syndrome of inappropriate antidiuretic hormone secretion (SIADH)

K Vomiting

L Water excess

6. A 72-year-old man visits his doctor for a check-up and repeat prescription. The doctor is concerned at the man's fluid status.

T 37.1°C, HR 110bpm, BP 90/60mmHg.

Capillary refill time (CRT): 4s; JVP: not visible; skin turgor: reduced; peripheral oedema: minimal.

Serum sodium 125mmol/L, urine sodium 33mmol/L.

7. A 72-year-old man has had severe abdominal pain for the past 48h. He has vomited twice but has begun passing small amounts of flatus. He is asked to stay nil by mouth and is treated with IV fluids (dextrose 5% 1L/6h).

T 37.3°C, HR 90bpm, BP 130/90mmHg.

CRT: <2s; JVP: not visible; skin turgor: normal; peripheral oedema: none.

Serum sodium 125mmol/L, urine sodium 32mmol/L.

8. A 72-year-old man is awaiting elective repair of his inguinal hernia. Prior to surgery, he is asked to remain nil by mouth overnight and given IV fluids (dextrose 5% 1L/12h).

T 36.6°, HR 80bpm, BP 125/85mmHg.

CRT: <2s; JVP: not visible; skin turgor: normal; peripheral oedema: none.

Serum sodium 109mmol/L, urine sodium 25mmol/L.

9. A 72-year-old man has been lethargic over the past week. He says it developed after he 'ran out' of his tablets 10 days ago. He is short of breath as he is assessed in the Emergency Department.

T 36.9°C, HR 85bpm, BP 130/80mmHg.

CRT: 2s; JVP: 4cm above sternal angle; skin turgor: normal; peripheral oedema: yes.

Serum sodium 124mmol/L, urine sodium 18mmol/L.

10. A 72-year-old man has been involved in a motor vehicle collision. The vehicle was ablaze when the emergency services rescued him. He is aggressively resuscitated with IV fluids (dextrose 5% 1L/4h, saline 0.9% 1L/6h, dextrose 5% 1L/8h).

T 38.8°C, HR 120bpm, BP 80/55mmHg

CRT: 5s; JVP: not visible; skin turgor: decreased; peripheral oedema: none.

Serum sodium 123mmol/L, urine sodium 16mmol/L.

Causes of deranged urea and electrolytes

For each scenario, choose the single most likely urea and electrolytes from the list of options below. Each option may be used once, more than once, or not at all. ★ ★ ★ ★

Reference ranges:

Sodium (Na⁺) 135–145mmol/L

Potassium (K⁺) 3.5–5.0mmol/L

Creatinine (Cr) 70–150μmol/L

Urea (Ur) 2.5–6.7mmol/L

Calcium (Ca²⁺) 2.12–2.65 mmol/L

Phosphate 0.8–1.5 mmol/L

A Na⁺134, K⁺ 3.0, Cr 66, Ur 2.2, Ca²⁺ 2.02, phosphate 0.41

B Na⁺130, K⁺ 6.0, Cr 88, Ur 9.6, Ca²⁺ 2.3, phosphate 0.8

C Na⁺124, K⁺ 4.4, Cr 90, Ur 5.6, Ca²⁺ 2.65, phosphate 0.87

D Na⁺142, K⁺ 5.7, Cr 264, Ur 18.2, Ca²⁺ 2.3, phosphate 1.2

E Na 138, K⁺ 4.2, Cr 96, Ur 7.4, Ca²⁺ 1.13, phosphate 0.9

F Na⁺142, K⁺ 2.8, Cr 79, Ur 4.2, Ca²⁺ 2.1, phosphate

G Na⁺128, K⁺ 5.2, Cr 301, Ur 15.5, Ca²⁺ 2.03, phosphate 0.5

H Na⁺142, K⁺ 5.6, Cr 458, Ur 42.6, Ca²⁺ 2.04, phosphate 2.4

I Na⁺126, K⁺ 4.2, Cr 67, Ur 2.2, Ca²⁺ 2.1, phosphate 1.4

J Na⁺134, K⁺ 6.2, Cr 78, Ur 2.6, Ca²⁺ 1.7, phosphate 2.1

11. A 24-year-old man has had diarrhoea and vomiting for the last 48h. He has not managed to eat anything over this period so has not used any of his regular insulin. His serum bicarbonate is 8mmol/L. He has type 1 diabetes mellitus.

12. A 52-year-old man has felt increasingly lethargic over the last 3 months. He has given up regular work and his family comment that he has become depressed and withdrawn. Despite the fact that he rarely leaves his house, he looks 'tanned' although has a few patches of much paler skin on his arms and legs.

13. A 58-year-old man has been drinking heavily for the last 10 days. He has woken this morning with severe central abdominal pain radiating to his back and has vomited several times. His Glasgow Coma Scale (GCS) score is 5.

14. A 54-year-old man has felt increasingly unwell over the last 6 months. He has lost his appetite and feels extremely tired, despite only minimal exertion. His ankles are swollen and he feels breathless at night, stopping him lying flat at night. He has had type 1 diabetes mellitus for the last 42 years.
Renal ultrasound scan: left 9.8cm and right 9.3cm in length.

15. A 48-year-old woman underwent an elective cholecystectomy 12h ago. She has a low blood pressure and is prescribed the following fluids: 5% dextrose IV STAT, 5% dextrose IV/2h, 5% dextrose IV/4h, normal saline 0.9%/6h.

ANSWERS

Single Best Answers

1. D ★

This woman has become acutely breathless. She is hypoxic and, as a reflex to this, is hyperventilating (as evidenced by the low pCO_2). As a result, she has developed an alkalosis.

A AND B These are both causes of a metabolic acidosis (with a raised anion gap).

C This does cause acute alkalosis via hyperventilation (and therefore low pCO_2 and a high pH), but tends to happen in the absence of hypoxia rather than as a response to it (as in pulmonary embolism).

E Vomiting causes a metabolic alkalosis (i.e. a high pH with a high HCO_3^-).

Williams A, (1998). ABC of oxygen: assessing and interpreting arterial blood gases. *BMJ* **397**:1213–1216.

→ http://www.bmj.com/cgi/content/extract/317/7167/1213

2. E ★   OHCM 8th edn → p699

This is Paget's disease. An increase in bone turnover followed by remodelling, bone enlargement, deformity, and weakness is typical. Calcium and PO_4^{3-} are normal with a markedly raised ALP.

3. E ★

Care needs to be exercised when hydrating certain groups of patients – the elderly and those with heart or liver failure in particular. This woman is 82 and is on two heart-failure medicines: she is unlikely to tolerate 3L of fluid in 18h without showing some signs of cardiac failure.

A This suggests a neurological deficit.

B This would indicate that she is dehydrated.

C A wheeze is unlikely to suggest fluid overload in combination with dry mucous membranes.

D These are the effects of overdiuresis.

4. B ★

This man has liver failure and therefore a total body sodium excess. Saline fluid therapies should therefore not be used during resuscitation (unless urgently required) to reduce the risk of worsening ascites and oedema.

5. D ★

Her potassium level is clearly raised, and if ECG changes were present, this would merit treatment with calcium chloride/gluconate. The most worrying findings would be decreased or absent P waves, PR-interval prolongation, widened QRS and atrioventricular dissociation. However, a high serum potassium with a normal creatinine raises the possibility that the sample has haemolysed and therefore the sample should be repeated. Other causes for pseudohyperkalaemia are prolonged tourniquet time or a 'drip-arm' sample while potassium-containing fluids are being infused.

A Although this does not reduce the potassium, it protects the cardiac membrane and an improvement is often seen within a few minutes. It can be repeated multiple times if needed.

B This is a polystyrene resin that binds the potassium in the gut, although it does have a slow (2h) onset of action and can cause faecal impaction.

C Actrapid insulin (10U) and 50ml of 50% dextrose shifts the potassium into the cells and can be repeated but blood glucose should be monitored.

E This is unlikely to have much effect on the overall potassium concentration.

→ http://www.gain-ni.org/Guidelines/hyperkalaemia-booklet.pdf

6. E ★   OHCM 8th edn → p692

This is a vague and rather uncommon presentation but is a useful reminder of some important physiology. Although the current complaints may seem disparate and benign, the clue lies in the past medical history: this man has insulin-dependent diabetes and gout and uses high-dose anti-inflammatory medications. He is almost certain to have a degree of chronic renal impairment and, as a result, some filtration imbalances.

The tingling around his mouth is perioral paraesthesia, which, in combination with depressive symptoms in someone with renal impairment, is suggestive of hypocalcaemia. The examination findings that illustrate this deficit are:

1) Trousseau's sign in which the wrist flexes and the fingers are drawn together in response to occlusion of the brachial artery.

2) Chvostek's sign in which facial muscles twitch in response to tapping over the parotid, revealing neuromuscular excitability due to the low calcium.

A This is a finding, especially in the setting of atrial fibrillation, that may support a transient ischaemic attack, i.e. loss of some neurological function, which resolves in <24h.

B This would support a putative diagnosis of hypothyroidism, which could present with symptoms of lethargy and depression as here but would not cause the distinctive perioral tingling.

C This is a non-specific finding, suggestive mainly of cerebellar disease or thiamine deficiency in prolonged alcohol use.

D Parotitis can be found in sarcoidosis; there is no suggestion of that here, the only link being the fact that it is the parotid that is tapped on to elicit Chvostek's sign in hypocalcaemia.

7. B ★

Potassium depletion is common in the setting of a high output from the stoma and should be monitored closely and replaced. If this continues once oral fluids are introduced and increased, medication to slow down the bowel transit can be used, i.e. loperamide. Fluid restriction (1–1.5L/day) and regular electrolyte solutions as part of this restriction can also be used.

8. E ★

The daily sodium requirement is ~100mmol. Each 1L bag of 0.9% saline contains ~150mmol, therefore this woman has received nearly five times the required amount. This is one of the reasons why a recommended 24h maintenance fluid regimen is 2L of 5% dextrose (each containing 30mmol sodium) + 1L of 0.9% saline supplemented over the 24h period with an additional 60mmol potassium.

9. E ★

The scenario suggests a patient in septic shock, with the source possibly from the gall bladder/biliary tree. This will need treatment with IV fluids and antibiotics. However, given the history of the metallic valve, there is a chance that any circulating sepsis may have settled here. In order to be able to treat this appropriately, it is vital to take blood cultures before any antibiotics are on board. This is a rule that can be applied generally in the investigation and treatment of infection: culture and then treat.

10. B ★   OHCM 8th edn → p688

The symptoms and drug history are suggestive of hypokalaemia. Apart from blood tests, a useful measure in suspected derangement of electrolytes is an ECG. There may be no changes, but severe hypokalaemia can cause an 'apparent prolonged QT interval' in which T waves are replaced by U waves, which are bigger and occur later.

If potassium is >2.5mmol/L and asymptomatic, it can be treated with oral supplements but if – as in this case – there are symptoms, treatment should be IV at no more than 20mmol/h and not more concentrated than 40mmol/L.

A This is used to treat acute atrial fibrillation (AF).

C This is used as a treatment for muscle cramps as occur, for example, in multiple sclerosis.

D This is used to treat paroxysmal AF.

E This is a potassium-sparing diuretic: it is not useful in the acute setting of hypokalaemia but is an option in the longer term to try and avoid a repeat.

Webster A, Brady W, and Morris F (2002). Recognising signs of danger: ECG changes resulting from an abnormal serum potassium concentration. Emergency Medicine Journal 19:74–77.

→ http://emj.bmj.com/cgi/content/abstract/19/1/74

11. E ★★   OHCM 8th edn → pp690, 526

This man has a malignancy and some neurological (confusion and lethargy) and renal (polydipsia) symptoms of hypercalcaemia. The speed of onset and the extent of symptoms should prompt treatment, even without knowing the serum calcium. If relying on laboratory results, calcium levels >3.0mmol/L are generally accepted as worth treating. In the first instance, patients need to be rehydrated before treatment with a bisphosphonate. These work by inhibiting osteoclastic bone resorption and have their maximal effect around a week after administration.

A Thiazide diuretics are contraindicated in hypercalcaemia as they increase absorption at the renal tubules. Loop diuretics, on the other hand, inhibit absorption at the loop of Henle, thus increasing urinary excretion of calcium, but – given the need for hydration – they need to be used with caution.

B This is used in the acute management of hyperkalaemia.

C This is used, among other things, used to control the symptoms of raised intracranial pressure caused by cerebral oedema.

D Whilst it is important to rehydrate, somewhere nearer 4 or 5L is usually required in the first 24h and 0.9% saline would be the fluid of choice.

→ http://cancerweb.ncl.ac.uk/cancernet/304462.html

12. C ★ ★   OHCM 8th edn → p684

This is metabolic acidosis, with a normal anion gap. Whilst it is organic acids that raise the gap, a normal gap in acidosis suggests a loss of HCO_3^- or ingestion of H^+ ions.

13. B ★ ★   OHCM 8th edn → p684

In cases like this that show a metabolic acidosis, it is important to work out the anion gap. It is easily done – just subtract the anions (Cl^- and HCO_3^-) from the cations (Na^+ and K^+) to get a measure of the organic acids on board. If the anion gap is high, there are more organic acids on board and they are responsible for the acidosis (e.g. lactic acid, ketones, phosphates).

14. D ★ ★   OHCM 8th edn → p698

This woman has all the features of osteomalacia – bone pain, a waddling gait (indicating proximal myopathy), fractures, and vitamin D deficiency (she is housebound). The hallmark of this condition is the poor mineral content of otherwise normal bones. In this case, it is actually the lack of sunlight that is the cause of the vitamin D deficiency and thus the bone pain. There are other causes of osteomalacia, such as liver disease, drugs, vitamin D resistance, but the most common is vitamin D deficiency, due to hermitude, poor diet, or malabsorption.

B This is Paget's bone disease.

E This is osteoporosis.

15. B ★ ★ ★   OHCM 8th edn → p526

Tumour lysis syndrome is associated with poorly differentiated lymphomas (e.g. Burkitt's lymphoma) and the leukaemias acute lymphoblastic leukaemia (ALL) and acute myeloid leukaemia (AML).

Combination chemotherapy and steroids trigger the death of large numbers of cancer cells leading to high potassium, high phosphate, and high uric acid with low calcium (which can lead to seizures). This leads to uric acid nephropathy and acute renal failure.

16.D ★ ★ ★

A T-score of less than −2.5 means osteoporosis is present. According to NICE guidelines, unless the T-score is dramatically low (less than −3), in women under 65, there needs to be another risk factor before treatment is started. Of those listed, only D qualifies.

B This needs to be the patient not the family with the disease.

C A BMI of <19kg/m² would qualify.

E This woman did not have an early menopause.

→ http://guidance.nice.org.uk/TA161

Extended Matching Questions

1. A ★

According to NICE guidelines (as with each of the answers to questions 1–5), women >75 years who present with a fracture should be started on a bisphosphonate without further investigations.

2. C ★

In the primary prevention of osteoporosis fragility fractures, bone density should be assessed in women over 70 years who have either an independent risk factor for fracture or an indicator of low bone mineral density.

3. C ★

Women aged 66–75 years who present with a fracture should have their bone density assessed.

4. A ★

In women >75 who have two or more independent clinical risk factors for fracture or indicators of low bone mineral density, treatment can be started without the need for a DEXA scan.

5. C ★

Women aged <65 years who present with a fracture need their bone density assessed. If the T-score is >3, there needs to be another risk factor before starting drug therapy. In this woman who had untreated early menopause, a T-score of <2.5 would be enough to warrant treatment.

General feedback on 1–5:

→ http://www.nice.org.uk/nicemedia/pdf/TA160guidance.doc

→ http://www.nice.org.uk/nicemedia/pdf/TA161guidanceword.doc

6. E ★

With any case of hyponatraemia, the keys to diagnosis are the hydration status of the patient and the urine 'spot sodium' concentration. In cases of hypovolaemia such as this, the urinary sodium is crucial. A value >30mmol/L suggests that sodium is lost renally, whilst <30 suggests it is being lost via other routes. The other possible cause of excess renal excretion of salts – Addison's disease – does not tally with the history: someone with Addison's and this level of hypovolaemia would be very unwell and symptomatic, as opposed to this man who is just about able to compensate.

Reynolds RM, Padfield PL, and Seckl JR (2006). Disorders of sodium balance. *BMJ* **332**:702–705.

7. L ★

This man is not dehydrated – far from it – and he has no signs of oedema. A look at his fluid chart is enough to see that excess dextrose is the cause of his hyponatraemia. If this was not the case, it would be worth checking his thyroid and later his pituitary function.

8. D ★

This is a common mistake and is evidenced by the very low sodium and examination findings suggesting euvolaemia.

9. B ★

The other possible cause of hypervolaemia in the setting of hyponatraemia is liver cirrhosis plus ascites. The examination findings may well be similar but the history is more suggestive of decompensated cardiac failure.

10. C ★

This man is dehydrated and, with a low urinary sodium, is losing salt other than via his kidneys. He has been in a fire so could have sustained burns and has a high temperature so will also be sweating.

11. G ★ ★ ★ ★

This patient has a metabolic acidosis due to diabetic ketoacidosis. Patients should be reminded to increase their insulin and not withhold it when they are unwell.

12.B ★★★★

This is Addison's disease associated with vitiligo. The lack of aldosterone results in the typical hyponatraemia/hyperkalaemia, and the loss of negative feedback results in an increase in adrenocorticotrophic hormone as well as melanocyte-stimulating hormone production, causing hyperpigmentation.

13.E ★★★★

This is severe acute pancreatitis with hypocalcaemia.

Corfield AP, Cooper MJ, Williamson RC, *et al.* (1985). Prediction of severity in acute pancreatitis: prospective comparison of three prognostic indices. *Lancet* **2**: 403–407.

14.H ★★★★

This is chronic renal failure, in comparison to acute renal failure, when kidney size is typically normal but the potassium is usually raised.

15.I ★★★★

Inappropriate use of 5% dextrose IV post-operatively can lead to a serious hyponatremia. The liver rapidly metabolizes the glucose to water and combined with the increase in antidiuretic hormone release intraoperatively results in hyponatraemia.

General feedback on 11–15:
A is refeeding syndrome, C is small-cell lung cancer, D is acute renal failure, F is Conn's syndrome, and J is tumour lysis syndrome.

Clinical chemistry

CHAPTER 12

EMERGENCIES

Being called to a clinical emergency is as nerve-wracking as it gets for many doctors. Being first on the scene and the most junior doctor only compounds this. The fear may be that one wrong decision could be crucial and that the recovery of the patient depends entirely on what is done at this moment.

The truth is that we are rarely – if ever – on our own for long and that senior help is for the most part just a few seconds away. It should also serve as some consolation that the approach to any clinical emergency should be much the same and depends heavily on the basic and advanced life support algorithms (Figures 12.1 and 12.2).

This chapter covers the focal points of the most common clinical emergencies with a view to raising confidence when encountering these scenarios. It is written in the spirit that any clinical encounter should be approached as if it is an emergency – this means resorting to the ABCDE (airway, breathing, circulation, disability, exposure) approach – clearly if the patient we are called to is sitting up in bed talking and drinking a cup of tea, then our expectations can be tailored accordingly.

As it is so hard to categorize what constitutes a clinical emergency, it is better that we go into every encounter expecting one. This is because it is easier to taper down one's level of urgency than it is to suddenly escalate treatment in the light of sudden surprising findings. In this way, the idiosyncratic situations – such as the call regarding the post-op thyroid patient – should be considered just as urgent as the seemingly clear cardiac arrest calls.

Having performed the systematic ABCDE assessment of each situation, the next stage is to develop the knowledge and confidence to go on and diagnose which specific emergency is unfolding and to apply appropriate

Adult Basic Life Support

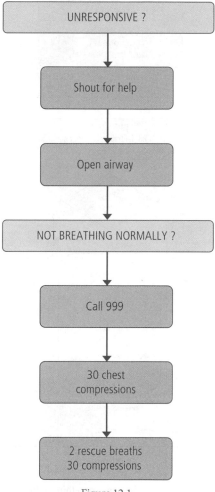

Figure 12.1

management plans. The questions in this chapter aim to reinforce the ability to perform this assessment, as well as outlining some of the specific therapies that are required to manage individual emergencies. The goal is that, just as the

Adult Advanced Life Support Algorithm

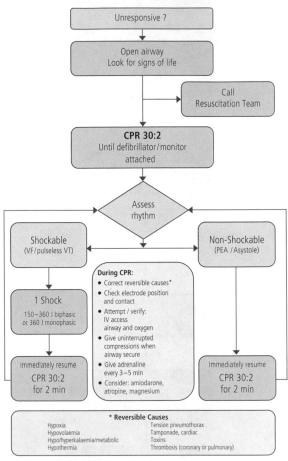

Figure 12.2

ABCDE approach should become something akin to second nature, so should the recognition and initial management of cases as diverse as acute asthma, hyperkalaemia, and paracetamol overdose. ■

SINGLE BEST ANSWERS

1. An on-call junior doctor responds to a crash call from an acute medical ward. She is the first to arrive at the bedside. The patient, a 56-year-old man, does not respond to voice or pain. His breathing is not audible from the end of the bed. On inspiration, his chest is drawn in while his abdomen expands, the opposite occurring on expiration. Which is the *single* most appropriate next step? ★

A Auscultate the chest

B Check position of the trachea

C Ensure airway is open and clear

D Give high-flow oxygen

E Percuss the chest

2. A 78-year-old man is found unresponsive and a doctor on the ward is called to the patient's bedside. The nurse has not been able to detect a blood pressure during routine observations. The patient is displaying no signs of life. He is not breathing and has no detectable pulse. Which is the *single* most appropriate next step? ★

A Get the resuscitation trolley from the nurses' station

B Give two rescue breaths immediately

C Go and check the notes for a Do Not Attempt Resuscitation (DNAR) order

D Insert two wide-bore cannulas into each antecubital fossa

E Start chest compressions at a rate of 30:2

3. An 18-year-old man has an acute episode of wheeze and chest tightness. He is unable to talk and is brought to the Emergency Department on high-flow oxygen. After back-to-back salbutamol 5mg NEB and one ipratropium bromide 500µg NEB, he remains breathless. Arterial blood gases are taken on arrival and 20min into treatment.

	Arrival	20min later
pH	7.37	7.32
pO$_2$ (kPa)	9.22	8.85
pCO$_2$ (kPa)	4.49	5.89
HCO$_3^-$ (mmol/L)	23	21

Which is the *single* most appropriate immediate management? ★

A Aminophylline 5mg/kg IV infusion

B Hydrocortisone 200mg IV

C MgSO$_4$ 2g IV infusion

D Refer to the Intensive Therapy Unit (ITU)

E Salbutamol 5mg NEB

4. A 44-year-old man is the victim of an assault, sustaining major head injuries. He is brought into the Emergency Department with a Glasgow Coma Scale (GCS) score of 3/15. During treatment by the resuscitation team, a chest X-ray is performed (Figure 12.3). Which is the *single* most appropriate immediate management? ★

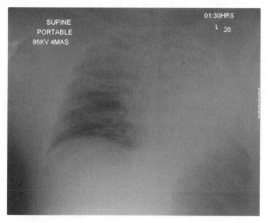

Figure 12.3

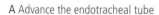

A Advance the endotracheal tube

B Insert a 14G cannula into the left second intercostal space

C Insert a 14G cannula into the right second intercostal space

D Insert a needle into the left posterior seventh intercostal space

E Retract the endotracheal tube

5. A 64-year-old man has tingling and weakness in his hands and arms. He has type 2 diabetes with chronic renal failure and 3 days previously underwent a prostatectomy. Bloods are sent to the laboratory and in the meantime, an ECG is performed (Figure 12.4). Which would be the *single* most appropriate course of action? ★

A Calcium gluconate 10mL IV

B Calcium resonium 15g PO

C Glucose 500mL + potassium 10mmol IV

D Refer for dialysis

E Salbutamol 2.5mg NEB

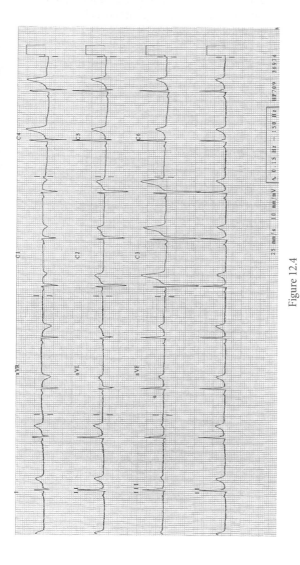

Figure 12.4

6. A 25-year-old man has been stabbed twice in the right-hand side of his abdomen. He is unsure what he was stabbed with but now has severe pain in his right upper quadrant with guarding. Warmed IV fluids are set up. He is very anxious and agitated.

T 36.5°C, HR 110bpm, BP 95/70mmHg, SaO₂ 97% on 10L O₂.

The Emergency Department doctor thinks his liver might have been damaged in the attack and calls the surgeons to assess him. Which is the *single* most appropriate initial management? ★

A Cross-match for packed red cells

B Diagnostic peritoneal lavage

C Focused Assessment with Sonography for Trauma (FAST scan)

D Immediate laparotomy

E Urgent CT scan of the abdomen

7. A 55-year-old man has collapsed. He has had abdominal pain and vomited several times in the last 3 days. He takes sodium valproate for generalized epilepsy. He is drowsy and clammy with cool peripheries.

T 37.2°C, HR 140bpm, BP 95/65mmHg.

Abdomen: epigastric tenderness.

Hb 9.1g/dL, WCC 12.5 × 10⁹/L.

Sodium 132mmol/L, potassium 4.9mmol/L, urea 9.8mmol/L, creatinine 89µmol/L.

Which *single* supplementary clinical examination would be the most informative at this stage? ★

A Chest

B Digital rectal

C Gait, arms, legs, and spine (GALS)

D Inguinal and testicular

E Neurological including cranial nerves

8. A 15-year-old girl has taken an overdose of 30 paracetamol tablets 3h ago. She is extremely anxious but otherwise asymptomatic. She has no past medical history. She weighs 45kg.

BP 125/65mmHg, HR 95bpm, SaO$_2$ 98% on air.

Which is the *single* most appropriate next step? ★

A Activated charcoal

B Gastric lavage

C *N*-Acetyl cysteine infusion

D Paracetamol plasma level at 4h

E Urgent liver function tests + clotting screen

9. A 21-year-old woman has been found unconscious by her partner. There are several packets of paracetamol and an empty bottle of vodka alongside her. When she comes to in the Emergency Department, she is confused and unable to estimate when she took the tablets.

Glasgow Coma Scale (GCS) score: 14/15.

Which is the *single* most appropriate next step? ★

A Observe the woman's GCS in the Emergency Department

B Refer her to the renal unit for haemodialysis

C Start *N*-acetyl cysteine immediately

D Start *N*-acetyl cysteine 4h after presentation

E Take paracetamol levels and treat if raised

10. A 66-year-old woman has suddenly become short of breath. She suffered no chest pain at the time but is now in discomfort with every deep breath in. Six days previously, she underwent the resection of a caecal carcinoma. Which is the *single* additional feature that should prompt the most urgent attention? ★

A BP 80/60mmHg

B Erythematous, swollen right calf

C HR 120bpm

D Raised JVP

E SaO$_2$ 95% on 5L O$_2$

11. A 61-year-old man has suddenly become very short of breath. In the last hour, he has had a CT guided biopsy of a mass in the right lung.

```
T 36.4°C, HR 120bpm, BP 100/60mmHg, SaO₂ 75%
on 15L O₂.
```

He looks cyanosed, his trachea is deviated towards the left, and breath sounds are much louder over the left hemi-thorax. Which is the *single* most appropriate course of action? ★

A Arterial blood gas

B Insertion of a cannula into the right second intercostal space

C Insertion of a chest drain

D Insertion of an airway adjunct

E Urgent chest X-ray

12. An 18-year-old woman has taken 80 paracetamol tablets. She was found at least 12h later by which time she was vomiting and confused. The on-call junior doctor is asked to assess her in the Emergency Department with a view to making a referral to the regional liver centre should it be necessary. Which *single* pair of investigations would be vital when making the referral? ★ ★

A Arterial blood gas + INR

B Albumin + lactate dehydrogenase

C Creatinine + blood glucose

D C-reactive protein + aspartate aminotransferase

E Prothrombin time + bilirubin

13. A 31-year-old woman has taken an overdose of paracetamol. She is very uncooperative but eventually tells you she took 24 tablets 6h ago. She feels nauseous and has vomited twice. She takes a number of regular medications. Which *single* regular medication would increase this patient's chance of severe liver damage? ★ ★

A Carbamazepine for mood stabilization

B Erythromycin for acne

C Fluoxetine for depression

D Propranolol for anxiety

E Xenical for obesity

14. A 24-year-old man has a painful right testis, lower abdominal pain, and nausea. The testis is swollen, hot, and extremely tender. The Emergency Department triage nurse contacts the junior doctor to discuss the patient over the telephone. Which is the *single* most appropriate question in the immediate assessment of this patient? ★ ★

A Are there associated rigors?

B Has there been vomiting?

C Has this happened before?

D How quickly did the pain come on?

E Is there pain on passing urine?

15. A 63-year-old man has been found by a neighbour collapsed on the floor of his flat. He is groaning and unable to give any information to the doctors, but the neighbour says he uses oxygen from cylinders even when he leaves the flat, which is very rarely. His peripheries are cold and he has numerous bruises on his arms and legs.

T 35.2°C, BP 70/40mmHg, HR 100bpm, SaO_2 90% on 35% O_2.

Glasgow Coma Scale (GCS) score: 11/15.

Capillary blood glucose: 3.5mmol/L.

Which is the *single* most appropriate next step? ★ ★ ★

A Arterial blood gas + titrated oxygen therapy

B Blood cultures + broad-spectrum antibiotics

C Cross-match + 2U O-negative blood

D Glucose 50% IV + capillary blood glucose monitoring

E Hydrocortisone 100mg IV + warmed IV fluids

?

16. A 55-year-old man has become increasingly short of breath in the 3h since returning to the ward after a thyroidectomy.

```
T 37.6°C, HR 110bpm, BP 100/60mmHg,
RR 35/min, SaO₂ 89% on air.
```

There are harsh inspiratory upper airway sounds and reduced air entry bilaterally. Which is the *single* most appropriate course of action? ★ ★ ★

A Cut the SC sutures

B Epinephrine 0.5mg IM

C Low-molecular-weight heparin 1mg/kg SC

D O₂ 15L via non-rebreather mask

E Salbutamol 5mg NEB

EXTENDED MATCHING QUESTIONS

Treatment of cardiac arrest

For each in-hospital cardiac arrest, choose the *single* most appropriate immediate next step from the list of options below options. Each option may be used once, more than once, or not at all. ★

A 150J biphasic shock

B Adrenaline 1mg IV

C Amiodarone 300mg IV

D Atropine 3mg IV

E Complete 2min of chest compressions at 30:2

F Continue cardiopulmonary resuscitation (CPR) and establish IV access

G Cool to 32–34°C for 12–24h

H Feel for a pulse/reassess the rhythm

I Give uninterrupted chest compressions

J Insert two wide bore cannulas

K Lidocaine 1mg/kg IV

L Praecordial thump

J Ventilate at 10 breaths/min

1. A 72-year-old man has collapsed and has no detectable cardiac output. Another doctor has already started to perform CPR. The defibrillator is attached to the patient and shows the rhythm in Figure 12.5.

2. A 56-year-old woman is found to be in asystole. She has been given some IV medication and her rhythm is reassessed a few minutes later. The ECG tracing has changed and is now as shown in Figure 12.6.

3. A 72-year-old man has been brought into the Emergency Department by the paramedics. He has had two complete cycles of CPR. The rhythm is reassessed and the ECG tracing is shown in Figure 12.7.

4. A 66-year-old man has collapsed on the ward. The cardiac arrest team have arrived and completed three complete cycles of CPR. The ECG tracing has changed but no pulse has been detected in the rhythm check (see Figure 12.8).

5. A 48-year-old man has a ventricular fibrillation (VF) arrest following a large anterior myocardial infarct. He has undergone one complete cycle of CPR and been shocked for the second time. Half way through the second cycle of chest compressions, his rhythm strip changes to an organized rhythm but he shows no signs of life.

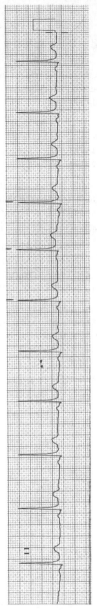

Figure 12.5

526

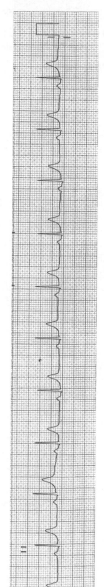

Figure 12.6

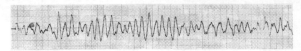

Figure 12.7

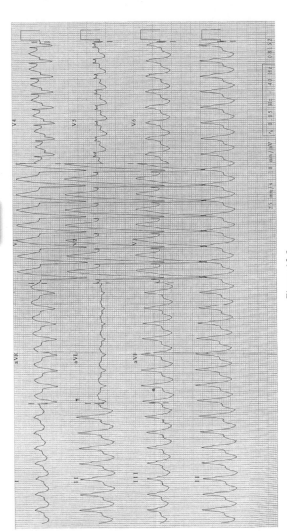

Figure 12.8

ANSWERS

Single Best Answers

1. C ★

The signs elicited by the junior doctor – silent breathing and 'see-saw' breathing – are those of complete airway obstruction. However, the key learning point here is that, even if the junior doctor failed to recognize these signs, the patient could be treated by sticking to the ABCDE mantra of resuscitation. Rather than second guessing what is going on (*'Maybe he's got a pneumothorax...'*), by working systematically from airway onwards, the problem may be treated without having to diagnose it. In this case, positioning, basic airway manoeuvres, airway suction, the insertion of an oropharyngeal airway, and then high-flow oxygen may be enough to alleviate the patient's breathing problems.

→ http://www.resus.org.uk/pages/guide.htm

2. E ★

This man has had a cardiac arrest. The new resuscitation guidelines published in 2005 state that after assessing ABC (airway, breathing, circulation) and calling for help (the cardiac arrest team), chest compressions should be started as soon as possible.

A The new ratio of compressions to breaths should be 30:2 and these should be started while waiting for the resuscitation trolley to arrive.

B This was part of the old guidelines.

C Resuscitation should always begin before clarifying DNAR status.

D The man has no cardiac output and, although this is indicated, this should not be the first thing to do.

→ http://www.resus.org.uk/

3. D ★

This man presents with severe asthma and does not respond to treatment (as evidenced by hypercapnoea on the arterial blood gases). According to British Thoracic Society guidelines, this meets the criteria for ITU referral. The rising pCO_2 suggests tiredness and thus the need for airway support to maximize ventilation: he may well need intubation. (Note: it would not be wrong to give this man another nebulizer, IV steroids, magnesium, or a theophylline, but the most pressing step at this time is to contact an anaesthetist with a view to securing the airway.)

→ http://www.brit-thoracic.org.uk/ClinicalInformation/Asthma/ AsthmaGuidelines/tabid/83/Default.aspx

4. E ★

The film shows complete collapse of the left lung with deviation of the trachea to the left. Following the endotracheal tube down the trachea, it is clear that, rather than stopping at the bifurcation, it actually continues down into the right main bronchus. It can therefore be assumed that this is the reason why the left lung has stopped being ventilated and has thus collapsed.

In busy, noisy resuscitation situations, it can be difficult to confirm that there is equal and bilateral air entry, which is why pictures like this exist. Treatment is simply to pull the tube back, auscultate the chest, and repeat the X-ray.

B AND C These would treat tension pneumothoraces.

D This is a possible approach to aspirating a pleural effusion for diagnosis.

5. A ★   OHCM 8th edn → p849

If there is clinical and ECG evidence of hyperkalaemia, as here, then urgent treatment is required to avoid progression into more unstable heart rhythms (ventricular fibrillation (VF)/ventricular tachycardia (VT)). The consensus is that patients with hyperkalaemia and ECG changes should be given IV calcium gluconate. This does not lower the potassium but should arrest the ECG changes within 1–3min.

B This increases gut losses of potassium but takes >2h to work. It should be employed but not as a first-line therapy.

C This is not a good idea. Glucose is used with potassium but also with insulin as an alternative to sliding scales to monitor blood glucose. It should also be used in the management of acute myocardial infarction in patients with diabetes. What this man needs in order to drive the potassium back into the cells is 50mL glucose 50% with 10U fast-acting insulin (the effects should be seen within 15min and last up to 6h).

D This is indicated if potassium is persistently >6mmol/L or in persistent acidosis (pH <7.2), but not in the first instance.

E This should be used alongside other measures but not alone and not as a first-line therapy.

Hollander-Rodriguez J and Calvert J (2006). Hyperkalaemia. *Am Fam Physician* 73:283–290.

→ http://www.aafp.org/afp/20060115/283.html

→ http://www.gain-ni.org/Guidelines/hyperkalaemia-booklet.pdf

(*Guidelines for the Management of Hyperkalaemia in Adults.* CREST, Northern Ireland Central Medical Advisory Committee, 2006.)

6. A ★

The patient must be resuscitated and stabilized before sending to the CT scanner.

B This is now rarely done.

C This will probably be carried out as part of the assessment of the circulation.

D This may well be the last step after all investigations are carried out.

E This is indicated but not until the patient is stable.

7. B ★

The initial clinical findings are that of shock. The blood results suggest acute blood loss. Against the background history – disregarding the distracting concurrent epilepsy – the likely source is the upper gastrointestinal tract. A digital rectal examination (DRE) provides vital information in this instance but remains underperformed in the acute setting.

8. D ★

Blood taken before 4h is unreliable because the drug is still being absorbed and distributed. The *N*-acetyl cysteine infusion does not need to be started unless the time of the overdose is unknown or has been staggered over a few hours.

Initial symptoms are often limited to nausea and vomiting but liver damage is possible in adults who have taken 10g or more (20 tablets) or as little as 5g in those with risk factors. These include those on liver-enzyme-inducing drugs, chronic alcohol abusers, and those who are likely to be deficient in glutathione such as people who have cystic fibrosis, human immunodeficiency virus (HIV) infection, or an eating disorder, or who are cachexic or starved.

A This should be considered if the overdose has been taken within 1h.

B The British Poisons Centres only recommend the use of gastric lavage in cases of overdose where activated charcoal is not effective (i.e. not paracetamol).

C This should not be started until the blood test has been taken at 4h and as long as the results are returned by 8h.

E There is often no change in these values acutely.

9. C ★

In cases like this where a serious overdose is suspected, it is advisable to give the paracetamol antidote *N*-acetyl cysteine immediately. The 4h figure refers to the time after ingestion at which plasma levels can be interpreted. If levels turn out to be below the treatment line, *N*-acetyl cysteine can be stopped without harm.

10. A ★

This woman has clearly suffered a pulmonary embolus (PE). However, the key for the doctor on call attempting to prioritize referrals is the patient's cardiovascular status: here, the systolic BP <90mmHg classifies this as a massive PE and therefore one that needs urgent assessment with a view to thrombolysis (if cardiac arrest is imminent). The other features may be useful in confirming diagnosis (apart from D, which cues pulmonary oedema rather than PE), but only A demands immediate attention.

British Thoracic Society Standards of Care Committee Pulmonary Embolism Guideline Development Group (2003). British Thoracic Society Guidelines for the Management of Suspected Acute Pulmonary Embolism. *Thorax* **58**:470–484.

→ http://www.brit-thoracic.org.uk/Portals/0/Clinical%20Information/Pulmonary%20Embolism/Guidelines/PulmonaryEmbolismJUN03.pdf

11. B ★

This man has rapidly developed the signs of a pneumothorax. Having just had a needle inserted into his chest, this is almost certainly an iatrogenic pneumothorax (the incidence of which outnumbers spontaneous pneumothoraces in several large studies). The deviation of the trachea suggests that it is under tension (i.e. the intrapleural pressure exceeds atmospheric pressure through both inspiration and expiration) and so needs urgent reversal. The British Thoracic Society advice is as follows:

If a tension pneumothorax occurs, the patient should be given high concentration oxygen and a cannula should be introduced into the pleural space, usually in the second anterior intercostal space mid clavicular line. Air should be removed until the patient is no longer compromised and then an intercostal tube should be inserted into the pleural space.

A AND E The tension that the right chest is under means the mediastinum is shifted to the left, causing compression of the great veins and impaired venous return. This is a serious situation that would lead to cardiorespiratory arrest unless addressed, leaving no time for any further investigations.

C A chest drain will be needed but not until the air has been removed.

D Whilst it is right to begin the management of this emergency situation by addressing the airway, there is no suggestion that this man is unconscious enough to tolerate either a Guedel or nasopharyngeal airway. He should be put on high-flow O_2 while attention is directed towards the air in his pleural space.

Henry M, Arnold T, and Harvey J (2003). BTS guidelines for the management of spontaneous pneumothorax. *Thorax* 58:ii39–ii52.

→ http://thorax.bmj.com/cgi/content/full/58/suppl_2/ii39

12.A ★★ OHCM 8th edn → pp856–857

The criteria for transfer to a specialist unit are:

- Encephalopathy/raised intracranial pressure: sustained BP >160/90mmHg or brief rises of systolic BP >200mmHg, bradycardia, decerebrate posturing, extensor spasms, or poor pupil response.
- INR >2.0 at 48h or >3.5 at <72h.
- Creatinine >200µmol/L.
- Blood pH <7.3.
- Systolic BP<80mmHg.

13.A ★★

Patient who have a regular excessive intake of alcohol, are taking enzyme-inducing medications (as in this case), or who have conditions causing glutathione depletion such as malnutrition, human immunodeficiency virus (HIV) infection, and cystic fibrosis should be treated as high risk. These patients can develop toxicity at lower plasma paracetamol concentrations and should be treated if the concentration is above the high-risk treatment line, which is 50% of the plasma paracetamol concentrations of the normal treatment line.

14.D ★★ OHCM 8th edn → p654

The key here is to explore the possibility of testicular torsion. The main differential is usually epididymo-orchitis in which the onset of pain is much more gradual. In a patient in whom the onset is dramatic and sudden, then torsion becomes the favourite. Whilst urinary symptoms (E) are also more common in epididymo-orchitis, they may overlap as part of the general extreme lower abdominal pain seen in torsion. Once torsion tops the list, the junior doctor's priority is getting a urological opinion: definitive treatment is surgery (for detorsion and orchidopexy) – the sooner this happens, the greater the chance of the testis being saved.

A Rigors cue an infective cause.

B Vomiting is rather too non-specific to be immediately useful.

C A previous similar episode may be suggestive of a hydrocoele.

→ http://emedicine.medscape.com/article/778086-treatment

15. E ★ ★ ★

This man has severe chronic obstructive pulmonary disease (COPD) (home and ambulatory oxygen) and with that degree of airways disease (and the bruising on the arms/legs), it is almost certain that he also uses steroids. This presentation is consistent with an Addisonian crisis due to long-term steroid use. In an emergency situation, it is often difficult to say what should happen first as many things are happening at the same time. However, giving IV steroids and IV fluids is the most important intervention that should occur and without which this man will probably die.

→ http://www.addisons.org.uk/info/manual/crisismanagement.pdf

16. A ★ ★ ★

This man has developed stridor soon after surgery near his airway. A rare complication of thyroidectomy is upper airway obstruction secondary to haematoma. To prevent the airway from being totally occluded, it is necessary to release the pressure this haematoma is causing by loosening the tightness of the compartment in which it is building up. If this does not improve his breathing, this man will very soon need intubation.

Whilst this is a rare scenario and not important per se, it is a reminder to take heed of breathing sounds and patterns and to pay respect to the fragility of the upper airway. All good emergency care starts with the airway: if a junior doctor detects unusual sounds causing respiratory compromise, he needs to act early – which may involve enlisting an anaesthetist's help – to secure it before damage is done.

B This is used in anaphylaxis, which is a reasonable differential in stridor (due to laryngoedema), but is less likely here than the local effects of the surgery.

C This is the treatment for a pulmonary embolus, which does cause sudden breathlessness, but not due to upper airway compromise.

D This is a reasonable response to dropping SaO_2 in someone with healthy lungs, but is not the treatment that is going to arrest this man's upper airway occlusion.

E This is useful to open smaller constricting airways (e.g. in asthma or COPD) but will not reduce the pressure effect of a haematoma on the trachea.

Savargaonkar AP (2004). Post-thyroidectomy haematoma causing total airway obstruction. *Indian J Anaesth* 48:483–485.

→ http://medind.nic.in/iad/t04/i6/iadt04i6p483.pdf

Extended Matching Questions

1. F ★

This man is in pulseless electrical activity (PEA) arrest consistent with the normal looking ECG trace but no detectable pulse. Chest compressions and ventilation should be continued and IV access established, after which a dose of adrenaline 1mg IV should be given every 3–5min. If the heart rate is less than 60bpm, a single dose of atropine 3mg IV should be given.

2. H ★

This woman's rhythm has changed from asystole to an ECG tracing that could be compatible with a pulse. Therefore, following the completion of the current cycle of CPR, the resuscitation team should feel for a pulse. On this occasion, there is no pulse and the resuscitation should continue down the non-shockable side of the algorithm.

3. B ★

The ECG trace shows ventricular fibrillation (VF) – a shockable rhythm. Resuscitation down the shockable side of the algorithm should proceed as follows: drug – shock – CPR – rhythm check sequence. Before the third shock, he should be given adrenaline 1mg IV, and before the fourth shock, amiodarone 300mg IV. The idea behind the order of the sequence is that the drugs given immediately before the shock will be circulated by the subsequent CPR.

4. C ★

The ECG has changed to pulseless ventriculat tachycardia (VT) and he needs to continue being treated down the shockable side of the algorithm. Therefore, just before the fourth shock, he needs to be given amiodarone.

5. E ★

It is always tempting to stop chest compressions when you see a rhythm check, but unless the patient shows signs of life compatible with a return of spontaneous circulation, the 2min cycle should be completed first.

General feedback on 1–5:
All answers are based on the Resuscitation Council (UK) 2005 guidelines.
→ http://www.resus.org.uk

INDEX